The Foot and Ankle in Rheumatoid Arthritis:
A Comprehensive Guide

For Elsevier:

Commissioning Editor: Robert Edwards
Development: Veronika Krcilova
Project Manager: Andrew Palfreyman
Design Direction: George Ajayi
Illustrations Buyer: Gillian Murray
Illustrator: Cactus

The Foot and Ankle in Rheumatoid Arthritis

A Comprehensive Guide

Philip Helliwell MA, PhD, FRCP

Senior Lecturer in Rheumatology, Academic Unit of Musculoskeletal Disease; University of Leeds, Leeds, UK

James Woodburn PhD, MPhil, BSc

Professor of Rehabilitation Studies, School of Health and Social Care and Health Qwest, Glasgow Caledonian University, Glasgow, UK
Formerly MRC Clinician Scientist Fellow, Podiatrist, Academic Unit of Musculoskeletal Disease School of Medicine, University of Leeds; Leeds, UK

Anthony Redmond PhD, MSc

Arthritis Research Campaign Lecturer, Academic Unit of Musculoskeletal Disease, University of Leeds; Leeds, UK

Deborah Turner PhD, BSc

Research Fellow Podiatrist, Academic Unit of Musculoskeletal Disease School of Medicine, University of Leeds; Leeds, UK, Senior Lecture, Department of Podiatry, University of Huddersfield

Heidi Davys MSc, BSc

Senior Rheumatology Podiatrist, Four Health Department Leeds Teaching Hospitals NHS Trust, Leeds, UK
Research Podiatrist, Academic Unit of Musculoskeletal Disease, University of Leeds

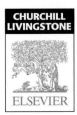

EDINBURGH LONDON NEW YORK OXFORD PHILADELPHIA ST LOUIS SYDNEY TORONTO 2007

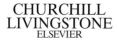

First published 2007

ISBN 10: 0 443 10110 8
ISBN 13: 978 0 443 10110 6

British Library Cataloguing in Publication Data
A catalogue record for this book is available from the British Library.

Library of Congress Cataloging in Publication Data
A catalog record for this book is available from the Library of Congress.

Notice
Knowledge and best practice in this field are constantly changing. As new research and experience broaden our knowledge, changes in practice, treatment and drug therapy may become necessary or appropriate. Readers are advised to check the most current information provided (i) on procedures featured or (ii) by the manufacturer of each product to be administered, to verify the recommended dose or formula, the method and duration of administration, and contraindications. It is the responsibility of the practitioner, relying on their own experience and knowledge of the patient, to make diagnoses, to determine dosages and the best treatment for each individual patient, and to take all appropriate safety precautions. To the fullest extent of the law, neither the Publisher nor the Authors assumes any liability for any injury and/or damage to persons or property arising out or related to any use of the material contained in this book.
Printed in China

The Publisher

Contents

Foreword

Rheumatoid Arthritis is a complex disease manifesting in a variety of different ways. Its impact on the foot and ankle can be devastating for the patient and a significant clinical challenge for healthcare practitioners. The authors of this text and associated interactive DVD have raised the profile of the foot and ankle in Rheumatoid Arthritis. As a multi-discilinary team they have been able to build an evidence base through a systematic research agenda designed around addressing clinical problems. Their contribution to our understanding of the effect of Rheumatoid Arthritis on the foot and ankle is significant. However, they would be the first to acknowledge that there is still much to research. Throughout the text they have been able to draw upon their clinical experience to add to the research base presented. This provides a rich resource for all healthcare practitioners concerned with the assessment, treatment and management of patients with rheumatoid arthritis impacting on foot and ankle function. The book gives a comprehensive guide taking the reader from the concepts of rheumatoid arthritis, diagnostic criteria, epidemiology and disease impact in respect of social, psychological, economically and clinical cost to evaluation and organisation and delivery of care.

Chapter 1 explores the epidemiology, natural history, genetic influence and pathogenesis of the rheumatoid arthritis. The authors focus on the epidemiology of foot disease and introduce podiatric concepts. In chapter 2 the application of gait analysis in the diagnosis and assessment of rheumatoid arthritis and the pathomechanics of the foot and ankle is explored. For many clinicians access to high quality gait and foot pressure laboratories is rare. The chapter highlights the benefit of such labs when assessing and treating complex foot and ankle pathologies. The authors draw upon their own fundamental research findings and clinical experience to guide the reader through key scientific findings linking pathomechanics and clinical observations. The value of gait analysis and foot pressure measurement is established and the benefit to patients through better diagnosis, care planning and treatment evaluation is clear.

Chapter 3 considers inflammatory joint disease and the way in which synovitis presents in the foot. The effect of synovitis is considered across the spectrum of rheumatoid disease, from early to late disease. Modifying intrinsic and extrinsic factors are considered in respect of the whole patient. The impact of rheumatoid arthritis on the pathology of joints, soft tissues, skin, vascular and nerve tissue is considered.

For any clinician Chapter 4 provides an overview of the clinical assessment. As already stated rheumatoid arthritis is a complex disease. Assessment of the musculoskeletal system is variable and often dependant upon the clinicians professional background. This has led to communication and coordination difficulties between clinicians and professional groups. In an attempt to reduce this the authors highlight the use of simple screening tools which then leads to greater consideration of screening tools specifically designed to assess the foot and ankle.

The role of imaging techniques in assessing bone, joint and soft tissue structures and disease progression is considered in Chapter 5. In Chapter 6 the treatment of rheumatoid arthritis is explored. The authors bring the clinician up-to-date in exploring the latest drug therapies available to treat rheumatoid arthritis. This includes the use of biological disease modifying drugs alongside the more familiar steroidal and non-steroidal anti-inflammatory systemic drugs. The chapter also explores intra-articular therapy providing the reader with helpful images and practical guidance in the techniques employed. The chapter concludes by highlighting the important and significant impact of podiatric interventions including footwear prescription, use of orthoses, callus debridement and skin and wound care management. The sections dealing with orthotic management and skin care draw on new research evidence generated by the authors and present findings in a clear and concise way.

Chapter 7 considers the surgical management of the foot and ankle. We are reminded of the importance of patient selection and assessment and the optimization of non surgical interventions prior to considering surgical solutions. Critically in this section the importance of multi-disciplinary assessment is highlighted. The evaluation of care in a disease characterised by being complex and multi-system with flares and remissions is critical to disease management. Chapter 8 provides an overview of how the clinician might approach the evaluation of disease activity, health and functional status and quality of life. The evaluation of the foot through the 'Leeds Foot Impact Score' is particularly exciting and should be considered by clinicians specialising in managing patients with musculo-skeletal foot disease.

The final chapter highlights the need to explore how care is organised. Throughout the text the authors reinforce the benefit of working in multi-disciplinary teams drawing on the expertise of different professional groups within clinical and research settings. The complexity of rheumatoid arthritis and its impact on foot and ankle function leaves no doubt that the organisation of care is critical. In England healthcare delivery is under-going radical and rapid change. The introduction of patient choice alongside plurality of providers and the shift towards increased primary care delivery presents both challenges and opportunities. It will be essential in these changes to preserve and develop multi-disciplinary clinics staffed by highly trained specialist staff. The danger will be the temptation to fragment and fracture care pathways in response to cost pressures. If this were to happen the adverse impact on patient care would be significant. The need to ensure services are connected, clinicians communicate and treatment interventions are coordinated is essential.

The Foot and Ankle in Rheumatoid Arthritis is a unique and valuable resource. It has been written by experts in the field drawing upon their considerable clinical and research experience. It presents the latest evidence base supporting the care of patients with rheumatoid arthritis in a clear and concise way. It should be a core text and reference manual for all clinicians wishing to specialise in the foot and ankle in rheumatoid arthritis.

Professor Steven West BSc, FChS, FRSM
Deputy Vice-Chancellor,
University of the West of England,
Bristol UK
Consultant Podiatrist

Foreword

A chance remark at the end of a Rheumatology conference in 2004, when I asked the Rheumatology clinicians present to pay more than lip service to the problems that patients experience with their feet, has given me the opportunity to write the foreword to this book.

Small joint inflammation is the hallmark of early Rheumatoid Arthritis, yet attention to the problems of the foot and ankle has been the Cinderella of the Rheumatoid world. As any clinician or health professional will tell you it is easier to look at the hands in an examination rather than the feet and consequently there appears to be a lack of attention paid to this problem.

Stylish shoes are an essential part of most women's wardrobe. In my cupboard there are still several pairs of fashionable shoes, remnants of the days when I was still working. They were to me a symbol of my position and authority when smart dressing was the vogue. I cannot wear them now, but somewhere in the back of my mind there is a possibility that just one day I might be able to. A friend of mine, another patient with Rheumatoid Arthritis, was invited to a rather 'posh' wedding. Much time was taken choosing an expensive outfit, and a pair of shoes that would not look too clumsy but would be comfortable. Several days before the wedding she experienced a 'flare' in her disease and on the morning of the 'looked-forward-to-day' was unable to wear the shoes because her feet were so swollen. The result, she stayed at home rather than spoil the outfit with her everyday but clumsy shoes.

There are over 8 million arthritis patients in the U.K., and the overall prevalence of females is far greater than men. Of course women are not the only ones to experience pain and discomfort in their feet. Rheumatoid Arthritis is a time consuming disease, everyday activities of work and leisure take longer to perform, particularly when your feet are swollen, painful and deformed. This often results in decreased capacity for paid and unpaid work. The cost of the disease is immense with many working days lost per year.

The book points out that there is no such thing as a typical 'rheumatoid' foot. As a patient I am always amazed at the variety of disabilities that Rheumatoid Arthritis can exhibit. Diagnosing the needs of an individual patient is paramount: there is a person connected to the foot! Many foot problems are under reported, and only 25% of patients have access to NHS care, and there is an even greater discrepancy amongst patients with Rheumatoid Arthritis. Foot health care service provision needs to be responsive to the varying needs of the patients throughout the course of their disease. As the disease progresses patients will need more than someone to deal with corns and calluses. A comprehensive foot care programme should lead to treatment for more demanding problems when needed, such as vasculitis, ulceration, neuropathy and necessary surgical intervention. Getting the timing right is so important. My Rheumatoid clinic has recently introduced the provision of a podiatrist to attend monthly clinics, an overdue luxury that is not available everywhere.

This book will draw attention to the varying needs of patients as their disease progresses, and to the need for multidisciplinary teams to improve patient care in the future, even though they may be difficult to establish. As a patient with increasing foot problems I am grateful that such a book now exists for clinicians and health professionals.

Mrs Enid Quest

Acknowledgements

The authors would like to pay tribute to the technical expertise and support of Mr Brian Whitham, Research Technician at the University of Leeds.

We would also like to thank the many patients whose images appear in this book and those who contributed to the case studies in Chapters 2 and 6.

Contributors

S J McKie
Consultant Musculoskeletal Radiologist,
Queen Margaret Hospital, Dunfermline

P J O'Connor
Consultant Musculoskeletal Radiologist,
Leeds General Infirmary, Leeds

N. J. Harris
Consultant Orthopaedic Surgeon,
Leeds FRSC (TR and Orth)

N. Carrington
Consultant Orthopaedic Surgeon,
York FRCS (TR and Orth)

Chapter 1

Current concepts in rheumatoid arthritis

INTRODUCTION

Rheumatoid arthritis (RA) is the commonest inflammatory arthritis seen in the UK, Europe and North America. It causes inflammation and destruction of synovial joints and, in many cases, has an additional systemic component that is associated with increased morbidity and mortality. The cost of the disease, both in individual and societal terms, is considerable. RA comprises the bulk of the work done by a general rheumatologist and is the commonest reason for referral from rheumatology to podiatry. The treatment of RA is rapidly changing and with new treatments has come new hope of preventing the deformities seen after many years of disease.

The foot remains a neglected area in rheumatology; it is far easier to look at the hands than to look at the feet. Examining the feet requires a certain amount of discomfort both for the examiner (who usually has to bend over from sitting to peer at these appendages) and the patient who has to struggle with footwear and socks or 'tights'. From our experience in post-graduate education we know that rheumatologists and podiatrists feel in need of more knowledge and skills with respect to the foot in RA and feel incapable of examining that part. We hope this book will fulfil this educational role.

It is our intention to make this book as evidence-based as possible. Inevitably, there will be areas where the evidence base is weak; in these instances we will be clear when we write from personal experience and practice. One point is clear from the existing literature in this field; the specialty of orthopaedics has contributed significantly to what we know about the foot in RA. In this context, we would make a plea that use of the term 'rheumatoid foot' is abandoned. Why? Well, there is no such thing as a typical 'rheumatoid foot'; RA is a complex disease that may manifest in several different ways. The term 'rheumatoid foot' is somewhat derogatory and demeaning. It tends to ignore the fact that there is a person connected to the (painful) foot (a person with the disease of RA) the impact of which will depend on many factors, including the other manifestations of the disease, personal and contextual factors. The WHO's International Classification of Functioning, Disability and Health enables health professionals to describe these aspects in a composite form, synthesizing different perspectives of health. These interactions and the protean manifestations of the disease should be addressed by anyone treating people with RA.

EPIDEMIOLOGY OF RHEUMATOID ARTHRITIS

The incidence of RA is falling. There are several reasons for this, briefly summarized below:

1. Changing diagnostic criteria
2. Changing methods of determining disease
3. Falling incidence of disease itself.

The diagnosis is usually made according to specific criteria. In RA, the criteria commonly used are those defined by the American College of Rheumatology (see Table 1.1) (Arnett et al. 1988). It is important to note that in the absence of a gold standard (such as a single clinical sign, radiological feature or pathological test) these criteria only reflect the clinical features used by clinicians in the clinic. They are used in general for classification purposes to allow comparison between different populations and to serve as entry criteria for clinical trials. They are not designed as criteria for diagnosing the individual patient in the clinic or at the bedside; these may be quite different. In this latter case clinical judgement is important, not the number of criteria the patient fulfils. Classification criteria do have an important role, nevertheless, and are designed to be specific rather than sensitive; although, ideally, criteria should have both high sensitivity and specificity. In reality, criteria are either very specific or very sensitive and the level of each can be manipulated during their development to serve the purpose required. The 1997 ACR criteria were reported to have a sensitivity of 91% and a specificity of 89%; this means that 9% cases of RA were not 'picked up' by the criteria and, conversely, 11% of cases diagnosed as RA were, in fact, some other arthropathy.

Just how well classification criteria perform will depend, as noted above, on the sensitivity and speci-

ficity, but these indicators can be changed, as already mentioned. The method of developing the criteria is also important. Usually, clinicians recruit people they regard as having typical disease, but, obviously, this may vary from clinician to clinician. More important are the cases used as 'controls' with whom the comparison is made and from which the criteria are derived. The criteria will perform best in populations of a similar composition to those on which they were developed. For example, if there were no cases of psoriatic arthritis in the control population at the time the criteria were developed it would be misleading to use these criteria to pick rheumatoid from psoriatic arthritis in a study using these criteria. Further, if the cases of RA used to develop the criteria were all of well-established disease then these criteria would have limited usefulness for early disease; in fact, this is exactly one of the limitations of the 1987 criteria as the average disease duration of the cases was 7.7 years.

Table 1.1 The 1987 revised criteria for the classification of rheumatoid arthritis

---

At least four of the following features should be present for at least 6 weeks:

1. early morning stiffness of the joints for at least 60 min
2. soft-tissue joint swelling observed by a physician of at least three of the following areas:
   a. proximal inter-phalangeal joints
   b. metacarpophalangeal joints
   c. wrist joints
   d. elbow joints
   e. knee joints
   f. ankle joints
   g. metatarsophalangeal joints
3. soft-tissue swelling observed in a hand joint in at least one of the following areas:
   a. proximal inter-phalangeal joints
   b. metacarpophalangeal joints
   c. wrist joints
4. symmetry of joint involvement of the following joint pairs:
   a. proximal inter-phalangeal joints
   b. metacarpophalangeal joints
   c. metatarsophalangeal joints
   d. wrist joints
   e. elbow joints
   f. knee joints
   g. ankle joints
5. the presence of subcutaneous rheumatoid nodules
6. the presence of rheumatoid factor in the serum
7. the presence of erosions on radiographs of wrists or hands.

To overcome this problem it has been suggested that alternative criteria be developed for early disease. In fact, an alternative classification tree method was developed for diagnosing RA using the same patients as the criteria given in Table 1.1. The advantage of this method is that a diagnosis can be made without features that often develop later in the disease, such as bony erosions. Harrison et al. have shown that the tree method is more sensitive for diagnosing early disease, but loses specificity; an inevitable trade off in this situation (Harrison et al. 1998). However, it may be futile to try and develop specific criteria for early RA if all early arthritis is undifferentiated. Berthelot has suggested that early arthritis may progress to whichever definitive arthritis (for example, RA or spondyloarthropathy) according to individual characteristics such as HLA status and cytokine polymorphisms. In a study of 270 cases of early arthritis (less than 1 year duration), the French group obtained longitudinal data for 30 months, relating the initial diagnosis to that given at the final visit (Berthelot et al. 2002). Over one-third of diagnoses changed in the follow-up period.

If a diagnostic biological marker were available diagnosis would be much more straightforward. A biological marker usually has pathological relevance, such as the finding of tubercle bacilli in the sputum of someone with suspected pulmonary tuberculosis. For some time it was thought that rheumatoid factor fulfilled this role in RA. But it later became clear that rheumatoid factor is present in only about 75% of cases of RA. Rheumatoid factor, however, may still have a pathological role (see section on aetiology) and certainly does have a role in predicting the course of the disease (see below).

Further biological markers have been sought. Antibodies to keratin, in particular anti-cyclic citrullinated peptide antibodies have been found to be more specific (95%) for RA than rheumatoid factor. However, this occurs at the cost of lower sensitivity (56%) (Bas et al. 2003). This test may, however, be of more use in situations where it is desired to have a very low rate of false positives. Other ways of looking at RA are under investigation. For example, magnetic resonance imaging (MRI) is a very sensitive technique for detecting inflammation. Joints not inflamed clinically may show extensive abnormalities. The same is true, but to a lesser extent, for ultrasound (U/S), especially power Doppler U/S. Both these techniques are discussed in the chapter on imaging. The point to be made here is that using these new techniques may change the way we diagnose and treat inflammatory diseases such as RA. MRI and U/S may permit much earlier diagnosis, but it is doubtful if they will be incorporated into diagnostic criteria until their cost and availability become more favourable.

Given the above considerations a number of studies have attempted to estimate the incidence and prevalence of RA. The prevalence of RA in the population is approximately 0.8%, a risk that is doubled for relatives of confirmed cases (Hawker 1997). The overall prevalence is higher in women (1.2%) than men (0.4%). Approximately two-thirds of new cases arise in females (Young et al. 2000) and the average age at onset is 55 years, although there is evidence that the average age of onset is rising in both women and men, and that new-onset cases in the elderly are equally male (Symmons 2002). Overall prevalence rates are falling, although this may, in part, be a fall in severity, as the criteria given above contain severity markers (such as rheumatoid factor, nodules and erosions). The prevalence of RA falls with latitude in Europe with the Italian prevalence about a half of that in Finland.

The incidence of RA, the number of new cases occurring in a defined time period (usually a year), is also falling. This fall is probably independent of the other factors outlined above (Uhlig & Kvien 2005). It is, however, a difficult statistic to obtain and true community incidence figures are uncommon. In the UK some of the best epidemiological data have come from the Norfolk Arthritis Register (NOAR), which 'captures' all cases of persistent early arthritis presenting to general practitioners in a well-defined and stable population (Symmons et al. 1994). The current estimate of incidence of RA is 25–50/100 000/year. In contrast, in the USA between 1955 and 1964 the incidence was 83/100 000/year (Doran et al. 2002).

KEY POINTS

- The overall prevalence of rheumatoid arthritis (RA) is 0.8% (1.2% in females, 0.4% in males)
- The incidence of RA in the UK is estimated to be 0.025–0.05%
- The prevalence and incidence of RA are falling

RISK FACTORS FOR DISEASE ONSET, PERSISTENCE AND SEVERITY

Whatever triggers the inflammation in early RA it is clear that a self-limiting inflammatory arthritis can occur, but may resolve spontaneously. It is those people in whom resolution does not take place that go on to develop established disease. The factors contributing to onset, persistence and severity are different, but may overlap. There is a strong genetic contribution to onset, with twin and other studies suggesting about a 60% contribution (see genetic factors). Other significant contributors to onset include:

- Age (the peak age of incidence for women is 55–64 years, for men 65–75 years. But for the absolute difference in incidence, the older you are the more likely you are to develop RA (Symmons et al. 1994))
- Smoking (smoking is not protective for this disease)
- Oral contraceptive pill (use of this female hormone is protective: the incidence of RA in women who have ever used oral contraceptives is about half that in women who have never used it) (Harrison et al. 2000)
- Diet (people with a diet high in polyunsaturates, i.e. olive oil and fish oil, have a lower incidence of disease, but coffee consumption may be a risk factor) (Symmons 2002).

The factors associated with persistence are less clear cut at this time. There is some experimental work using a rat model that suggests the hypothalamo-pituitary axis may be an important factor, but there is no equivalent evidence from humans (Sternberg et al. 1989).

In contrast, the factors associated with disease outcome are well researched. These include:

- Age (the disease course is more severe, the older the age of onset)
- Health Assessment Questionnaire score at diagnosis (this is a self-completed measure of function and higher scores, indicating worse disability, indicate a less favourable prognosis)
- The presence of rheumatoid factor (rheumatoid factor is a key marker for subsequent disease severity and is found in about 60% of new cases) (American College of Rheumatology Subcommittee on RA 2002, Young et al. 2000)
- Delay in instigating therapy
- Smoking (people who smoke are more likely to develop extra-articular disease)
- The presence of immunogenetic markers such as the shared epitope (Sanmarti et al. 2003, Young et al. 2000) and some TNF polymorphisms (Fabris et al. 2002) (see also section on genetic factors below)
- Social deprivation is also an important factor.

NATURAL HISTORY

In the 1980s Fries developed the Stanford Health Assessment questionnaire (HAQ) and pioneered the assessment of outcome in RA (Fries et al. 1980). Fries

noted that the five main outcomes of any chronic disease were:

- Death
- Disability
- Direct costs
- Discomfort
- Drug side-effects.

It is important to distinguish between *process* and *outcome* indicators. In RA process indicators reflect the activity of the inflammatory process and include such things as the CRP or the swollen joint count. Outcome indicators are the result of the disease activity and include joint damage, work disability and the five 'D's given above. Discomfort, or pain, is slightly problematic in that it can result from active joint inflammation or from secondary osteoarthritis due to joint damage (the same is probably also true for functional limitation; the HAQ can work as a process measure in early disease). It is generally believed that in RA if the inflammatory activity of the disease can be controlled then the outcome will improve, but data such as these do not yet exist over a long period of time: 20 years or more.

It is surprisingly hard to obtain reliable data on the long-term outcome of any chronic disease. The main reason for this is the difficulty of setting up a study that may last some 30 years and where what is known about the disease and its treatment are likely to have changed dramatically over that period of time. Thus, factors that were thought important (and, thus, were part of the baseline information) at the onset of the study become less significant whereas others, not included in baseline information, achieve greater importance or even emerge during the follow-up period. The logistics of setting up (with appropriate long-term funding) such studies and achieving complete follow-up data are immense. People die, move away, lose interest, get better and stop responding: all factors that confound such studies and may bias the results.

Another important factor is the disease progression untreated; we all know of people who never went to their doctor until they had developed devastating deformities in many of their joints, but we don't know whether this would occur in an unselected sample of people at disease onset if they had been followed for a long period. Spontaneous remission of established disease obviously occurs and some people will just be wrongly diagnosed using established criteria.

It is also worth noting that clinical trials of new drugs that obviously aim to change the course of the disease are almost always conducted on selected groups of patients and not a representational cross section of people attending rheumatology clinics. People such as the elderly and those with co-morbidity (such as heart and lung disease) are often excluded from these studies. Other indicators of disease severity are rarely, if ever, controlled for in clinical trials: these include many of those mentioned above such as socio-economic status, smoking and immunogenetic status. According to one estimate, only 5% of people attending rheumatology clinics with a clinical diagnosis of RA fulfil the usual eligibility criteria for intervention studies in this disease (Wolfe 1991). A direct result of this is that it becomes difficult to generalize the results of the studies to the general rheumatology population and, equally importantly, the reported side-effect profile of the intervention is not applicable to everyone with the disease. A consequence of the latter is that a true idea of side-effects can only be appreciated when the drug has been in use for some time and post-marketing surveillance data are available; this is particularly true for a side-effect with a very low incidence, cancer for example.

Therefore, there are a number of epidemiological difficulties with identifying true and modified natural history in chronic diseases such as RA. Nevertheless, it is clear that overall the outcome of RA is not good. Mortality is increased in RA with the median age of death in males and females being 4 and 10 years earlier than in the general population (Mitchell et al. 1986). There appears to be shortening of the lifespan for those with the more severe disease associated with seropositive RA (Hawker 1997) and, indeed, with the other markers for disease severity noted above. The commonest causes of death attributed to RA are infections, renal disease, respiratory disease and gastrointestinal disease. It is also becoming clear that there is an increased cardiovascular morbidity and mortality in RA as, not only do the usual risk factors for disease (such as obesity, hypertension and hyperlipidaemia) occur, but there is also an additional risk from the disease itself, linked to inflammation in blood vessels. On top of all these factors are the risks of treatment where deaths occur due to side-effects; avoidable and tragic, but a calculated risk with any treatment.

Estimates of disability over time are beset with the difficulties already mentioned, in addition to the (hopefully) improved outcomes that follow from new treatments. One study stands out in particular, from Droitwich, in the Midlands of the UK (Scott et al. 1987). A cohort of 112 patients were originally documented in the 1960s and subsequently followed up for a period of 20 years. Unfortunately, only 46 people had complete follow-up data, although many more had partial data; 37 (35%) people had died. At the 20 year point 19% of people were severely disabled and 27% had some form of joint arthroplasty. But this was not a group of people who were treated in the same manner

as we would today; the main DMARDs were penicillamine, gold, chloroquine and prednisone, this was the days before methotrexate, leflunomide and biologics. So we could fairly reasonably assume that today's outcome after 20 years would be better. Against this is the risk of serious adverse effects from the treatment; the controversy over the withdrawal of rofecoxib (Vioxx) in 2004 exemplifies this (see Chapter 6).

RA is associated with decreased capacity of both paid work and unpaid work, such as domestic chores (Backman et al. 2004), and has been described as a time-consuming disease because everyday activities of work and leisure take longer to perform (March & Lapsley 2001). Work disability increases with disease duration and approximately 20% of people with RA report significant work disability within 1 year of diagnosis, one-third by 2 years, and up to 60% within 10 years of onset (Barrett et al. 2000). Some one-third of people with RA will leave the workforce entirely within 3 years of diagnosis (Barrett et al. 2000), although work disability is a product of type of work and sedentary workers, unsurprisingly, will fair better than manual workers (Young et al. 2002).

The costs of RA are immense and can't all be measured. Costs are usually classified into three main groups: direct, indirect and intangible. Direct costs are obvious and would include, for example, the costs of medical care and loss of income. These are easily and usually measured in any cost–benefit analysis. Indirect costs are resources lost due to the disease, such as loss of production at the person's work: these may not always be assessed in such studies. Intangible costs represent those costs of disease that can't be measured; within this rubric would be included such things as the suffering due to the disease and the marital stress that might result from one partner having the disorder. Clearly, to the individual the intangible costs might far outweigh the other costs, but to society, to health economists and to planners, the direct and indirect costs are the most important.

The overall costs of RA are considerable, considering that the prevalence of the disease is only 1 in a 100 people. They may exceed those of osteoarthritis, a disease that is much more prevalent in the community. The reason for this is clear in the rheumatology clinic; well over two-thirds of the work done by a rheumatologist is RA, as patients need to be seen frequently over the course of their (lifetime) of disease. McIntosh estimated the total cost burden of the disease to be 1.3 billion pounds annually, roughly divided half and half into direct and indirect costs (McIntosh 1996). However, even allowing for inflation, the direct costs of the disease are now likely to be increasing rapidly with the advent of new and expensive treatments, although it has been argued that savings in other areas as a result of better disease control offset these costs (see Chapter 6 for further discussion of this).

In the USA in 2003, the costs of the disease were estimated to be about eight times those in the UK (Dunlop et al. 2003). Indirect costs were estimated at 10.2 billion dollars, direct costs at 5.5 billion dollars. In the USA it is estimated that the total costs of arthritis are 2.4% of the gross national product (GNP), whereas in the UK this equates to 1.2% GNP for RA alone. Some examples of lost days in a 2-week period due to RA are given below (from the Dunlop paper):

- 0.5 days of work
- 2.4 days of restricted activity
- 1.1 days in bed.

KEY POINTS

- Mortality is increased in rheumatoid arthritis with shortening of lifespan of up to 10 years
- Morbidity is a significant factor in contributing to disability and the costs of the disease – estimated to be 1.2% of the GNP in the UK

PATHOGENESIS OF RHEUMATOID ARTHRITIS

What follows is a simplified account of recent developments. The reader interested in further detail is advised to consult more detailed review publications (Choy & Panayi 2001, Firestein 2003).

The cause of RA remains a mystery. However, several recent developments provide an insight into the mechanisms responsible for the initiation and maintenance of the disease, in addition to providing clues for treatment. The basic pathology is an abnormal synovium: the layer of cells to be found in the tissue lining the joint cavity. The synovium in RA is thickened and inflamed owing to an increase in blood vessels and inflammatory cells. These cells comprise synoviocytes, but also neutrophils, lymphocytes (both T and B cell lines) and macrophages. The T lymphocytes have migrated to the joint from elsewhere after stimulation by dendritic cells the mechanism of which is described below.

The immune system relies on two major mechanisms to combat foreign proteins such as bacteria. The innate immune system can recognize these foreign proteins without any previous contact; they do so via cell-surface receptors encoded in the cell DNA. The adaptive immune system is more complex, but much more powerful when fully activated. Foreign protein is engulfed and 'digested' by antigen presenting cells, such as dendritic cells; these cells then display fragments of the protein on their cell surface along with class II HLA molecules: a complex that can be 'recognized' by equivalent receptors on lymphocytes. Lymphocytes (mainly T lymphocytes) thus activated will undergo clonal selection and development, and act powerfully in response to fragments of the same protein subsequently encountered.

The trigger to these events remains unknown. It may be a bacterium or more likely a virus such as Epstein–Barr virus (EBV) that initiates the event. These pathogens are ubiquitous and most of us will 'meet' them at some point; the real question is why some respond with an autoimmune response and others don't. The answer to the last question may be in the specific cell-surface proteins that control the body's ability to recognize self: the HLA antigens. The trigger may even be a self protein, such as collagen, or it may be some other molecule or a combination of antigens. These events may be taking place long before the arthritis manifests itself. For example, we now know that some abnormalities are present in the serum of people long before they develop RA: rheumatoid factor and the more specific anti-cyclic citrullinated peptide antibodies.

Whatever the initiating event, once the immune system becomes activated and targets the joint (or rather the synovium), the events become self-perpetuating and, again, depend on factors particular to the host. Several susceptibility and severity markers have been identified including cytokine polymorphisms and HLA class II molecules. Activated T lymphocyte cells migrate to the synovium and release pro-inflammatory cytokines, notably, and interferon gamma (INFγ) and interleukin-17 (IL-17). In turn, these cytokines stimulate other cells; important among these are macrophages that release tumour necrosis factor alpha (TNFα), and interleukin 1 (IL-1). Macrophages can also release chemicals that are toxic to cartilage, including free oxygen radicals, nitric oxide, prostaglandins and matrix metalloproteinases (MMPs). Macrophages and their products are, therefore, important 'players' in the inflammatory processes seen in the joint in RA. However, they are not the only cells causing problems: B lymphocytes, neutrophils, fibroblasts and chondrocytes are all capable of producing harmful cytokines and chemicals that contribute to joint inflammation, bone absorption and cartilage destruction. Within this inflammatory tissue it now seems likely that TNFα plays a major role both in stimulating other cells and in promoting the release of other important pro-inflammatory cytokines.

The importance of rheumatoid factor has tended to be overshadowed by these other mechanisms. However, rheumatoid factor is still used as a diagnostic and prognostic marker in RA. The precise role of rheumatoid factor remains unknown, but immune complexes are found in the joint. The immune complexes consist of rheumatoid factor and are capable of combining with complement. These complexes attract and are engulfed by neutrophils that subsequently release inflammatory molecules similar to those noted above. Important among these are bone-specific cytokines, such as osteoprotegerin (OPG), and receptor activator of nuclear factor ligand (RANKL), which mediate osteoclast activation.

All these changes are well developed by the time the patient presents to the clinic. Without treatment they will cause bone loss and cartilage destruction. This is manifest radioligally as the appearance of bone erosions and joint space narrowing. The end point of this process is secondary osteoarthritis with complete loss of cartilage and joint destruction. The aim of treatment is to prevent these changes developing. As control of disease activity may, for many reasons, not be ideal there is a further role for treatment: that of rehabilitation and adaptation.

THE ROLE OF GENETIC FACTORS

A higher concordance in monozygotic twins suggests the importance of genetic factors in the aetiology of RA. In RA, estimates of monozygotic twin disease concordance range from 12% to 15% (Macgregor et al. 2000). An alternative way of describing this is as an estimate of the genetic contribution to the variance in liability to RA, which suggests that up to 60% of disease is likely to be explained by genetic factors. It has been estimated that first-degree relatives of RA cases are 10 times more likely to develop the disease than individuals in the population without an affected relative.

The prominent role of T lymphocytes in the synovium provides a possible mechanism for this association. T lymphocytes recognize HLA class II molecules on antigen presenting cells and an association between HLA DR subtypes and RA has been found. The link between presentation of a (possibly) ubiquitous antigen and the immune response has not been fully elucidated, but the association of these susceptibility and severity genes, which code for cell surface antigens involved with the process of antigen presentation, is certainly a step forward. Interestingly, there are only a restricted number of subtypes of these HLA antigens associated with RA – HLA DRβ 0401/4; common to these is a particular five amino acid sequence in the

third hypervariable region, the so-called 'shared epitope'. The HLA molecule is expressed on the surface of the cell and consists of an antigenic 'groove'. In fact, the shared epitope amino acids actually point away from this groove so the mechanism is obviously not entirely related to specific antigen presentation.

THE INTERNATIONAL CLASSIFICATION OF FUNCTIONING, DISABILITY AND HEALTH (ICF)

The World Health Organization (WHO) has introduced a novel system for recording the personal impact of disease. Formerly, the International Classification of Impairments, Disabilities and Handicap (ICIDH), this new framework permits a more comprehensive description of the health state and the interaction of the person with their environment, shifting the emphasis from cause to impact. It is intended for use by health workers, but may also be used in research and in planning for health. The WHO regards this new approach as being much more widely applicable to the whole of society, not just a minority with disabilities. The ICF is intended to complement the International Statistical Classification of Diseases and Related Health Problems (ICD-10). ICF classifies health, ICD-10 classifies diseases. It is useful to consider the ICF as based on a biopsychosocial model and the ICD-10 on a medical model of disease. A useful summary of the biopsychosocial model is provided by Waddell (Waddell 1987) (see Fig. 1.1).

An introduction to the ICF is available and further documents can be ordered from the WHO website (http://www3.who.int/icf/icftemplate.cfm). In use it is fairly complex, but there are efforts to concentrate

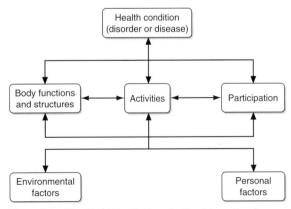

Figure 1.1 The World Health Organization International Classification of Functioning, Disability and Health (ICF): outline structure (see http://www3.who.int/icf/icftemplate.cfm).

on particular diseases; for RA there has been some pre-liminary work published (Stucki & Cieza 2004), but much further work remains to be done. It is, of course, possible to apply this system to any part of the body for any disease; the Leeds Foot Impact Scale (LFIS) for RA was constructed around the domains of 'impairments', 'activities' and 'participation' with a special category for 'footwear' (Helliwell et al. 2005) (see Chapter 8). The ICF was designed as a tool that could be used in a variety of different situations, including the personal and institutional level. However, the ICF is not a measurement tool; it is a system for classifying human function and disability. For a specific disease such as RA it determines *what* should be measured, not *how* it should be measured. It is easy to see how it could determine what is important to measure in different situations, such as a study designed to define the level of functioning and disability for surgery to the forefoot. A tool such as the LFIS, based on some aspects of the ICF, can capture the essence of the impact of the disease on the individual and can help identify the aspects that are more likely to respond to simple interventions such as orthotics.

A very simple explanation of how the ICF can be used follows. The ICF works from four lists: body function, body structure, activity/participation and environment. Within each of these domains are chapters, and within the chapters further subdivisions. For example, for the ankle joint, the descriptor would be: body structures (s), chapter 7; structures related to movement (s7); structure of lower extremity (s750); structure of foot and ankle (s7502); ankle joint and joints of foot and toes (s75021). However, a weakness

is that pain in the ankle cannot be specifically described: body functions (b); sensory functions and pain (b2); pain (b280); pain in body part (b2801) and pain in lower limb (b28015) (see Fig. 1.2).

A further element of uncertainty concerns the introduction of qualifiers. The qualifiers are intended to provide additional information, coded on a five-point scale, common to all descriptors that allow an assessment of the degree of impairment, from 'no impairment' to 'complete impairment'. Thus, in the first example given above, the complete code would be s75021.1 for 'mild' impairment of the ankle joint. Much more work is required to examine the meaning of these qualifiers as there is yet no evidence for their reliability or external validity.

The qualifiers for activity/participation are slightly different and more difficult to conceptualize. The *performance* qualifier describes the individual's existing solutions in their own environment, including any assistive devices used. The *capacity* qualifier describes an individual's highest achievable level of functioning, always acknowledging that some environments are more 'permissive'. This approach, comparing capacity and performance, does enable an assessment of how much the environment facilitates (or obstructs) the individual. As indicated above, the fourth domain is the environment, with which this can be described. Here is an example of the latter, where a hospital fails to provide an orthotic service for people with foot problems due to RA: environment (e), chapter 5; services (e5); health services systems and policies (e580) and health services (e5800). The qualifier in this case indicates the extent to which this provides a barrier to

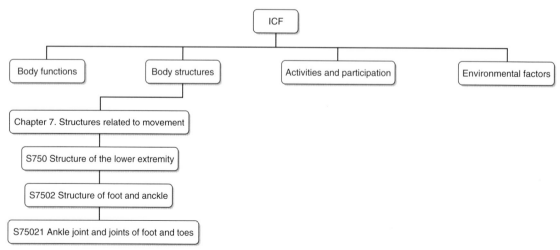

Figure 1.2   The ICF classification for the ankle and foot.

function; in this case a 'moderate' barrier (25–49%) making the complete code e5800-2 (the minus sign indicating that this is a barrier. A facilitator is indicated by a plus sign).

The ICF, therefore, provides a comprehensive system with which to classify functioning and disability. It permits a synthesis of the issues relevant to health professional and patient alike and permits the integration of environmental and contextual factors (Stucki & Ewert 2005). A lot more work is required on the classification and on the core sets, but it seems likely that it will become the norm for health workers in this field. Therefore, in defining the elements of impairments, function, disability and handicap this book will utilize the structure proposed by the ICF.

THE EPIDEMIOLOGY OF FOOT DISEASE IN RHEUMATOID ARTHRITIS

Symmetrical small joint polyarthritis is the hallmark of early RA; metacarpophalangeal and proximal inter-phalangeal joints in the hand, and metatarsophalangeal and proximal inter-phalangeal joints (although difficult to distinguish clinically, often causing 'painful toes') in the foot. This is the common clinical impression of how the disease starts and is reflected in the criteria for diagnosis put forward by the American College of Rheumatology (Arnett et al. 1988). As already discussed, however, these criteria were developed using cases of established disease and, thus, may not function well in early disease, nor may they reflect the actuality of everyday cases seen in the clinic. It is, therefore, clinical surveys of early and established disease that give us the best indication of the patterns and frequency of joint involvement in this disorder.

It is worth noting again the importance of methodology (see section on Natural History). Longitudinal surveys give better quality information about progression and risk factors for progression, but are difficult to perform and have their own limitations. More often, studies are of the cross-sectional type making it impossible to infer causal associations with indicators identified at the time. A comparison of cross-sectional data at two different time points in two different populations is useful, but still limited in terms of data quality.

Another important point concerns the method of assessment. If we are concerned with patterns and prevalence of joint and soft-tissue involvement then, clearly, the method of assessment is important. Clinical examination is probably the least sensitive method of detecting joint and soft-tissue involvement yet this is the method used in most of the classic studies. With modern imaging techniques, such as U/S and MRI, clinically undetectable abnormalities are being found: this is likely to change the way that we look at patterns of joint and soft-tissue involvement in both early and late disease (see Chapter 5 on imaging the foot and ankle).

Early disease

As already mentioned, small joint inflammation in the hands and feet is the hallmark of early RA. Although symptoms may be prominent, signs are often more subtle and synovitis may be difficult to detect especially in the metatarsophalangeal joints and in the rearfoot (Maillefert et al. 2003). The metatarsal and metacarpal squeeze test has been identified as a clinical sign of inflammation in these joint groups, but the sensitivity and specificity of this test in RA is not exceptional (sensitivity 67%, specificity 89%; compare these with the 1987 revised criteria where the sensitivity is 82% and the specificity 78%) (Rigby & Wood 1991). Occasionally, the 'daylight sign' is seen (see Clinical Features in Chapter 4) and this is reported as an early sign of RA due to inflammation of the inter-metatarsal bursa (Dedrick et al. 1990).

One of the first studies of early disease was conducted by Fleming and colleagues at the Middlesex Hospital in London, UK published in 1976. They found that RA more commonly occurs in the winter and they listed the site of onset as follows: hand 28%, elbow 3%, knee 8%, foot 13% and ankle 6%. It is often difficult for patients to remember and exactly locate the site of their first symptoms; sometimes joint symptoms occur simultaneously in several areas. Fleming and colleagues found this to be the case in 29% of cases (Fleming et al. 1976a). This group also recorded individual joint involvement: in the foot and ankle the prevalence of joint involvement at onset was as follows: right ankle 25%, left ankle 23%, both ankles 18% (the talo-crural and sub-talar were not separately identified), right mid-tarsal 8%, left mid-tarsal 13%, both mid-tarsal 6%, right metatarso phalangeal joints 48%, left 47%, both 43% (compare these with the metacarpophalangeal joints: right 65%, left 58%, both 52%) (Fleming et al. 1976b). Interestingly, these authors went on to perform factor analysis of patterns of joint involvement finding that early metatarsophalangeal involvement was associated with a younger age group and better prognosis (Fleming et al. 1976c).

Although the hand, particularly the metacarpophalangeal joints in the hand, are considered to be earliest joints involved in RA, it has been shown that MRI-detectable synovitis is present in the metatarsophalangeal joints in the absence of synovitis in the hand

(Ostendorf et al. 2004). In this study of early disease the abnormalities detected in the metatarsophalangeal joints consisted of bone oedema, synovitis and erosions: the longer the disease the more abnormalities were found.

Metatarsophalangeal joint involvement (or the metacarpophalangeal joints in the hand), identified by a positive squeeze test, is one of three criteria (including ≥3 swollen joints and morning stiffness of ≥30 min) in an early referral algorithm for newly diagnosed RA (Emery et al. 2002). If effective treatment requires early diagnosis, then health professionals have an important role in identifying potential patients. None more so than podiatrists who are often referred patients with metatarsalgia that has failed to respond to initial treatment in primary care. Where no obvious mechanical cause can be identified, suspicions should fall on other causes and testing for the three criteria above is easily achieved and should be widely taught.

Historical aspects

The paper of Vainio, looking at a group of almost 1000 patients with RA, has achieved almost iconic status (Vainio 1956). In fact, the original paper was published in such an obscure journal that most people (including the current authors) now rely on a facsimile of the original, published in honour of Vainio in a symposium on the foot in 1991 (Vainio 1991). The facsimile unfortunately does not do justice to the original paper, giving little original data. Vainio was a Finnish orthopaedic surgeon who pioneered surgery of the foot in RA and who published extensively on this topic and travelled widely lecturing on surgery of the hand and foot. Vainio indicates a prevalence of 89% of 'foot troubles' in RA with slightly higher prevalence in females than males. (It is interesting to note that in terms of the ICF classification, this may be more contextual than a true reflection of the prevalence as the footwear demands of females are generally different to those of males.) Vainio's is essentially a cross-sectional survey; indeed, it could be called a cumulative survey, as these cases were amassed and reported on as time progressed. Involvement of the forefoot was reported to be common with abnormalities of the hallux predominating and increasing with duration of disease. The rearfoot was also reported to be commonly involved excluding the talo-crural joint (9%), the sub-talar joint being involved in 70% of cases and often occurring early, causing significant disability. Vainio also indicated the frequent involvement of soft-tissue structures such as the long tendons and their sheaths (6.5%), the forefoot and rearfoot inter-articular ligaments, and the sesamoid bones of the foot.

The method of selection of Vainio's patients remains obscure, but there is no doubt about the way that Michelson and colleagues collected patients in their survey that, essentially, reproduced that of Vainio. Michelson and colleagues systematically examined the feet of an unselected group of 99 patients with RA for an average disease duration of 13 years. They confirmed Vainio's figures for prevalence of foot symptoms (93%) (Michelson et al. 1994). Michelson also looked at the frequency of symptoms in different parts of the foot and, in contrast with Vainio, found that ankle symptoms were more common than forefoot symptoms (42% v 28%; a further 14% had both ankle and forefoot symptoms and a further 3% had midfoot and forefoot symptoms). Interestingly, for podiatrists, very few patients had special shoes or 'inserts' provided.

Review of established disease at the rearfoot (Fig. 2.18)

One of the few prospective studies looking at the rearfoot was designed to assess the radiological progression of disease at the ankle joint complex over a 20-year period (Belt et al. 2001). Follow-up was, of course, incomplete with only 68/103 of the original cohort having assessment at 20 years. For this reason the figures quoted, based on the original sample size, are difficult to interpret, but what does seem clear is that sub-talar joint disease exceeds and precedes talo-crural disease. Further, many patients may not have any ankle involvement at 20 years. Cross-sectional studies generally support the observation that sub-talar disease occurs earlier and is more severe than talo-crural involvement; one exception is a study reported by Spiegel and Spiegel who found (clinically) more frequent disease in the talo-crural joint (Spiegel & Spiegel 1982).

There are, of course, other important extra-articular structures at the rearfoot, notably the tendon of tibialis posterior. This structure has been the subject of numerous studies, particularly following the advent of ultrasound and MRI. The association between the 'typical' pesplanovalgus deformity and dysfunction in the tibialis posterior tendon has received a lot of attention and, although there may be an element of co-morbidity in this association (the coincidence of severe disease in several adjacent areas – see Fig. 1.3), the pesplanovalgus deformity is generally associated with tenosynovitis, longitudinal tears or even complete rupture of this important structure (Jernberg et al. 1999). Surprisingly overlooked, is the contribution from Keenan and co-workers, who demonstrated that tibialis posterior dysfunction may be secondary to

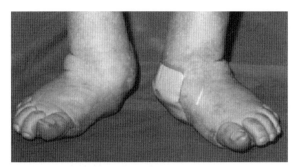

Figure 1.3 Typical rear-foot deformity in established rheumatoid arthritis. Note the valgus heel position, loss of longitudinal arch and prominence of navicular bone.

gastrocnemius-soleus muscle weakness (Keenan et al. 1991). This group combined electromyography and kinematics with radiographic and clinical data and the pathomechanical model they proposed is eloquent, yet requires updating. Encouragingly, techniques that combine gait and imaging are emerging and can be applied in prospective cohort studies to investigate this area (Woodburn et al. 2005, Turner et al. 2003, Woodburn et al. 2003).

The prevalence of pesplanovalgus deformity increases with increasing duration of disease. Spiegel and Spiegel reported a prevalence of 46% of 'flat feet' in their cohort, although it was difficult to see what definition had been applied (Spiegel & Spiegel 1982). Shi et al. performed serial radiographs of the feet in a cohort of patients with RA and found an increasing prevalence of flat foot as measured by the calcaneal pitch, the deformity being worse in a group with more severe disease (Shi et al. 2000). Clearly, the aetiology of rearfoot deformities in RA is more complex than just tibialis posterior tendon dysfunction (see biomechanics section in Chapter 2) but this is nevertheless an important structure with a vital role in rearfoot stability.

Vainio also indicated that the heel may be commonly involved in RA; an important observation since it is now commonly thought that involvement of the heel is the hallmark of seronegative spondylo arthropathies. Vainio recorded the presence of Achilles bursitis (presumably retrocalcaneal bursitis), calcaneal spurs and the presence of painful rheumatoid nodules in the heel pad (Vainio 1991).

Bouysset and colleagues looked closely at new bone formation on the calcaneus finding 'spurs' on the posterior aspect of the heel in 31% of 397 feet and inferior spurs in 30% of feet (Bouysset et al. 1989). In fairness, Bouysset report that only a minority of these 'spurs' were inflammatory, most being the sort of mechanical

spur found in the general population with advancing age. The inferior 'spurs' were most often related to 'flat' feet and calcaneo-valgus deformity. Despite all these abnormalities the patients in Bouysset's study reported very few symptoms in the heel.

Michelson, on the other hand, found frequent symptomatic heels in his cohort, with 29% of patients complaining of heel pain. Generally, the worse the functional grade the more prevalent were the symptoms in the foot, particularly the forefoot, again emphasizing that many foot problems do not occur in isolation and often reflect severity and duration of disease.

Review of established disease at the midfoot

The mid-tarsal joints are frequently neglected both clinically and experimentally yet the talo-navicular joint, in our experience, is involved early in RA and may cause significant pain and disability. The work of Bouysett and colleagues in France supports this; this orthopaedic group has reported on the progression of foot disease in RA including patients with varying disease duration (Bouysset et al. 1987). Talo-navicular joint involvement occurred early and ultimately most frequently in an unselected population of 222 patients. The frequency of mid-tarsal joint involvement, according to the findings of this group, is given in Table 1.2.

Michelson also found the mid foot to be a common site for symptoms: although 27% of patients reported mid-foot symptoms, only 5% said they were their most important foot symptom (Michelson et al. 1994). From a clinical and epidemiological aspect detection of synovitis in the mid-tarsal joints is difficult and may tend to underestimate the true prevalence of involvement. A systematic study of mid-tarsal involvement using ultrasound or MRI has yet to be undertaken. It is our belief that the talo-navicular

Table 1.2 Frequency of mid-tarsal joint involvement at 15 years in 222 patients with rheumatoid arthritis (adapted from Bouysset 1987).

Joint	n	Percentage
Talo-navicular joint	133	60
Cuneo-navicular joint	98	44
Cuneo-metatarsal joint	69	31
Talo-crural joint(*)	53	24
Sub-talar joint (*)	120	54

* Talo-crural and sub-talar joints included for comparison.

joint is an important and frequently involved joint in the mid foot and is important in the evolution of the common foot deformities seen in RA. Preliminary studies are encouraging and data from Leeds have shown an association between sites of midtarsal joint inflammation and deformity when the region is reconstructed in 3D from MRI images (Woodburn et al. 2002). Furthermore, biomechanical studies have demonstrated the important torsion control mechanism of the talonavicular joint (Lundberg et al. 1989) and, using a cadaver model, change in midtarsal orientation, consistent with medial longitudinal arch collapse, when important supporting structures were selectively attenuated (Woodburn et al. 2005). Work of this nature certainly deserves further study with a view to elucidating biomechanics and considering treatment approaches.

Review of established disease at the forefoot

Forefoot deformity is not uncommon in the general population so that prevalence figures for disease must be interpreted in the context of the 'background' of deformity. Complaints of foot pain rise with age to a peak prevalence of almost 16% for women in the 55–64 age group and toe deformity occurs in 15% of the population (Garrow et al. 2004). By comparison hallux abducto valgus occurs in 80% of patients with established RA, the prevalence increasing with increasing duration of disease (and age) (Spiegel & Spiegel 1982). Vainio found a similar prevalence of deformity at the great toe, again increasing with disease duration, and a high prevalence of mallet toe deformity.

Early RA, as already mentioned, is clinically felt to be an early site of inflammation and, although difficult to detect clinically, may be manifest by a positive metatarsal sqeeze test. Now studies using MRI suggest that synovitis may be present in the metatarsophalangeal joints before disease in the hand is apparent (Ostendorf et al. 2004).

One of the consequences of synovitis of the metatarsophalangeal joints is capsular and ligamentous attenuation, particularly if the joint is repeatedly or continuously stressed. Inflammation in the forefoot is a prime example of this: when involving the deep transverse metatarsal ligament then the metatarsophalangeal joints will tend to drift apart, the forefoot will clinically 'spread' and the head of the metatarsal will sublux ventrally (Stainsby 1997). This common forefoot deformity also increases with increasing disease duration, but may be an early symptom along with metatarsophalangeal pain. The role of anatomy and biomechanics is an important one and an analogue model for the MCP joints of the hands has recently

been proposed (Tan et al 2003). Both synovitis and bone erosion have a predilection for the radial side of the metacarpophalangeal joints associated with collateral ligament damage and abnormal flexor tendon alignment and action. Since we tend to see 'fibular' drift of the toes the same relationship may exist at the MTP joints, but this has yet to be tested. The relationships between these factors are not insignificant and yet a lack of understanding prevents solutions to current treatment dilemmas. For example, in forefoot reconstruction the traditional arthroplasty based on resection of the metatarsal head and a portion of the proximal phalanx is favoured, whilst others argue to protect the metatarsal head and undertake soft-tissue revision with relocation of the plantar plate (Stainsby 1997). Of course, one functional role of custom orthoses is 'soft-tissue substitution' where cushioning materials are used to off-load and protect prominent metatarsal heads and overlying callus. How well these materials achieve this is not known, although pressures can be reduced and symptoms improved (Hodge et al. 1999). In both examples, a greater understanding of the structure and function of the forefoot will allow current treatment approaches to be better appraised and new approaches developed, and both these themes will be developed in later chapters.

In the 1970s Jacobi and colleagues studied the commoner varieties of hallux abnormalities in RA (Jacoby et al. 1976). In a population of 200 consecutive inpatients they described:

- Hallux valgus (deviation of the great toe by more than 20°) in 58%. This they distinguished from hallux valgus in people without RA where there is often associated bony exostoses and bursa formation. Although no precise figures were given the latter two features were reported to be 'rare' in their population of patients. An associated varus deformity of the first metatarsal was seen in most of these cases and may contribute to the forefoot spead.
- Hallux tortus. A medial rotational deformity of the great toe associated with hallux valgus (defined as a rotation of more than 20°). This deformity was often associated with an area of high pressure over the inter-phalangeal joint. The deformity was found in 29% of feet (Fig. 1.4).
- Hallux rigidus. The group defined this as less than 20° of passive dorsiflexion of the first metatarsophalangeal joint and this was found in 78% of feet. The 'mobile' and 'rigid' groups were distinguishable on the basis of disease duration, the 'rigid' group having a disease duration on average 13 years longer.

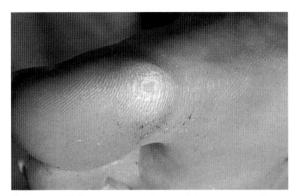

Figure 1.4 Hallus tortus et abductus with prominent callus formation overlying the interphalangeal joint of the great toe.

- Chisel toe. This was defined as a symptom complex comprising hyperextension of the inter-phalangeal joint, a pressure effect between the nail plate and the overlying shoe, and a plantar callosity under the inter-phalangeal joint. This triad occurred in 22% of feet.
- Hallux elevatus. This was defined as an absent range of plantar flexion at the hallux and was seen in 10% of feet.
- Inter-phalangeal claw, defined as an inability to dorsiflex the distal phalanx of the great toe associated with a limited range of movement (in the range of 10–30°) and an associated dorsal callosity over the joint. This was found in 7% of toes.

There were a number of other deformities noted but these were of diminishing prevalence. Many of the deformities occurred in the same foot. Some discussion was devoted to the management of such deformities, stressing the importance of appropriate footwear. In a

KEY POINTS

- Foot involvement occurs in 90% of people with rheumatoid arthritis (RA)
- The metatarsal (or metacarpal) squeeze test, more than three swollen joints and early-morning stiffness of more than 30 min are strong indicators of early RA
- Pes planovalgus occurs in up to 50% of affected people
- The talonavicular joint is a common source of symptoms
- Early involvement of the deep transverse metatarsal ligament causes widening of the fore-foot and difficulty with footwear

further publication this group noted the presence of symptoms, deformities and radiological abnormalities in the same patient group (Vidigal et al. 1975). Interestingly, they noted that clinical symptoms usually exceeded radiological abnormalities, except in the midfoot joints, where the opposite occurred. This group also found a high prevalence of ankle and mid-tarsal symptoms in their patient group, and a relatively high prevalence of enthesopathy at the heel (31%). However, it was disappointing that further efforts were not made to look at the association between symptoms, deformities, generic data and disease specific associations, other than duration of disease.

FACTORS ASSOCIATED WITH THE PREVALENCE AND PROGRESSION OF FOOT DISEASE IN RHEUMATOID ARTHRITIS

There is a dearth of good epidemiological data making assertions and observations very difficult. Most studies report an increasing prevalence of foot deformities with advancing duration of disease and age, both of which factors are obviously closely related. Specific data looking at the relationship between bodily function, structure, activities/participation and the environment, as suggested by the ICF, are not available. Given the proposed mechanism of early deformity in RA, external force on inflamed and attenuated articular stabilization mechanisms, it would not be surprising to find a positive relationship between body mass index and the prevalence of foot deformity. Other factors may be important. For example, rear-foot pronation is fairly common in the general (non-diseased) population and this may be a risk factor for accelerated rear-foot deformity in people with inflammation of the sub-talar joint. The field is rich in potential for further studies.

One important study has looked at the relationship between lower limb pain, structural deformity and function (as measured by questionnaire and by direct measurement of gait parameters) (Platto et al. 1991). This study had limitations, it was a small sample size ($n = 31$) and the instruments used were fairly crude, but the results were interesting in that the gait parameters were largely a function of pain, rather that structural deformity. When analysed by individual areas there was a relationship between pain and structural deformity, and this relationship carried over to the between area comparisons in some cases. Thus, rear-foot deformity was correlated with fore-foot pain, as might be expected. Rear-foot deformity appeared to have the largest impact on gait and mobility. There is now an opportunity to carry out much more sophisticated studies of this kind, using MRI and U/S to quantify inflammation on a regional basis, and using detailed multi-segment foot analysis to quantify gait (see Chapter 2).

The relationship between disease severity and severity of foot involvement has been mentioned in a number of publications, but we must be careful to make sure we are comparing like with like. As already mentioned, disease severity can be measured as a process item or as an outcome item. Someone with very active disease classified as 'severe' but in the early stages may have very few foot deformities. On the other hand, someone in remission (no disease activity) who has had the disease for 30 years may have extreme foot deformities. As these concepts become accepted into medical outcomes, aided by the OMERACT process (Bellamy 1999), further meaningful information on the relationship between these domains will become available.

Meanwhile, we are only just beginning to develop the tools to look at the impact of foot disease on the individual, aside from their disease elsewhere. The LFIS should enable us to decode the different aspects of foot involvement and further careful studies with this instrument should help measure the differential impact of the disease and the effect of treatments on the different domains of assessment. Once this information is available it should be possible to obtain a clearer idea of the costs and burden of foot involvement in RA. We already know that the impact is considerable. For example, in the study by Vidigal of established disease lower-limb symptoms were four times more frequent than those in the upper limb, and the foot second to the knee in symptom severity (Vidigal et al. 1975).

SUMMARY

RA is a complex multi-system disorder that commonly affects the foot and ankle. This chapter has provided background reading on the pathogenesis, epidemiology and genetics of this disorder, in addition to describing the epidemiology of foot pathology in RA. Finally, novel podiatric concepts are introduced. This chapter has provided an introduction to the topic, in preparation for the chapters to come.

References

American College of Rheumatology Subcommittee on Rheumatoid Arthritis. Guidelines for the management of rheumatoid arthritis: 2002 Update. [see comment]. Arthritis & Rheumatism 2002; 46(2): 328–346.

Arnett FC, Edworthy SM and Bloch DA The American Rheumatism Association 1987 revised criteria for the classification of rheumatoid arthritis. Arthritis and Rheumatism 1988; 31(3): 315–324.

Backman CL, Kennedy SM, Chalmers A and Singer J Participation in paid and unpaid work by adults with rheumatoid arthritis. Journal of Rheumatology 2004; 31(1): 47–56.

Barrett EM, Scott DG, Wiles NJ and Symmons DP The impact of rheumatoid arthritis on employment status in the early years of disease: a UK community-based study. Rheumatology 2000; 39(12): 1403–1409.

Bas S, Genevay S, Meyer O and Gabay C Anti-citrullinated peptide antibodies, IgM and IgA rheumatoid factors in the diagnosis and prognosis of rheumatoid arthritis. Rheumatology 2003; 42(5): 677–680.

Bellamy N Clinimetric concepts in outcome assessment: the OMERACT filter. Journal of Rheumatology 1999; 26(4): 948–950.

Belt EA, Kaarela K, Maenpaa H, Kauppi MJ, Lehtinen JT and Lehto MU Relationship of ankle joint involvement with subtalar destruction in patients with rheumatoid arthritis. A 20-year follow-up study. Joint, Bone, Spine: Revue du Rhumatisme 2001; 68(2): 154–157.

Berthelot JM, Saraux A, Le Henaff C, Chales G, Baron D Le, Goff P and Youinou P Confidence in the diagnosis of early spondylarthropathy: a prospective follow-up of 270 early arthritis patients. Clinical & Experimental Rheumatology 2002; 20(3): 319–326.

Bouysset M, Bonvoisin B, Lejeune E and Bouvier M Flattening of the rheumatoid foot in tarsal arthritis on X-ray. Scandinavian Journal of Rheumatology 1987; 16(2): 127–133.

Bouysset M, Tebib J, Weil G, Noel E, Colson F, Llorca G, Lejeune E and Bouvier M The rheumatoid heel: its relationship to other disorders in the rheumatoid foot. Clinical Rheumatology 1989; 8(2): 208–214.

Choy EHS and Panayi GS Cytokine pathways and joint inflammation in rheumatoid arthritis. New England Journal of Medicine 2001; 344: 907–916.

Dedrick DK, McCune WJ and Smith WS Rheumatoid arthritis presenting as spreading of the toes. A report of three cases. Journal of Bone & Joint Surgery – American Volume 1990; 72(3): 463–464.

Doran MF, Pond GR, Crowson CS, O'Fallon WM and Gabriel SE Trends in incidence and mortality in rheumatoid arthritis in Rochester, Minnesota over a forty year period. Arthritis and Rheumatism 2002; 46: 625–631.

Dunlop DD, Manheim LM, Yelin EH, Song J and Chang RW The costs of arthritis. Arthritis and Rheumatism 2003; 49: 101–113.

Emery P, Breedveld FC, Dougados M, Kalden JR, Schiff MH and Smolen JS Early referral recommendation for newly diagnosed rheumatoid arthritis. evidence based development of a clinical guide. Annals of Rheumatic Diseases 2002; 61: 290–297.

Fabris M, Di PE, D'Elia A, Damante G, Sinigaglia L and Ferraccioli G Tumor necrosis factor-alpha gene polymorphism in severe and mild–moderate rheumatoid arthritis. Journal of Rheumatology 2002; 29(1): 29–33.

Firestein GS Evolving concepts of rheumatoid arthritis. Nature 2003; 423: 356–361.

Fleming A, Crown JM and Corbett M Early rheumatoid disease I Onset. Annals of the Rheumatic Diseases 1976a; 35: 357–360.

Fleming A, Crown JM and Corbett M Incidence of joint involvement in early rheumatoid arthritis. Rheumatology & Rehabilitation 1976b 15: 92–96.

Fleming A, Benn RT, Corbett M and Wood PHN Early rheumatoid disease II. Patterns of joint involvement. Annals of the Rheumatic Diseases 1976c; 35: 361–364.

Fries JF, Spitz P, Kraines RG and Holman HR Measurement of patient outcome in arthritis. Arthritis and Rheumatism 1980; 23(2): 137–145.

Garrow AP, Silman AJ and Macfarlane GJ The Cheshire Foot Pain and Disability Survey: a population survey assessing prevalence and associations. Pain 2004; 110(1–2): 378–384.

Harrison BJ, Silman AJ and Symmons DP Does the age of onset of rheumatoid arthritis influence phenotype? A prospective study of outcome and prognostic factors. Rheumatology 2000; 39(1): 112–113.

Harrison BJ, Symmons DP, Barrett EM and Silman AJ The performance of the 1987 An RA classification criteria for rheumatoid arthritis in a population based cohort of patients with early inflammatory polyarthritis. Journal of Rheumatology 1998; 25(12): 2324–2330.

Hawker G Update on the epidemiology of the rheumatic diseases. Current Opinion in Rheumatology 1997; 9(2): 90–94.

Helliwell PS, Reay N, Gilworth G, Redmond A, Slade A, Tennant A and Woodburn J Development of a foot impact scale for rheumatoid arthritis. Arthritis Care Research 2005; 53(3): 418–422.

Hodge MC, Bach TM, Carter GM Orthotic management of plantar pressure and pain in rheumatoid arthritis. Clinical Biomechanics 1999; 14: 567–575.

Jacoby RK, Vidigal E, Kirkup J and Dixon AJ The great toe as a clinical problem in rheumatoid arthritis. Rheumatology & Rehabilitation 1976; 15(3): 143–147.

Jernberg ET, Simkin P, Kravette M, Lowe P and Gardner G The posterior tibial tendon and the tarsal sinus in rheumatoid flat foot: magnetic resonance imaging of 40 feet. Journal of Rheumatology 1999; 26(2): 289–293.

Keenan MA, Peabody TD, Gronley JK and Perry J Valgus deformity of the feet and characteristics of gait in patients who have rheumatoid arthritis. J Bone Joint Surg 1991; 73A: 237–247.

Lundberg A, Svensson OK, Bylund C, Goldie I and Selvik G Kinematics of the ankle/foot complex—Part 2: Pronation and supination. Foot Ankle 1989; 9: 248–253.

Macgregor AJ, Sneider H, Rigby AS, Koskenvuo M, Kaprio J, Aho K and Silman AJ Characterising the quantitative genetic component to rheumatoid arthritis using data from twins. Arthritis and Rheumatism 2000; 43(1): 30–37.

Maillefert JF, Dardel P, Cherasse A, Mistrih R, Krause D and Tavernier C Magnetic resonance imaging in the assessment of synovial inflammation of the hindfoot in patients with rheumatoid arthritis and other polyarthritis. European Journal of Radiology 2003; 47(1): 1–5.

March L and Lapsley H What are the costs to society and the potential benefits from the effective management of early rheumatoid arthritis? Best Practice & Research in Clinical Rheumatology 2001; 15(1): 171–185.

McIntosh E The cost of rheumatoid arthritis. British Journal of Rheumatism 1996; 35: 781–790.

Michelson J, Easley M, Wigley FM and Hellmann D Foot and ankle problems in rheumatoid arthritis. Foot & Ankle International 1994; 15(11): 608–613.

Mitchell DM, Spitz PW, Young DY, Block DA, McShane DJ and Fries JF Survival, prognosis, and causes of death in rheumatoid arthritis. Arthritis and Rheumatism 1986; 29: 706–714.

Ostendorf B, Scherer A, Moreland LW and Schneider M Diagnostic value of magnetic resonance imaging of the forefoot in early rheumatoid arthritis when findings on imaging of the metacarpophalangeal joints of the hands remain normal. Arthritis and Rheumatism 2004; 50: 2094–2102.

Rigby AS and Wood PHN The lateral metacarpophalangeal/metatarsophalangeal squeeze: an alternative assignment criterion for rheumatoid arthritis. Scandinavian Journal of Rheumatology 1991; 20: 115–120.

Sanmarti R, Gomez A, Ercilla G et al. Radiological progression in early rheumatoid arthritis after DMARDS: a one-year follow-up study in a clinical setting. Rheumatology 2003; 42(9): 1044–1049.

Scott DL, Coulton BL, Symmons DPM and Popert AJ Long-term outcome of treating rheumatoid arthritis: results after 20 years. Lancet 1987; 1: 1108–1111.

Shi K, Tomita T, Hayashida K, Owaki H and Ochi T Foot deformities in rheumatoid arthritis and relevance of disease severity. Journal of Rheumatology 2000; 27(1): 84–89.

Spiegel TM and Spiegel JS Rheumatoid arthritis in the foot and ankle – Diagnosis, pathology, and treatment. The relationship between foot and ankle deformity and disease duration in 50 patients. Foot & Ankle 1982; 2(6): 318–324.

Stainsby GD Pathological anatomy and the dynamic effect of the displaced plantar plate and the importance of the integrity of the plantar plate–deep transverse metatarsal ligament tie-bar. Annals of the Royal College of Surgeons of England 1997; 79: 58–68.

Sternberg EM, Young WS, Bernardini R, Calogero AE, Chrousos GP, Gold PW and Wilder RL A central nervous system defect in biosynthesis of corticotrophin releasing hormone is associated with susceptibility to streptococcal wall induced arthritis in rats. Proceedings of the National Academy of Science (USA) 1989; 86: 4771–4775.

Stucki G and Cieza A The International Classification of functioning, disability and health (ICF) core sets for rheumatoid arthritis: a way to specify functioning. Annals of Rheumatic Diseases 2004; 63(supplement II): 40–45.

Stucki G and Ewert T How to assess the impact of arthritis on the individual patient: the WHO ICF Annals of Rheumatic Diseases 2005; 64: 664–668.

Symmons DP, Barrett EM, Bankhead CR, Scott DG and Silman AJ The incidence of rheumatoid arthritis in the United Kingdom: results from the Norfolk Arthritis Register. British Journal of Rheumatology 1994; 33(8): 735–739.

Symmons DPM Epidemiology of rheumatoid arthritis: determinants of onset, persistence and outcome. Best Practice and Research Clinical Rheumatology 2002; 16(5): 707–722.

Tan AL, Tanner SF, Conaghan PG et al. Role of metacarpophalangeal joint anatomic factors in the distribution of synovitis and bone erosion in early rheumatoid arthritis. Arthritis and Rheumatism 2003; 48: 1214–1222.

Turner DE, Woodburn J, Helliwell PS, Cornwall ME, Emery P Pes planovalgus in rheumatoid arthritis: a descriptive and analytical study of foot function determined by gait analysis. Musculoskeletal Care 2003; 1: 21–33.

Uhlig T and Kvien TK Is rheumatoid arthritis disappearing? Annals of Rheumatic Diseases 2005; 64(1): 7–10.

Vainio K The rheumatoid foot: a clinical study with pathological and roentgenological comments. Annals of Chirurgiae et Gynaecologiae 1956; Suppl 45(Suppl 1): 1–110.

Vainio K The rheumatoid foot. A clinical study with pathological and roentgenological comments. Clinical Orthopaedics & Related Research 1991; 265: 4–8.

Vidigal E, Jacoby RK, Dixon AS, Ratliff AH and Kirkup J The foot in chronic rheumatoid arthritis. Annals of Rheumatic Diseases 1975; 34(4): 292–297.

Waddell G A new clinical model for the treatment of low back pain. Spine 1987; 12: 632–644.

Woodburn J, Cornwall MW, Soames RW, Helliwell PS Selectively attenuating soft tissues close to the sites of inflammation in the peritalar region of patients with rheumatoid arthritis leads to development of pes planovalgus. Journal of Rheumatology 2005; 32: 268–274.

Woodburn J, Nelson KM, Lohmann Siegel K, Kepple TM, Gerber LH Multisegment foot motion during gait: proof of concept in rheumatoid arthritis. Journal of Rheumatology 2004; 31: 1918–1927.

Woodburn J, Udupa JK, Hirsch BE et al. The geometrical architecture of the subtalar and midtarsal joints in rheumatoid arthritis based on MR imaging. Arthritis and Rheumatism 2002; 46: 3168–3177.

Wolfe F Rheumatoid arthritis. In Bellamy NJ (ed) Prognosis in the rheumatic diseases, 1st edn, Kluwer Academic Publishers, Dordrecht, 1991; 37–82.

Young A, Dixey J, Cox N et al. How does functional disability in early rheumatoid arthritis affect patients and their lives? Results of 5 years of follow-up in 732 patients from the Early Rheumatoid Arthritis Study (ERAS). Rheumatology 2000; 39(6): 603–611.

Young A, Dixey J, Kulinskaya E et al. Which patients stop working because of rheumatoid arthritis? Results of five years' follow up in 732 patients from the Early Rheumatoid Arthritis Study (ERAS). Annals of the Rheumatic Diseases 2002; 61(4): 335–340.

Chapter **2**

Pathomechanics and the application of gait analysis in rheumatoid arthritis

INTRODUCTION

Gait analysis is the study of human walking. The walking pattern of patients with rheumatoid arthritis (RA) has been described as one that is slow and modified to lessen pain, and features changes to the pattern and range of joint motion, altered muscle activity and stress distribution to the plantar region. As clinicians, we get the opportunity to observe the patient walking as they enter the consulting room, but too often this is brief and unrewarding as well as impractical as the lower limb and foot is often obscured by clothing and footwear. A formal qualitative approach is recommended as part of the GALS locomotor screening system (see Chapter 4) and this is helpful, but this chapter covers quantitative gait analysis using instrumentation in a laboratory setting. In Leeds, over the past few years, we have been developing a gait analysis 'toolkit' to permit analysis of the lower limb and specifically the foot. Our laboratory, shown in Figure 2.1, comprises a short flat 10 m walkway and our 'toolkit' contains an instrumented walkway to measure the basic spatial and temporal parameters of gait; force and pressure plates are embedded into the floor to measure those quantities and an arrangement of six cameras record motion.

Gait analysis is carried out following referral from the multidisciplinary team that may include:

- The podiatrist requesting plantar pressure measurement to assist the design of a custom off-loading foot orthosis for an RA patient with forefoot ulceration.
- The physicians may request gait analysis to help explain foot mechanics for a patient with persistent unresolved tibialis posterior tenosynovitis after recognizing the foot was pronated.

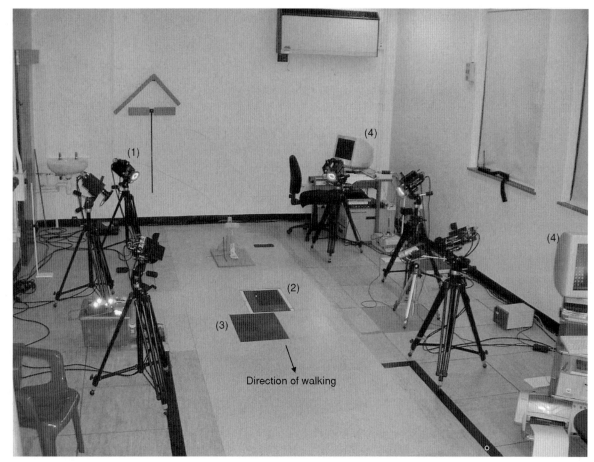

Figure 2.1 Gait Analysis Laboratory, Academic Unit of Musculoskeletal Disease, University of Leeds. Situated in the Rheumatology Outpatient Department the laboratory comprises (1) six-camera motion capture system; (2) plantar pressure distribution analysis system; (3) force plate; (4) computer workstations. Not shown are optical timing device, in-shoe pressure analysis system and instrumented walkway.

- The orthopaedic surgeon, planning a total ankle replacement, may request an analysis of the ankle 3D kinematics and kinetics as a baseline to evaluate prospectively any restoration of ankle function.
- Finally, the orthotist may request simple spatial and temporal measurements to check the gait symmetry when prescribing orthopaedic footwear and orthoses.

Our laboratory strategy uses gait analysis to understand more fully the relationship between inflammatory joint disease, impairment to foot structure and function and the compensatory gait strategies patients adopt to overcome painful and disabling deformity. Gait analysis is, therefore, aided when we have prior knowledge of the nature and severity of foot/lower limb impairments, and the general and localized inflammatory status. It adds to our patient history, extends our clinical examination by quantifying joint function during activities of daily living and complements other investigations, particularly imaging that aims to localize and quantify joint pathology and impairment. Indeed, there are only a handful of gait-related publications in RA and the most useful are those that explore these relationships, albeit in small study sizes (Siegel et al. 1995, O'Connell 1998).

Applying gait analysis techniques to the study of foot function is challenging. These challenges include elements of the following dilemmas:

- Past studies have modelled the foot as a single rigid body that tells us little about the small, interdependent and functionally important small joints of the foot.
- The disease itself presents problems: in our kinematic foot model, anatomical landmarks, where tracking motion markers are placed, can often be obscured by localized joint or soft-tissue swelling introducing error to our motion calculations.
- Most techniques require barefoot walking, something patients with RA and painful feet rarely do, so it is difficult to verify the true walking pattern in some cases.

These problems are not insurmountable and we have already introduced multi-segment foot models to study functional groups of small joints, employed ultrasound to measure localized swelling to improve our marker site placement error and measure, where possible, patients shod and barefoot.

Critics of gait analysis often cite the length of time to capture and process data and the challenge of deciphering multiple variables at multiple joint sites in 2- or 3D. Our laboratory employs techniques that mostly automate these processes so we are now in line, in terms of time, with, for example, magnetic resonance imaging (MRI) as a special investigation. As you will see throughout the chapter and from the CD, software visualization of motion from rendered models enables better gait interpretation and clinical reports can be easily standardized. Future challenges include establishing normal values for the common gait parameters measured in relationship to the gender and age distribution of the patients we see with RA, and to introduce prospective studies that enable predictive and prognostic gait variables to be identified with regard to their relationship with underlying disease processes and foot impairment. Finally, continued development of these techniques as potential outcome measures for clinical trial is required (Fransen et al. 1997, Woodburn et al. 2003).

Approximately 90% of our gait laboratory workload is clinical research and we are aware that gait analysis is not commonly undertaken in rheumatology centres. For that reason, this chapter will aim to briefly describe the gait analysis techniques used in Leeds, outline the application to foot disease in RA, assimilate the research evidence and present appropriate case histories to highlight selected areas. Throughout the chapter, abnormal gait features will be related to underlying pathological processes, primarily inflammation and foot anatomy and biomechanics.

KEY POINTS

- Gait analysis is the systematic study of human walking
- Useful parameters to measure in RA include spatial temporal features, 3D joint kinematics and kinetics and plantar pressure distribution
- Given the complex anatomy, the application of gait analysis techniques in the foot is challenging
- Gait analysis can be used alongside the clinical history, examination and other special investigations to gain a better understanding of the relationship between inflammatory joint disease, impairment and compensatory gait mechanisms.

GAIT ANALYSIS TECHNIQUES AND THEIR APPLICATION IN RHEUMATOID ARTHRITIS

There are a number of gait analysis techniques that have been previously employed to study foot function in RA. Over time, these techniques have evolved from 2- to 3D analyses, with data integrated to provide simultaneous measurement of joint angles, electromyographic muscle activity signals and foot pressure distribution, for example. Foot models have increased in their complexity (Woodburn et al. 2004). It is beyond the scope of this book to describe all of these techniques and we focus on those currently employed in our own laboratory. Suggestions for further reading are provided at the end of the chapter.

Observational gait analysis

Observational gait analysis is a qualitative visual description of human walking. It forms part of the GALS system described earlier in the book. Our approach is to observe the patient on the walkway over several trials noting major functional deficits in a systematic way from the head to foot. Initial impressions include walking speed, symmetry, balance, and protective mechanisms for painful joints. We note the posture and movement for the head, neck and shoulders and arm swing through the walking sequence. We observe spine, hip, knee and ankle motion. For the foot we comment on the movement between the rearfoot relative to the leg and the forefoot relative to the rearfoot and the rise and fall of the medial longitudinal arch during the stance phase. We note the position of the hallux and the weight-bearing capacity of the lesser toes. We classify each defect by predominant direction of motion, e.g. flexed/extended or varus/valgus, and quality of the range of motion on a nominal scale – hypermobile, within-normal-limits, stiff, rigid. These observations are made in the sagittal and frontal planes with the patient barefoot and in their current shoes, including any orthoses, or using normal assistive gait devices. Care should be taken to avoid a prolonged session as comorbidities such as cardiovascular disease may impair valid observations.

In our patients, we regularly observe slow antalgic gait patterns which are asymmetrical and feature motion defects at a number of lower limb joints and the feet, in a variety of patient specific patterns. We regularly note wide arm swing to aid balance, and a forward-tilted head where the patient, keen to avoid painful obstacles, checks the path immediately ahead. The 'rheumatoid shuffling gait' has been well-described and is fairly easy to characterize as will be seen later.

As an aid to observational gait analysis, many groups record walking on video media and use slow motion playback to facilitate the qualitative analysis. This can be time consuming and lacks precision and reliability. Our approach is to record video during our instrumented gait analysis because our motion analysis software allows us to synchronize the two formats so we can combine at once our gait metrics with the direct observations. Discordance is common so it is ensured that the quantitative 3D data drives our interpretation of the observed 2D video images. Foot motion appears too complex and occurs too quickly about small ranges of motion to rely on video alone.

KEY POINTS

- Observational gait analysis is a qualitative visual description of human walking
- Initial impressions in our RA patients can be gained for walking speed, symmetry, balance, and compensatory antalgic patterns including limp and the shuffling gait
- In RA patients we systematically observe alignment and motion in the upper and lower limbs and spine in the frontal and sagittal planes
- Video recording facilitates review and can be integrated with quantitative techniques.

Spatial and temporal gait parameters

The overall gait style can first be considered by its basic spatial (distance) and temporal (timing) parameters. Historically, a single temporal parameter – the 50-foot walking time – featured as an outcome measure in over one-quarter of therapeutic trials of anti-rheumatic drugs in the mid 1970–80s (Grace et al. 1988). However, the test lacked responsiveness; only 41% of studies detected statistically significant differences, with a mean difference of only 2 s improvement, mostly of interventions tested for 6 weeks or less. Despite respectable reliability, this simple temporal measure lost favour as disease driven outcomes were established and the HAQ became the gold standard functional outcome. Nevertheless, Fransen and Edmonds (1999) revived interest in these gait parameters as outcomes for therapeutic trials, this time for orthopaedic footwear in rheumatoid arthritis, implementing electronic timing and footswitches to record walking speed, cadence and stride length (Fransen & Edmonds 1999). When shortened to three averaged trials of 8 m, these variables were highly reliable and responsive. These shorter walking distances are much simpler to measure and have the benefit of reducing the co-morbid effects of cardiovascular and pulmonary disease and minimizing fatigue.

Tethered electric footswitch systems, video analysis and pencil and paper exercises where sequential chalked or inked footprints are measured by hand, are amongst the techniques used to measure spatial and temporal gait parameters. Some are manually timed, cumbersome and time-consuming, whilst others involve tethered devices and body-placed sensors. Indeed, the latter require patients to adapt to the techniques and Fransen further concluded that for therapeutic trials two assessment sessions were necessary for a superior baseline (Fransen & Edmonds 1999).

In the modern gait laboratory, there is now a preference for instrumented walkways; solid or portable mat walkways with grids of embedded pressure sensors that record each footfall and automatically calculate and display spatial and temporal parameters via dedicated computer software. Algorithms permit analysis of standard parameters, such as walking speed, cadence, cycle-time, stride length and double-support, and other features such as the timing of stance and swing as a percentage of the gait cycle, toe-in/out angles (angle of gait) and heel-to-heel distance (base of gait). Walkway systems have the advantage of portability and can measure patients barefoot and shod and using assistive walking devices. Independent evaluation shows they are valid and reliable tools for clinical gait analysis (McDonough et al. 2001, Bilney et al. 2003).

Looking at the footfall pattern in the CD and depicted diagrammatically in Figure 2.2, we can delineate the sequence by periods when the foot is in ground contact (stance phase), when the foot is airborne (swing phase) and when both feet are on the ground (double-support time). These variables can be represented in absolute units (s) or as a percentage of the time taken for one complete gait cycle. The number of steps taken over the measurement period can be counted and cadence established and if the time and distance measurements are known, average walking speed can be calculated. Five key variables, routinely reported in studies of people with rheumatoid arthritis, are defined in Table 2.1 and summary data presented for a cross-sectional sample of patients and a cohort of able-bodied subjects. Our data support that of others showing that patients with rheumatoid arthritis typically walk at a slower speed with a lower step rate and a longer cycle time. Stride length is shorter and the double-support period lengthened. These changes are associated with a number of disease related factors including impairments in the lower limb and foot, primarily pain, stiffness and deformity. Consider the following case.

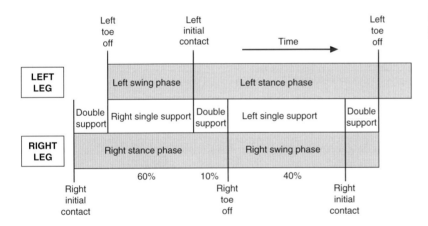

Figure 2.2 A schematic diagram of the phases of gait.

Table 2.1 Definition of five spatial and temporal gait parameters used in rheumatoid arthritis (RA) gait analysis and mean (SD) data for able-bodied subjects and RA patients

Variable (unit of measurement)	Definition	Typical findings in RA	Able-bodied[1] (n=45)	RA[2] (n=40)
Walking speed (m/s)	Distance per unit of time	Slow	1.26 (0.15)	0.88 (0.23)
Cadence (number of steps per min)	Step rate per min	Reduced	115 (9)	103 (10)
Cycle time (s)	The elapsed time between the first contact of two consecutive footfalls of the same foot	Longer	1.05 (0.08)	1.17 (0.12)
Stride length (m)	The distance between the sequential points of initial contact by the same foot	Shorter	1.33 (0.13)	1.03 (0.22)
Double-support time (% of gait cycle)	Part of the gait cycle characterized by both feet on the ground simultaneously. There are two double-support periods during one gait cycle	Longer	16.5 (2.9)	21.4 (5.4)

[1] Forty-five able-bodied control subjects (20 males/25 females) with a mean age of 54.9 years (SD 11.9) and [2] forty RA patients (9 male and 31 female), with a mean age of 56.2 years (SD 12.7) and a mean disease duration of 13.7 years (SD 10.9) (unpublished data from the University of Leeds).

Case study

This 55-year-old female patient with 18 years' disease duration underwent gait analysis in 2001. She presented with marked stiffness and 15° of fixed flexion deformity in the right knee and extensive impairment in the forefoot including pain and stiffness from severely eroded MTP joints. Observing the overall footfall pattern (Figure 2.3) we can see that the gait pattern is asymmetrical with stride-to-stride variability and lateral drift from the forward line of progression. Her spatial-temporal parameters are abnormal (Table 2.2, column A). Three years later her gait parameters remain unchanged against a background history of quiescent disease and stable drug management (Table 2.2, column B). She underwent an intensive footcare programme including orthopaedic footwear, customized foot orthoses and physical therapy. One month later (Table 2.2, column C) we note good improvement in her walking parameters, which were associated with self-reported improvements in pain and stiffness.

The case reported above highlights a number of important relationships between gait parameters, disease activity and impairment of structure and function in the lower limb and foot. Pain is perhaps the most significant factor related to altered gait function and so we may expect changes not only in well-established disease as highlighted above, but in early disease as well. The relationship is complex but interesting to study in individual cases and five are presented in Table 2.3 to illustrate this point:

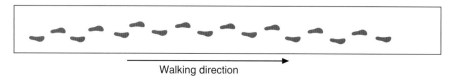

Walking direction

Figure 2.3   Overall footfall pattern from one pass on the instrumented walkway.

Table 2.2   Spatial and temporal gait parameters for a rheumatoid arthritis patient measured on three occasions over a 36-month period.

Variable	A – gait analysis 2001	B – gait analysis 2004 (pre-treatment)	C – gait analysis 2004 (1 month post-treatment)	Change B–C
Walking speed (m/s)	0.78	0.77	0.93	21% faster walking speed
Cadence (steps/min)	101	100	108	8% increased step rate
Cycle time (s)	1.18	1.20	1.11	8% shorter cycle time
Stride length (m)	0.92	0.92	1.06	15% longer stride length
Double-support (% gait cycle)	18.9	17.5	15.1	14% reduction in double-support time

Table 2.3   Summary demographic, disease, foot impairment and gait parameters from five selected rheumatoid arthritis cases of different disease duration.

Patient/ sex/age	Disease duration (years)	DAS (2–10)	LFIS (0–51)	Foot deformity (0–19)	SJC (0–14)	TJC (0–14)	Speed (m/s)	Cadence (steps/min)	Cycle time (s)	Stride length (m)	Double-support time (% gait cycle)
1/F/43	<1	7.29	33	0	14	14	0.86	95	1.27	1.09	18.4
2/F/29	<1	4.13	19	0	1	5	1.30	122	0.98	1.29	12.7
3/M/72	5	5.73	35	11	12	12	0.54	96	1.26	0.68	24.4
4/F/60	7	3.49	13	11	0	6	0.63	85	1.42	0.90	24.5
5/F/53	14	5.48	47	13	8	8	0.90	115	1.05	0.94	19.4

DAS: Disease Activity Score; LFIS: Leeds Foot Impact Scale; SJC: Swollen Joint Count for the foot; TJC: Tender Joint Count for the foot.

Patient 1 is a newly diagnosed case who has just started DMARD therapy. Her disease activity is high (elevated DAS) and locally very active in the feet (high number of swollen and tender foot joints) with marked foot impairment (high Leeds Foot Impact Scale [LFIS] score), but no deformity noted. Her inflammatory status and pain drive the functional changes characterized by slow walking speed, reduced cadence and stride length, and longer cycle time and double-support phase. By contrast, patient 2, a younger female patient who has started her DMARD therapy, has less disease activity, less foot impairment, fewer tender or swollen foot joints and also no foot deformity. Her gait parameters are well within normal limits. Patient 3 is an older male RA patient entering disease flare, determined by a high DAS score (5.73) and a high number of swollen and tender joints, with active disease in the feet. He also has significant foot impairments as identified by his high LFIS score and his forefeet are markedly deformed. These combinations of factors give rise to the classic shuffling gait of RA characterized by very slow walking speed, the very short stride length and the very long double-support phase. By contrast, patient 4 is a 60-year-old female patient with severe and painful forefoot deformity. Her disease was relatively quiescent and only her MTP joints were tender on palpation, but not swollen. She reported a 'guarded' gait to avoid walking on her MTP joints hence the long double support time, short stride and slow walking speed. So, although she was tender on examination, her foot impact scores were low and we

conclude that this may be the result of her compensatory antalgic gait. Finally, patient 5 represents a typical female RA patient with long-standing disease who has both active disease, marked rigid foot deformity at which a high number of joints are swollen and tender and high self-reported foot-related impairment and disability. Her gait parameters are abnormal yet not as marked as some of the other patients. She has slowed her walking down, shortened her stride length with a subsequent increase in contact time but still maintains a normal step rate.

These cases serve to illustrate the complex relationship that exists between disease related factors, impairment and the basic spatial and temporal parameters of gait. Disease duration alone is not predictive of change as we can see from Figure 2.4, a trend towards decreased walking speed and stride length with increased disease duration. However, the relationship is not strong with a correlation coefficient of around 0.4. When grouped by the LFIS scores, no differentiating clusters emerged so foot impairment may have a limited effect. Intuitively, change in basic gait parameters are probably influenced by factors such as disease activity, age, impairment, co-morbid disease and proximal limb joint involvement amongst others.

Across a range of studies where patient cohorts have differed by disease duration, impairment and disability, spatial and temporal gait parameters in RA are consistently reported as abnormal. For example, Isacson and Brostrom (1988) studied 17 female RA patients less than 50 years of age, with average disease duration of 17 years and found the mean velocity to be

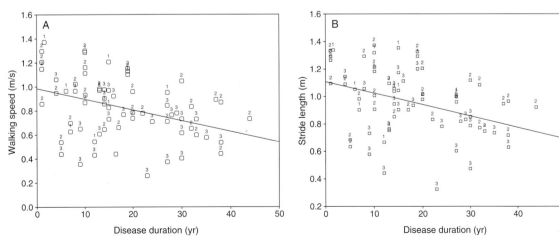

Figure 2.4 The relationship between disease duration and walking speed (A) and stride length (B) for 71 rheumatoid arthritis cases. Individual cases are identidied by severity of foot impact as determined by the Leeds Foot Impact Scale where 1=mild impact, 2=moderate impact and 3=severe impact (University of Leeds, unpublished data).

0.6 m/s, stride length 0.9 m and gait cycle duration 1.4 s. These findings are typical and as a general rule these gait parameters fall between 50 and 90% of normal values when adjusted for age and sex (Locke et al. 1984, Isacson & Brostrom 1988, Kennan et al. 1991, Platto et al. 1991, O'Connell et al. 1998, Fransen & Edmonds 1999).

The association between specific foot impairments and gait parameters has also been investigated. In the rearfoot, Locke and colleagues (1984) demonstrated that five patients with isolated and untreated ankle and subtalar joint pain had a walking speed of 0.69 m/s and a single limb support time at 72% of normal (Locke et al. 1984). Hindfoot pain and deformity are important in rheumatoid arthritis and Platto et al. (1991) showed stronger correlations between these impairments and gait parameters, including speed, stride length, double-support and cadence, than those for the forefoot. Keenan et al. (1991) supported these observations in a study of 10 patients with pes planovalgus confirmed by standard radiographic measurements. They found walking speed and cadence to be 51% and 84% of normal, respectively, whilst the stride length was 0.86 m. These cases had long-standing disease averaging 25 years, but matched to a similar group (with rheumatoid arthritis) by age and sex without flatfoot deformity, changes to gait parameters were markedly worse. We have also studied 23 patients with earlier disease averaging 7 years who had acquired pes planovalgus and found gait cycle times longer on average by 0.15 s, stride length shorter by 0.31 m, double-support times increased by 8.1%, speed slower by 0.39 m/s and cadence reduced by 17 steps/min in comparison with normal (Turner et al. 2003).

Impairments associated with forefoot disease in RA are well documented and O'Connell's group measured the gait of 10 patients with symptomatic disease (O'Connell et al. 1998). Using the Sickness Impact Profile subsection for ambulation they showed a strong correlation between increasing disability and reduced walking speed ($r= -0.74$) and stride length ($r= -0.72$). In this middle-aged group with average disease duration of 12 years, the average walking speed (0.97 m/s) was 71% of normal; stride length (1.06 m) 77% of normal and cadence (112 steps/min) 96% of normal.

Spatial and temporal gait parameters have featured as the main gait outcome in around eight intervention studies. The trend is towards short-term improvements across all the gait variables and this is summarized for walking speed in Figure 2.5. In the majority of these studies, relief of pain and foot-related disability accompanied improved walking parameters.

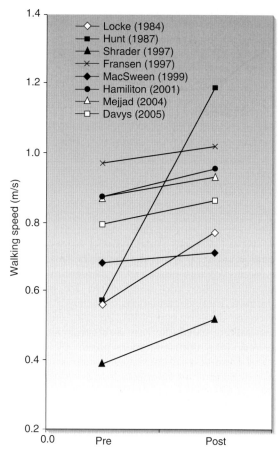

Figure 2.5 Pre- and post-treatment walking speeds for eight intervention studies. Locke (1984): five cases treated with custom foot orthoses; Hunt (1987): single case study of ankle-foot orthosis; Shrader (1997): single case study of custom foot orthosis and shoe modification; Fransen (1997): small randomized controlled trial (RCT) of off-the-shelf orthopaedic footwear (n=30) [data taken from repeated measures trial]; MacSween (1999): before/after study of custom foot orthoses in eight rheumatoid arthritis patients; Hamilton (2001): 24 cases with early disease (<1 year) assessed after 6 months of DMARD therapy; Mejjad (2004): small RCT of custom foot orthoses (n=16) [data summarized as average from reported left and right values]; Davys (2005): RCT of plantar forefoot callus debridement (n=38).

However, no generalizable conclusions can be drawn because of the variation in the nature and conduct of each study. Nevertheless, the overall trend is encouraging since these interventions are often adjunct to systemic treatment as well as other ongoing therapy and educational care. These small-to-medium effects are well recognized in rehabilitation therapy (Ottenbacher 1989).

Joint kinematics

Joint kinematics describes the relative motion between two adjacent bones, but ignores the causes of that motion. Kinematic measurement allows us to quantify the range and pattern of motion during gait. In RA, since we know repeated episodes of synovitis weaken and eventually destroy joints, change in motion parameters should be expected and these changes may be associated with laxity in early disease and stiffness and deformity later. Furthermore, we know

patients develop antalgic gait patterns and may position and hold joints in a certain pose to lessen symptoms and this compensatory strategy may also be characterized by joint kinematics. However, it is widely acknowledged that measuring joint kinematics in the foot is challenging: a combination of the complex anatomy and the technical limitation of measurement systems.

To briefly explain, in Figure 2.6, a severely deformed foot is presented (Fig. 2.6A) and we must consider how to define the joints of interest. The measurement system uses passive retroflective markers whose positions are tracked by cameras as the patient walks. Three markers are required to track each segment to allow 3D measurement and others markers are required to define specific landmarks to enable the geometry of the segment to be defined. It is clear from the size of the markers, the geometry and tight packing of the foot bones that studying, for example, the small inter-tarsal joint would be extremely difficult (Fig. 2.6B). Furthermore, bones such as the talus are locked in the ankle mortise and have inaccessible surface landmarks to place skin sensors or markers. To overcome this, we combine groups of bones into larger and more accessible segments with relevant functional meaning. In our case (Fig. 2.6C), we have created segments for the shank, rearfoot, forefoot and hallux.

Because of these limitations, only a small handful of studies have reported kinematic parameters from the foot in RA (Table 2.4). In six RA patients with

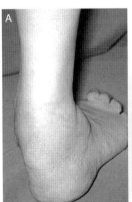
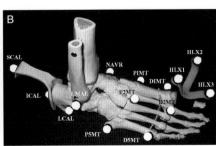
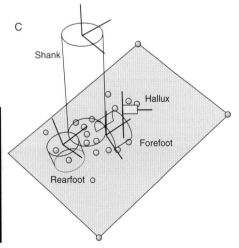

Figure 2.6   (A) severe foot deformity in rheumatoid arthritis; (B) skeleton foot model showing anatomical landmarks for skin-surface markers and tracking markers for a typical multi-segment kinematic foot model used in rheumatoid arthritis; (C) the same patient with segments (geometry defined by cones) for the shank, rearfoot, forefoot and hallux segments from standing foot pose.

Table 2.4 A summary table of foot kinematic studies in rheumatoid arthritis with reference to measurement technique, defined foot model and kinematic parameters measured.

Authors	Measurement technique	Model	Kinematic parameters
Marshall et al. (1980)	Digitized cine film (1D)	Shank and foot	Ankle joint in sagittal plane
Locke et al. (1984)	Two single axis electrogoniometers	Ankle joint complex*	Ankle dorsiflexion/plantarflexion Hindfoot inversion/eversion
Isacson & Brostrom (1988)	Tri-axial electrogoniometer	Shank and foot	Ankle joint motion in all three planes
Keenan et al. (1991)	Two single axis electrogoniometers	Ankle joint complex (tibiotalar and subtalar joints)	Ankle dorsiflexion/plantarflexion Hindfoot inversion/eversion
Siegel et al. (1995)	3D video-based motion analysis system	Shank and foot	Joint angular displacement of the foot relative to the leg in all three planes
O'Connell et al. (1998)	3D video-based motion analysis system	Shank and foot	Joint angular displacement of the foot relative to the leg in all three planes
Woodburn at al (1999, 2002, 2003) and Turner (2003)	Electromagnetic tracking	Ankle joint complex	Joint angular displacement of the rearfoot relative to the leg in all three planes
Woodburn et al. (2004)	3D video-based motion analysis system	Shank, rearfoot, forefoot and hallux	Joint angular displacement of the rearfoot relative to the leg, the forefoot relative to the rearfoot in all three planes and the hallux in flexion/extension relative to the forefoot

*The ankle joint complex comprises the tibiotalar and subtalar joints

advanced subtalar disease and pes planovalgus deformity, Marshall et al. (1980) detected a more plantarflexed foot prior to ground contact to assist the foot in landing flat accompanied by prolonged ankle dorsiflexion and delayed heel-rise. These sagittal plane features about the ankle joint were consistent with a slow shuffling gait and prolonged double-support, mechanisms thought to lessen pain and enhance stability. Similarly, Locke et al. (1984) showed that increased dorsiflexion was accompanied by more valgus (eversion) motion in the frontal plane during stance in five patients with painful ankle and hindfoot joints.

In pes planovalgus, these abnormal motion patterns are consistent with the observed deformity and we confirmed these early findings in larger cohorts with early and more flexible foot deformity (Woodburn et al. 1999, 2002, Turner et al. 2003). Furthermore, we undertook 3D measurements and were, therefore, able to demonstrate the coupled motion pattern between excessive ankle joint complex eversion and internal leg rotation (Woodburn et al. 2002, Turner et al. 2003) (Fig. 2.7). In all of these studies, however, measurement is restricted to the ankle joint or the ankle joint complex (ankle and subtalar

joint) using active marker systems based on electrogoniometry or electromagnetic tracking.

The utility of gait analysis has been well demonstrated by the National Institutes of Health group in the USA (Siegel et al. 1995, O'Connell et al. 1998). Starting with a single rigid body model of the foot, they were able to relate forefoot disease to altered foot function and separate two cases by severity. The contrast in foot function between cases with near-rigid hindfoot varus and flexible pronated foot was also clearly demonstrated, the former showing < 5° of total movement about an inverted position, the latter showing 10° of total movement about an everted position (Siegel et al. 1995). This group then focused specifically on forefoot disease and showed diminished ankle plantarflexion in late stance and delayed heel rise, deficits associated with loss of forefoot rocker function (O'Connell et al. 1998).

In 2004, the first proof of concept for a multisegment kinematic foot model for RA, based on the Oxford foot model (Carson et al. 2001) was presented (Woodburn et al. 2004). This provided a more complete description of foot motion deficits in RA adding to the work already presented for patients with fore-

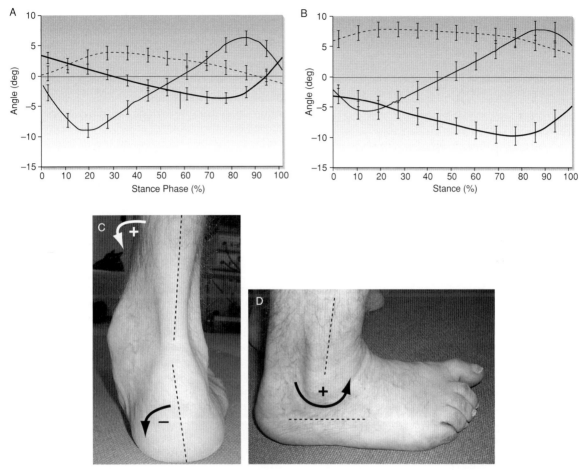

Figure 2.7   Motion curves for the ankle joint complex in (A) able-bodied control group (*n*=45) walking barefoot; (B) rheumatoid arthritis group with painful valgus heel deformity (*n*=50). The solid line represents dorsiflexion (+)/plantarflexion(–), the solid line with markers represents inversion(+)/eversion(–) and the dashed line represents internal(+)/external rotation(–). Bars represent the 95% confidence interval of the mean. Clinical interpretation from a selected case, (C) eversion (–) of the calcaneus relative to the leg, which is internally rotated (+) and (D) dorsiflexion (+) of the rearfoot relative to the leg.

foot pain and pes planovalgus. In the current model, presented in Figure 2.6, we are now able to measure 3D motion between four foot segments and record the rise and fall of the medial longitudinal arch by tracking a marker on the highest point of the arch at the tuberosity of the navicular. For RA, this is a functionally relevant model since we can expect motion deficits to occur between the rearfoot and shank, and forefoot and rearfoot segments associated with disease in and around the ankle and tarsal joints. The need to extend markers off a wand to enable reliable tracking precludes measurement at all five metatarsophalangeal joints. Nevertheless, the hallux is an important segment to track given the prevalence, severity and

impact on function of 1st MTP disease in RA (Spiegel & Spiegel 1982, Shrader & Siegel 2003). This model is currently used at Leeds in clinical gait analysis to assist treatment planning and evaluation in complex cases and in clinical research to understand more fully dysfunctional movement in the foot joints.

In the Leeds gait laboratory, a real-time 3D motion capture (MOCAP) system is used and this is summarized in Figure 2.8. Briefly, we start by palpating and marking surface landmarks on the leg and foot to which we attach small reflective markers. Some markers are attached directly to the skin, others on wands extending from the heel and the hallux and four attached to a rigid plate mounted on a Velcro ankle

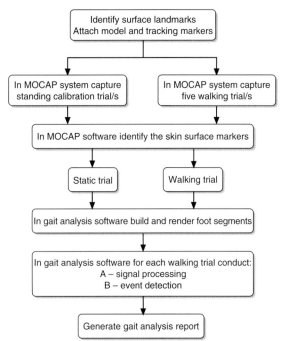

```
┌─────────────────────────────────────┐
│     Identify surface landmarks        │
│  Attach model and tracking markers    │
└─────────────────────────────────────┘
        │                    │
        ▼                    ▼
┌──────────────────┐  ┌──────────────────┐
│ In MOCAP system  │  │ In MOCAP system  │
│ capture standing │  │ capture five     │
│ calibration      │  │ walking trial/s  │
│ trial/s          │  │                  │
└──────────────────┘  └──────────────────┘
        │                    │
        ▼                    ▼
┌─────────────────────────────────────┐
│ In MOCAP software identify the skin   │
│ surface markers                       │
└─────────────────────────────────────┘
        │                    │
        ▼                    ▼
┌──────────────┐      ┌──────────────┐
│ Static trial │      │ Walking trial│
└──────────────┘      └──────────────┘
        │                    │
        ▼                    ▼
┌─────────────────────────────────────┐
│ In gait analysis software build and   │
│ render foot segments                  │
└─────────────────────────────────────┘
                  │
                  ▼
┌─────────────────────────────────────┐
│ In gait analysis software for each    │
│ walking trial conduct:                │
│     A – signal processing             │
│     B – event detection               │
└─────────────────────────────────────┘
                  │
                  ▼
┌─────────────────────────────────────┐
│   Generate gait analysis report       │
└─────────────────────────────────────┘
```

Figure 2.8 Schematic diagram for kinematic data capture using a multi-segment foot model. MOCAP – motion capture system. Signal processing is undertaken to smooth the motion trajectories. Event detection uses force plate data to identify heel-strike (start) and toe-off (stop) to normalize the kinematic variables in the time domain.

wrap. The patient is carefully positioned in a calibration frame to standardize the standing pose and capture a static trial. Five or more walking trials are conducted in such a way that the patient's foot lands on dual mounted force and pressure plates embedded in the walkway. As the cameras track the markers they are automatically identified for both the static and walking trials. Each trial is then processed in a proprietary motion analysis software package. The standing trial with the anatomical markers is used to build the four segments with the relevant geometry, correct orientation and segment embedded reference frames defined. These reference frames provide a local coordinate system that is fixed and moves with each segment (assumed to be rigid). For each frame of the captured walking sequence, computations are made of the orientation of the coordinates of two segments forming each joint in the software and the joint angles determined. Different computational processes are available for this but the joint angles are finally expressed in clinically meaningful terms such as dorsiflexion/plantarflexion. Intermediate steps in the process include filtering of the raw motion data to

remove noise, and data reduction using averaging across trials for the stance period only (heel-strike to toe-off) using the onset and end of the force signal recorded as the foot strikes and leaves the force-plate. Finally, a standard report is generated that provides time normalized angle diagrams for each segment by axis of rotation and summary data, including minimum and maximum joint angles, range of motion and angles and their timings at key events such as heel-strike, mid-stance, heel-rise and toe-off (Fig. 2.8).

Since the process described above is mostly automated, routine application of multi-segment foot kinematics as a clinical investigation tool is now feasible. Our approach uses gait analysis to understand more fully the relationship between inflammatory joint disease, impairment to foot structure and function and the compensatory gait strategies used by patients. For example, in Figure 2.9, a 54-year-old male with long-standing resistant RA presented with severe pes planovalgus and marked forefoot deformity. Managed on anti-TNF therapy his treatment was problematic because of recurrent plantar MTP ulceration. Bed rest followed by custom orthoses and off-the-shelf extra-depth shoes eventually healed the ulcers, but no improvement was noted for his extremely painful and disabling rearfoot and forefoot deformities. Using a multi-segment kinematic foot model the change in the motion parameters could easily be detected and explained in the context of the clinically detected joint stiffness (reduced range of motion) and deformity (altered joint position from which motion occurs).

The rearfoot (Fig. 2.9A), was dorsiflexed at initial foot contact and continued in this direction to late stance. Heel-lift was delayed and plantarflexion severely limited during propulsion, characteristic of the loss of the forefoot rocker function. In the frontal plane the rearfoot was excessively everted and stiff and the motion pattern is closely related to the observed valgus heel deformity. The rearfoot was also more externally rotated than normal and this represents the coupled internal leg rotation with rearfoot eversion described earlier. The forefoot (Fig. 2.9B) was dorsiflexed relative to the rearfoot and this is consistent with the collapsed medial longitudinal arch and no plantarflexion of the forefoot was measured during the propulsion phase. The 'twisting' about the forefoot is characterized by the large inverted forefoot position relative to the everted heel position with only a small amount of forefoot eversion during terminal stance. In the transverse plane the forefoot abduction, characteristic of a pronated foot type, was identified as a fixed deformity because of the absence of late stance forefoot adduction. In Figure 2.9C, we can see the collapse of

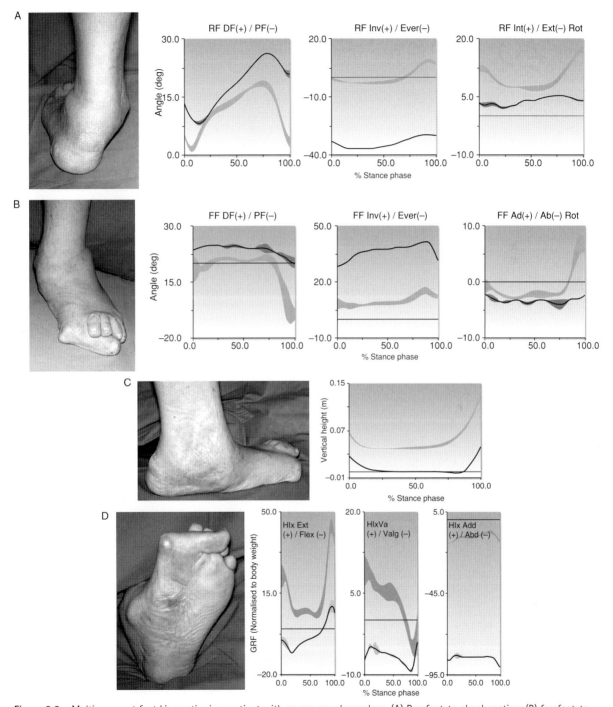

Figure 2.9 Multi-segment foot kinematics in a patient with severe pas planovalgus. (A) Rearfoot-to-shank motion; (B) forefoot-to-rearfoot motion; (C) vertical height of the medial longitudinal arch and (D) hallux-to-forefoot motion. Grey shaded area represents mean±1 SD for five age- and sex-matched able-bodied persons. The represent motion in the sagittal, frontal and transverse planes respectively. In (C), the line represents the vertical arch height for the patient.

the medial longitudinal arch, confirmed in walking by the ground contact made by the motion marker on the tuberosity of the navicular from the foot-flat to heel-rise period of stance. Finally, in Figure 2.9D, the gross deformity of the hallux is captured well during walking with evidence that the toe is slightly flexed and stiff in flexion/extension, rotated in valgus in the frontal plane and abducted ~90° to the forefoot.

This set of motion patterns is typical for pes planovalgus in rheumatoid arthritis, although extreme in this case. The multi-segment approach shows the extent of the functional impairment arising from persistent inflammation in the foot joints and this patient had evidence of synovitis in the ankle and tarsal joints and MTP joints. It could be argued that such close agreement between clinically detected impairment and the abnormal motion patterns negates the need for gait analysis. However, it was eventually decided that the patient undergo forefoot reconstruction surgery and triple arthrodesis in the rearfoot, and the information assisted the surgical planning. Moreover, the findings improve our understanding of foot function in this disease. What effect does arthroplasty and arthrodesis procedures have on foot function in rheumatoid arthritis? Our post-surgery repeat analysis may help us determine this and further assist design and evaluation of new orthoses and footwear.

The real benefits for gait analysis will emerge if we can identify abnormal function in early disease. In terms of joint motion in the foot, the current challenge is fraught with difficulties, as we have already identified considerable variation in able-bodied adults. Given that the motion also has a temporal element over the walking cycle we also need to identify the key parameter, be it a peak value, the timing of that peak value, or the duration a certain value persists above a normal level or a combination of these. At the moment, in early cases, it is not possible to diagnose abnormal motion on the basis of identifying any one parameter which lies outside two standard deviations for the mean value in normal subjects. Pragmatically, we currently look for a combination of factors, including localization of disease activity within the foot, clinical red flags and an overall trend in the motion pattern towards abnormal function.

For example, in the following case – a 31-year-old female patient with well-controlled disease (3 years) but persistent right foot problems – three features stand out:

1. MRI confirmed synovitis of the ankle and subtalar joint and tenosynovitis of tibialis posterior and flexor digitorum longus.
2. Patient self-reported change to foot posture, 'I can feel my foot rolling in.'

3. Pain and swelling localized to the tendons passing the ankle medially with increased subtalar joint eversion on passive examination, tender when stressed at end range of motion.

In Figure 2.10, swelling can be detected along the course of the medial ankle tendons and the heel is in valgus when standing. Passive range of motion during the examination of the subtalar joint tended towards an increased range of motion, especially in eversion. The MRI findings are consistent with the clinical picture. From our current understanding of normal function, the motion pattern is within normal limits, according to standard diagnostic criteria based on means and standard deviation. However, we believe the foot posture has changed according to the self-reported evidence and it is that change which may be of more interest in terms of a biomechanical factor associated with the persistent soft-tissue pathology. Cause and effect is not clear, but the association between the pathology, the clinical picture and the associated movement pattern is notable. Furthermore, the preserved range of motion should facilitate foot orthotic therapy using corrective devices aimed at reducing the amount of eversion and its timings through stance.

Excessive and prolonged rearfoot eversion is the hallmark motion pattern in patients with progressive pes planovalgus and it has been demonstrated in a number of kinematic studies (Locke et al. 1984, Keenan et al. 1991, Siegel et al. 1995, Woodburn et al. 2002, Turner et al. 2003). It is characterized by progressive shift towards an eversion motion envelope as the subtalar joint becomes unstable. Keenan et al. (1991) described three subtalar motion abnormalities for 10 patients with a mean disease duration of 25 years: abnormal eversion of the calcaneus at heel-strike, everted subtalar alignment through the entire stance phase of gait and insufficient inversion motion during propulsion to establish a neutral or inverted subtalar joint alignment. Importantly, we have found strong evidence to support early motion changes (disease duration ~5 years) in patients with active peri-talar disease (Woodburn et al. 2002) (Fig. 2.11). Here, the inversion/eversion motion patterns were consistent with the observations of Keenan and others, but with less severe deformity. The frequency of tibiotalar joint involvement in RA is less than the subtalar or midtarsal joints (Lehtinen et al. 1996, Bouysset et al. 1987), but reports show decreased ROM and change in motion pattern favouring dorsiflexion (Locke et al. 1984, Woodburn et al. 2002). This may be associated with secondary stresses from other joints, particularly when the subtalar joint is abnormally aligned (Klenerman 1995).

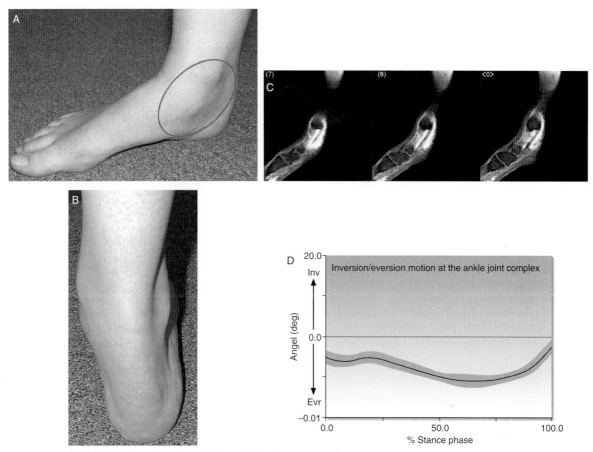

Figure 2.10   (A) Swelling along the course of the medial ankle tendons; (B) valgus heel deformity on weight bearing; (C) post-gadolinium fat-suppressed T1 weighted MRI sequence showing enhancement, in three consecutive slices, of tibialis posterior consistent with tenosynovitis; (D) the inversion/eversion motion pattern during walking (mean ±1 SD from five trials).

The subtalar joint has a 'torque converter' role, which couples subtalar joint inversion with external leg rotation, and eversion with internal leg rotation. The pronated foot is associated with excessive motion for the latter two and frequently propagated as an injury mechanism for a number of common musculoskeletal complaints in the lower limb and foot. This coupling effect has been demonstrated in the pes planovalgus foot, showing that the ankle joint complex failed to reach a neutral or inversion alignment and that leg rotation reached a neutral or externally rotated alignment, under the barefoot walking condition (Turner et al. 2003). As a potential injury mechanism, interestingly, valgus heel and knee deformities are frequently observed together in RA and a distal-proximal causal relationship has been proposed but never studied seriously.

What is happening inside the RA foot to cause these motion pattern changes? The medial ankle and tarsal joint ligaments have important motion guiding and stabilizing functions and tibialis posterior is considered the major muscle maintaining the medial longitudinal arch. Persistent or repeated inflammation at these sites may lead to collapse of the arch (pes planus) or valgus of the hindfoot (pes valgus) or both (pes planovalgus) depending on the patterns of joint and soft-tissue involvement. Under physiological loads, the largest tarsal joint rotations are found at the talonavicular joint, especially in the frontal plane (Lundberg et al. 1998). This joint remains stable because the inferior calcaneonavicular (the spring) ligament and the superomedial calcaneonavicular ligament are force-bearing and resist medial and plantar displacement of the talar head, assisted by the expansive insertion and blending of the tibialis posterior to the tuberosity of the navicular.

Histopathological analysis suggests this region is an 'enthesis organ' comprising the osteotendinous

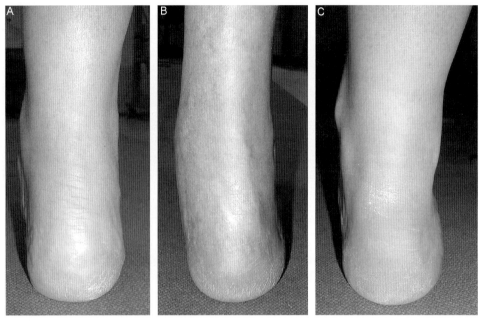

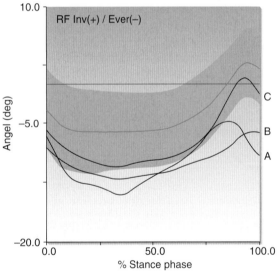

Figure 2.11 Three patients with disease duration of <1 year and all presenting with self-reported ankle/rearfoot or medial longitudinal arch instability and clinical evidence of active peri-talar joint disease. In (D) the frontal kinematics of the rearfoot are shown for each patient Patient A had the mildest deformity and motion approaching the outer one standard deviation from the mean pattern (shaded zone). Patient B shows abnormal motion outside one standard deviation from normal to foot flat to toe-off. Patient C had the most significant deformity with abnormal motion most prominent shortly after loading through to heel lift, but shows good inversion motion through the propulsive phase.

junction (the enthesis), the superomedial part of the calcaneonavicular ligament (which may fuse with the tendon), the tendon sheath, and associated accessory bones (Morrigl et al. 2003). Rich in fibrocartilage, degenerative changes associated with inflammation in RA may target the enthesis itself or adjacent locations. Indeed, MRI studies confirm coexisting insufficiency in the inferior calcaneonavicular ligament and chronic tibialis posterior dysfunction (Yao et al. 1999). Using stab incisions in this region to represent longitudinal fibre tears and focal degeneration, frontal plane changes in talonavicular joint orientation were found in a cadaver foot experiment (Woodburn et al. 2005). Combined with similar attenuation to the medial ankle tendons, followed by cyclic loading at physiological levels, the simulated damage resulted in gross postural changes consistent with pes planovalgus. When tibialis posterior is dysfunctional, the midfoot loses its rigidity and stability during the latter part of stance (Coakley et al. 1994, Yao et al. 1999). The powerful gastro-soleus complex then acts across the talonavicular joint as well as the forefoot during propulsion and the resultant motion is thought to stretch the calcaneonavicular and medial plantar ligaments (Coakley et al. 1994, Yao et al. 1999). Visualization of these structural changes in foot geometry was demonstrated through 3D MRI reconstruction of the tarsal joints in pes planovalgus feet (Woodburn et al. 2002). In the talonavicular joint region, very accurate measurement of bone–bone orientation and separation showed an increased distance between the calcaneus and navicular with plantar drift of the talar head. There was strong evidence of ligamentous insufficiency, and half the patients had synovitis, about one-quarter erosive joint changes and over one-third tenosynovitis of tibialis posterior. A reconstruction is shown in Figure 2.12.

Although tibialis posterior tendon rupture is uncommon (a series of three imaging studies found the prevalence to be < 5% amongst cases with pes planovalgus due to rheumatoid arthritis), the tendon may attenuate within its structure through inflammatory damage, and thus become dysfunctional (Coakley et al. 1994, Masterton et al. 1995, Jernberg et al. 1999, Premkumar et al. 2002). The gait changes presented earlier show coupled motion around the joints of the rearfoot. In the cadaver study reported earlier, the tibionavicular, anterior tibiotalar and tibiocalcaneal portions of the medial deltoid ligament were also attenuated on the basis that the tibiotalar and subtalar joints are also involved in rheumatoid arthritis (Lehtinen et al. 1996). This resulted in further changes in eversion orientation and small amounts of internal tibial rotation through the tibiotalar and the tarsal joints. More recently, attention has been paid to degeneration of the interosseous talocalcaneal and cervical ligaments associated with inflammation in the sinus tarsi region (Jernberg et al. 1999, Bouysset et al. 2003). These ligaments are important stabilizers of the talocalcaneal joint and when diseased may contribute to the valgus heel

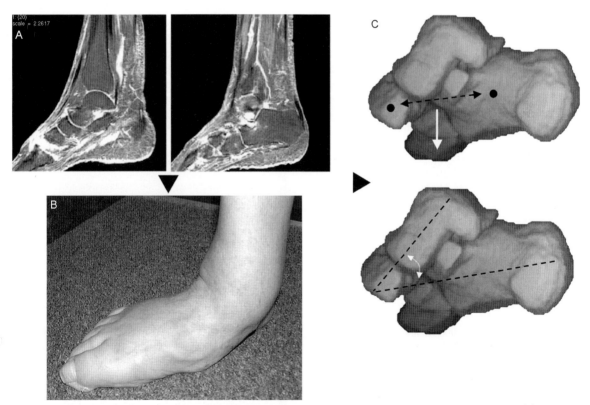

Figure 2.12   Two sagittal slices of a post-gadolinium MR sequence showing disease activity in the tarsal joint region (A). The clinical picture is that of severe pes planovalgus (B). In (C) the 3D rendition of the calcaneus, cuboid, talus and navicular is presented. The distance between the geometric centroids of the calcaneus and navicular is significantly greater than normal owing to the insufficiency of the plantar calcaneonavicular ligament and this creates a gap into which the talar head accommodates. This can be measured by an increase in the angle formed between the principle axes of the talus and calcaneus.

deformity described earlier (Kjaersgaard-Andersen et al. 1988). The potential for widespread changes in tarsal structure and function does exist as soft-tissue compromise on the medial side of the foot resulted in small changes in joint orientation at the calcaneocuboid joint (Woodburn et al. 2005). The 3D MRI reconstructed model confirms this, as do the measurements showing flattening also along the lateral aspect of the foot (Woodburn et al. 2002).

The approach to foot kinematics described so far relate only to barefoot walking conditions. Using an electromagnetic tracking technique that allows sensors to be applied to the skin through 'windows' cut in a set of laboratory shoes, 3D ankle joint complex kinematics have been measured in-shoe (Woodburn 1999, 2002). Less variability was reported between repeated trials possibly related to improved patient comfort when wearing shoes. The standard shoe had a heel height of 4 cm and served to increase the anterior-posterior pitch of the shoe so that plantarflexion motion was increased for the groups studied. Joint range of motion was not appreciably changed and a small decrease in dorsiflexion was noted. Most interestingly, the stiff medial counter in the test shoe served to invert the subtalar joint and externally rotate the leg, bringing about partial correction of the valgus deformity. No assumptions could be made on the closeness of match between the laboratory standard shoe and those worn by patients day-to-day. Nevertheless, the observed motion control has some interesting implications towards the design of therapeutic footwear.

The final clinical scenario for RA is the acutely painful foot and a patient is featured in whom rheumatoid arthritis was suspected, but where the diagnostic classification criteria had not been fulfilled. This lady presented with an acutely painful and stiff right ankle and exquisitely tender MTP joints 1–3. On examination, synovitis was suspected at the ankle and subtalar joint and she was markedly tender behind the lateral malleolus along the course of the peroneal tendons and in the sinus tarsi. Tenosynovitis of both peroneal tendon sheaths was confirmed by ultrasonography. Her ankle was stiff and very painful when moved into dorsiflexion and her heel was in mild varus when standing. All MTP joints were tender on palpation, notably the medial three. Her spatial and temporal gait parameters were within normal limits, but she commented that she was: 'Putting up with it but holding . . . (her) . . . foot out the way to make the ball of . . . (her) . . . foot less painful.'

In Figure 2.13, the lateral ankle and medial forefoot swelling is obvious. The peroneal tendon sheath pathology is evident on ultrasound. Her heel is in varus on standing and during walking a ~10° inverted position was measured during the entire stance phase. Careful attention to the chronological order of the symptomology suggests her gait pattern is a compensatory effort to avoid loading the medial MTP joints. The complete picture, mapping the disease process to clinical history and the impairment of structure and function provides a more complete understanding of foot function in this case and the information was used to plan the conservative treatment plan as an adjunct to the medical intervention, following subsequent confirmation of the diagnosis.

There has been limited use of joint kinematic analysis as a functional outcome in rheumatoid arthritis. Using a modified standard shoe ankle joint complex, 3D kinematics were measured with and without a custom functional foot orthosis in patients with painful correctable valgus heel deformity (Woodburn et al. 2003). The devices changed the motion pattern towards normal with the main effect being a statistically significant change in eversion motion throughout the stance phase. The orthoses re-established a normal inverted heel-strike position, allowed eversion though the mid-stance phase and increased inversion though propulsion. The devices had no significant effect on reducing internal leg rotation or ankle joint complex dorsiflexion. Beneficially, the changes in kinematic parameters were sustainable over a 30-month period accompanied by improvement in symptoms.

KEY POINTS

- Kinematics describes the motion in the joints of the foot regardless of the forces causing that motion
- It is not possible to simultaneously measure the movement in all the small joints of the foot during walking. Joints must be grouped into functional units typically comprising the shank, rearfoot, forefoot and hallux
- In pes planovalgus, excessive and prolonged eversion coupled with internal leg rotation and dorsiflexion are notable features. Medial longitudinal arch collapse and forefoot inversion, dorsiflexion and abduction are components of the abnormal motion patterns
- It is possible to demonstrate, in individual cases, close association with sites of inflammation, clinical symptoms, impairment to structure and function and abnormal foot joint motion patterns
- In RA, foot motion can be changed through the use of custom orthoses.

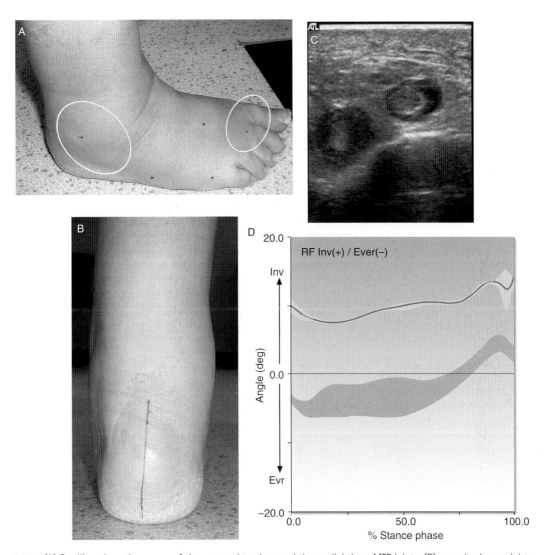

Figure 2.13   (A) Swelling along the course of the peroneal tendons and the medial three MTP joints; (B) varus heel on weight bearing; (C) tenosynovitis on high-resolution ultrasound of peroneus longus and brevis; (D) the inversion/eversion motion pattern in walking (mean ±1 SD from five trials) indicated by the line in comparison with normal range in able-bodied subjects (grey region).

Joint kinetics

Imagine patients with RA walking to the shops to undertake an errand, each time the foot strikes the ground the patient applies a force to the ground. At the same time the ground applies to the patient a reaction force of the same magnitude, but in the opposite direction (the ground reaction force). In the gait analysis laboratory we use a force platform set flush with the floor to measure the ground reaction forces (GRF). Our system allows us to visualize the GRF vector in relationship to the 3D geometry of the leg and

foot and to study the three orthogonal components of the force vector designated F_X, F_Y and F_Z (Fig. 2.14). During stance phase, the path of the point of application of the force vector within the area of foot contact can be tracked and this is referred to as the centre of pressure (COP). For all these variables, the data can be normalized from 0 to 100% of stance.

The vertical F_Z component shows a spike immediately after initial foot contact and the characteristic double hump separated by a middle valley. The two peaks are approximately 110–140% body weight because of the added effect of vertical acceleration on body weight.

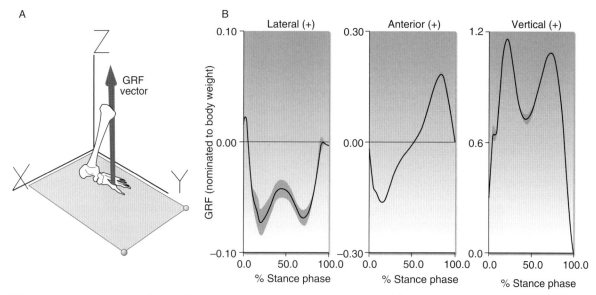

Figure 2.14 A single pose of the right foot captured during the walking sequence. In (A) the location of the ground reaction force vector can be visualized in relationship to the geometry of the leg and foot and where it passes relative to the ankle joint. In (B), the Fx, Fy and Fz orthogonal components of the GRF are shown normalized in the time domain from 0 to 100% of the stance phase.

The forces generated parallel to the walking surface, sometimes referred to as the shear forces, also exhibit typical patterns during stance. During initial contact, as the foot comes down and inwards onto the ground, the plate pushes outwards in a lateral direction on the foot; therefore, the initial signal is positive in F_x. For most of stance phase the plate pushes inwards acting in a medial direction (negative F_x). For the first half of stance phase, the anterior-posterior F_y component is negative for the first half of the cycle as the foot drives forward and into the plate. In the second half, the force becomes positive as the patient drives the foot backwards on the plate during the propulsive phase. The magnitude of the F_x and F_y forces is approximately one-tenth and one-third of the vertical GRF respectively. As noted earlier, walking speed in patients with RA is often slow and this serves to flatten the F_z pattern since momentum and vertical acceleration are both reduced. This is a typical finding in patients with well-established forefoot pain with accompanying short stride-length and slow walking speed (O'Connell et al. 1998). This group showed a diminution of both the F_y and F_z force components during stance phase. For F_y, the negative force component directed towards the heel was significantly less negative, particularly at the 2nd peak occurring near 90% of the stance phase. Both the double peaks for the F_z component were blunted in early and late stance and the COP tended to be closer to the ankle joint and was delayed in anterior progression. This is illustrated for a typical case in Figure 2.15.

In RA as the number and severity of lower limb and foot impairments increase, gait is adapted to compensate, and the GRFs change. GRF data are used in a further calculation, known as inverse dynamics, to determine the internal forces and moments that act across all the lower limb joints in response to external forces including the GRFs. However, the force plate acts as a single force sensor and the spatial distribution of the GRF on different segments of the foot cannot be determined. Therefore, until recently, a major limitation in this approach is that the foot has to be modelled as a single rigid body restricting analysis to the ankle joint. Furthermore, armed with estimates of internal moments and forces and image sequences, such as an ankle MRI, it may be tempting to infer cause and effect between abnormal joint loading and diseased tissue. However, net joint forces and moments cannot tell us how loading is shared amongst important structures that bridge a joint such as the capsule, ligaments and muscle-tendon units and are ultimately diseased in RA. The major structures that contribute to the net moments of force, or torque, are the muscle forces, so our data tell us something about the mechanical output of the controlling muscles. How well these muscles act to produce and control limb movement can be determined from joint power analysis. Joint power is calculated by multiplying the net moment of the force by the joint angular velocity. When profiled over stance, the time integral of the power curve tells us the positive and negative mechanical work done. Our

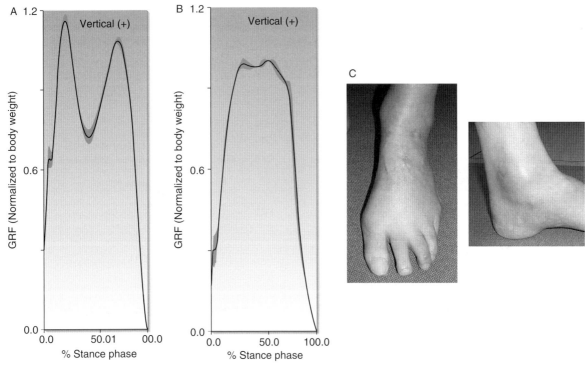

Figure 2.15   Fz vertical component of the GRF for (A) normal able-bodied adult, age and sex matched to a rheumatoid arthritis patient shown in (B). The patient, aged 69 years and disease duration of 5 years, had active disease on day of gait assessment. His walking speed was 0.54 m/s, stride length 0.68 m and double-support time 24.4% of stance. He was markedly tender and swollen over all five MTP joints (C) and the midtarsal, subtalar and tibiotalar joint with probable medial tendon inflammation. Consequently, his GRF profile fails to show the characteristic peaks and mid-stance trough demonstrated in normal gait.

assumption is that all bone and muscle forces are reduced to a single vector resultant force and moment and that these can be expressed, in a 3D analysis, about each axis of rotation. Power and work are scalar terms but for the purposes of clinical relevance can also be conveniently partitioned by each body plane.

The net torque generated by the muscles crossing the ankle joint, the internal moment, is predominantly plantarflexion for most of stance phase. Initially, however, a small dorsiflexion torque is developed during initial contact as the GRF vector is located posterior to the ankle joint centre (Fig. 2.16). Here, the ankle rapidly plantarflexes under control from the ankle dorsiflexor muscles acting eccentrically. This is the first rocker function of the foot and ankle. The COP then rapidly advances from its initial point of contact towards the ankle joint centre coinciding with a reduction of the dorsiflexor moment to zero and the onset of a plantarflexor moment. As the COP advances forward from the ankle joint centre, the moment arm increases and the plantarflexor moment increases to a peak in late terminal stance (~60% stance). During this

period the plantarflexor muscles act eccentrically to control the forward rotation of the leg over the foot (the second rocker function) and then concentrically to generate a rapid push-off where the COP, located at the MTP joints, is furthest from the ankle centre (the third rocker function). Towards toe-off, a small but functionally important third peak occurs, a small dorsiflexor moment to effect toe clearance from the ground. The power profile shows the typical power absorption phase from initial contact (80% of stance) where typically ~ −10 J of negative work is undertaken through to the large and rapid power generation phase towards toe-off, where typically ~ 30 J of positive work is undertaken (Buczek et al. 1994).

These normal ankle moments are shown in Figure 2.16, contrasted with a patient who presents with markedly swollen and tender MTP, midtarsal, subtalar and tibiotalar joint and probable medial tendon tenosynovitis consistent with a flare in his disease (DAS score was 5.73). His walking speed was slow (0.54 m/s), stride length short at 0.68 m and double support time prolonged at 24.4% of the stance phase.

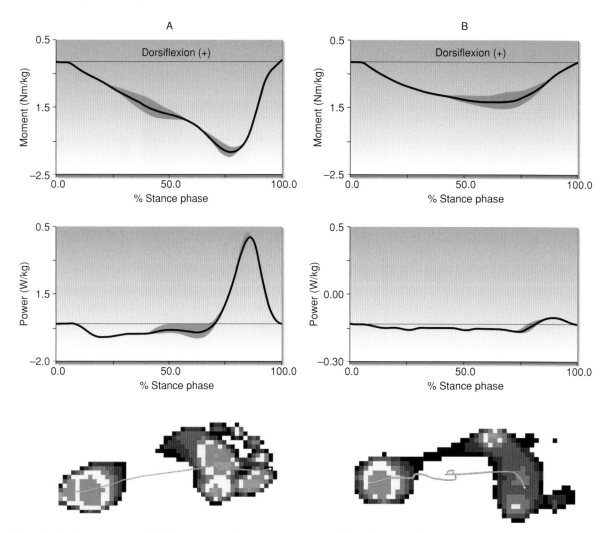

Figure 2.16 Sagittal plane ankle joint net muscular moments, power profiles and pressure distribution pattern with COP overlaid in (A) able-bodied adult matched with (B) rheumatoid arthritis case (as presented in Figure 2.15).

His impairments are closely related to underlying gait function; his foot is placed carefully on the ground, with loss of first rocker function. The COP remains in the heel and midfoot region for a prolonged period during stance (notice the dither and posterior progression in the midfoot) and towards toe-off the COP remains posterior to the location found in otherwise healthy individuals such that the moment arm during stance is much reduced. The sagittal plane moments are significantly lower than normal and the power generated in terminal stance is about one-fifth the normal value. These findings are typical in RA patients, especially those with forefoot pain and this has been clearly demonstrated by the work of O'Connell et al. (1998). This group hypothesized that the third rocker function

of the foot would most likely be affected in RA patients with symptomatic forefeet disease. They confirmed this by showing a significant reduction in the peak plantarflexion moment accompanied by a delay in the anterior progression of the COP in comparison with normal, as typically demonstrated by the case presented within.

Similarly, changes can be detected in the moment and power profiles in both early and well-established disease. In Figure 2.17A, this patient was assessed prior to total ankle joint replacement and demonstrated characteristic reduction in both the moment and power profile. By contrast, in Figure 2.17B, this patient with early disease has adopted an antalgic gait in response to forefoot pain and subsequently developed inflammation in the subtalar joint and peroneal

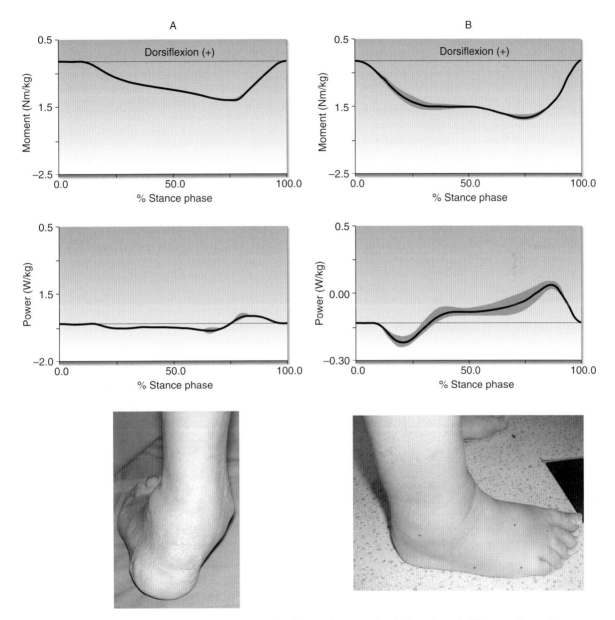

Figure 2.17 Sagittal plane ankle moment and power profiles for two rheumatoid arthritis patients. In (A) this patient underwent gait analysis prior to total ankle joint replacement surgery. Patient B had peroneal tendon tenosynovitis and a stiff inverted heel. During stance ankle dorsiflexion was absent.

tenosynovitis. We noted in the clinical examination severe pain on ankle dorsiflexion and to avoid this, the patient is maintaining the foot in a plantarflexed pose during gait. This is captured by the near normal plantarflexion moment and the generation of power from about 30% of stance through to toe-off, indicating active plantarflexion of the gastrocnemius-soleus complex to maintain the compensatory joint pose.

In a complete 3D model, reference should also be made to the internal moments and power profiles about the secondary plane axes, but these are less reliable than the sagittal plane. The frontal plane is important in RA as we have previously seen the kinematic changes associated with pes planovalgus and varus heel deformity. Eng and Winter (1995) showed an evertor moment during initial contact and terminal stance, with an invertor moment during mid-stance. In the transverse plane, a small external rotation moment was observed during initial contact, then again with a higher peak during propulsion. In both planes, small and highly variable power phases, accounting for ~7% of the total work for the ankle joint, were observed. Interestingly, Siegel et al. (1995) compared two cases with rigid varus and mobile valgus rearfoot deformity. The patient with the varus deformity showed an evertor muscular moment for ~75% of stance phase, opposing the inverted foot position in comparison with a large invertor moment controlling the everted foot position, with the COP remaining lateral to the midline of the foot in the mobile valgus rearfoot case. No data for the transverse plane were presented. In Figure 2.18, the frontal plane moments and power are shown for a patient with a flexible collapsing pes planovalgus. The net muscular moment in the frontal plane is predominantly invertor, opposing the everted position of the foot during stance. Currently, we have made no observation on transverse plane net muscular moments or power profiles in feet of people affected by RA.

KEY POINTS

- The ground reaction force (GRF) is equal and opposite in direction to force applied to the ground each time a patient's foot strikes the ground
- In the gait laboratory this can be measured using a force plate.
- The GRF vector has three orthogonal components designated F_x, F_y, F_z.
- In RA each component of the GRF can be affected according to impairments encountered.
- The internal moment is the net torque generated by the muscles crossing the ankle joint. From this joint power can be calculated.
- In RA, the sagittal net muscular torque and joint power can be significantly reduced where the ankle is stiff, or the forefoot is impaired, primarily by pain and deformity.

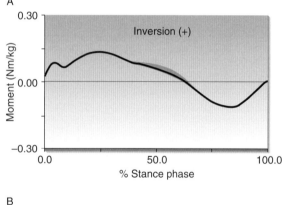

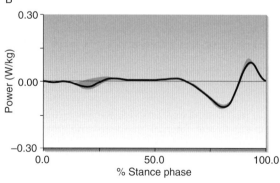

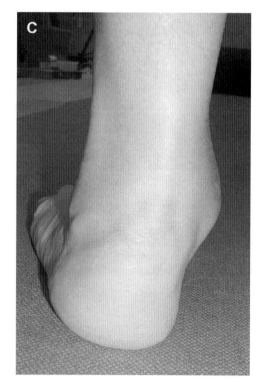

Figure 2.18 Frontal plane ankle joint moment (A) and power (B) profile in a 43-year-old patient with 9 years' disease duration. His disease was active on the day of gait assessment and he presented with a collapsing but flexible pas planovalgus deformity (C) and probable tenosynovitis of the medial ankle tendons located around tibialis posterior and flexor digitorum longus.

$$\text{Pressure (Ncm}^2) = \text{Force (N) / Area (cm}^2)$$

Figure 2.19 Pressure is defined as the force (Newtons) per unit area (cm²). It is more appropriate to express pressure using SI units: the kilopascal (kPa).

Plantar pressure distribution

Plantar pressure distribution measurement is the most frequently used gait analysis technique employed in the study of RA. The equipment is readily available, relatively easy to install and use, and it provides information that can be both visually interpreted for clinical use and processed for more robust analyses. As described earlier, the GRF has a COP point location within the area of contact of the foot that changes though the stance phase of gait. If the contact area is known over which the force vector is distributed we can calculate pressure, defined as the force per unit area and expressed in kPa (Fig. 2.19). In the Leeds laboratory two pressure measurement systems are used: a plate device, similar to our force plate, but with a matrix array of small (5 × 5 mm) capacitance-based transducers or sensors, and, using the same technology, a flexible in-shoe pressure sensing insole (sensors in the array vary in size ~10 × 5 mm). The former permits higher resolution measurement at the foot/plate interface and is able to detect pressure over small discrete anatomical regions such as the metatarsal heads. In-shoe measurement is useful to study step-to-step variability within a walking sequence, to analyse pressure distribution during activities of daily living such as walking, standing and stair climbing, and, importantly, it permits measurement at the interface between the foot and the shoe or foot and shoe-orthosis. Measurements are generally undertaken using both systems to allow assessment of foot function and to assist planning or evaluating some therapeutic interventions as part of the overall assessment protocol. In each case, the visual output also serves as a powerful education tool to explain to patients how their foot shape has changed, why certain regions of the foot are tender if located at a site of prominent deformity and high pressure, or why a callus or ulceration is present and how a shoe or orthosis is working to redistribute pressure from these sites (Fig. 2.20).

Most pressure distribution measurement systems have software tools to permit detailed analysis of foot function. The walking footprint can be used to study the geometry of the foot: the algorithm overlaying a series of lines determined from subdivisions of the foot contact area defined by anatomical landmarks. In Figure 2.21, one of these footprints is shown for a

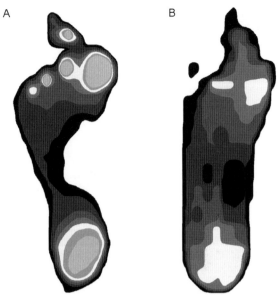

A   B

Figure 2.20 Plantar pressure distribution pattern from a typical patient with rheumatoid arthritis recorded from (A) platform device and (B) in-shoe device. Both techniques capture the lack of lesser toe contact, Pressure distribution is similar over the metatarsal head region, but the superior spatial resolution of the platform device captures the sharp focal pressure in the middle three metatarsal heads. Furthermore, the in-shoe system is measured at the interface of the foot and contoured custom orthosis, hence, the reduced forefoot pressures and the increased contact are in the midfoot region in comparison with the platform-based technique.

patient with a severe pes planovalgus foot. In comparison with normal (Fig. 2.21A), the collapsed medial longitudinal arch and severely abducted forefoot can easily be visualized (Fig. 2.2B) with a significant increase in the subarch angle (case 148° versus 105° in able-bodied subject), defined by the angle formed between the points RLN (see Figure 2.21). Other parameters are useful in relation to typical forefoot changes in RA and include the hallux angle (case 72° versus 8° in able-bodied subject), and spreading of the metatarsals using a co-efficient of the forefoot width/foot length (case 0.4 versus 0.36 in able-bodied subject). In a preliminary analysis, several of these footprints parameters were correlated with 3D structural variables derived from MRI reconstructions in pes planovalgus (Woodburn 2002). These findings are encouraging and suggest that important structural information may be gained from simple footprint parameters avoiding the unnecessary use of radiographic techniques.

Having gained information on the overall foot shape, analysis can then determine how pressure is

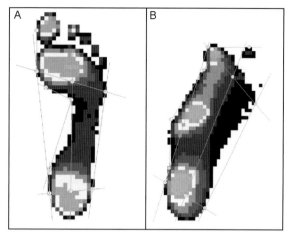

Figure 2.21 Foot geometry parameters taken from the footprint of (A) able-bodied subject and (B) patient with severe pes planovalgus. A standard algorithm defines each parameter as a distance or angle measurements taken from anatomically relevant reference lines overlaid on the pressure pattern.

distributed, in terms of magnitude and timing, in plantar regions of interest. This can be simply visualized in 'playback' mode and in Figure 2.22 a profile is shown for a patient with sharp focal pressures over the MTP joints. The diagram depicts the profile across the whole foot every 0.06 s for 15 frames (foot contact time = 0.90 s). A small spike of pressure appears in the second frame located at the medial calcaneal tubercle, which was prominent when directly palpated. In the midfoot a normal medial arch profile is present for the entire stance phase duration. Peak pressure values can be determined for each region of interest when masks are overlaid on the footprint. The major abnormality, in this case, existed in the forefoot with sharp spikes of pressure, in excess of normal upper limits, across the 2nd-to-5th MTP regions (Fig. 2.23). Not only are these pressures abnormally high, but they develop around 0.36 s and last until 0.84 s, a contact time of 0.48 s, representing over 50% of the stance phase. Lesser toe

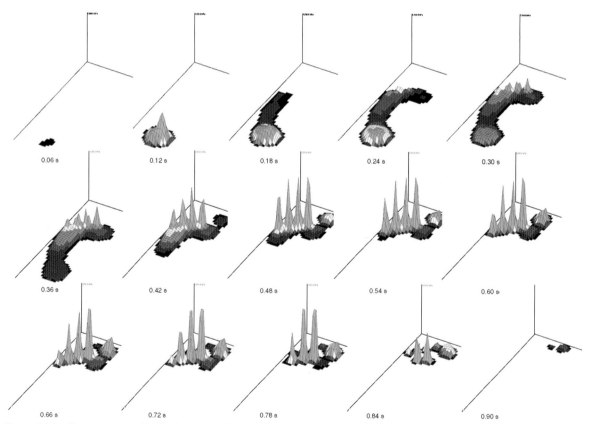

Figure 2.22 Plantar pressure distribution pattern in a patient with rheumatoid arthritis. The first frame in the upper left corner is recorded shortly after heel-strike (0.06 s) and then presented every 0.06 s until toe-off in the lower right frame (0.09 s).

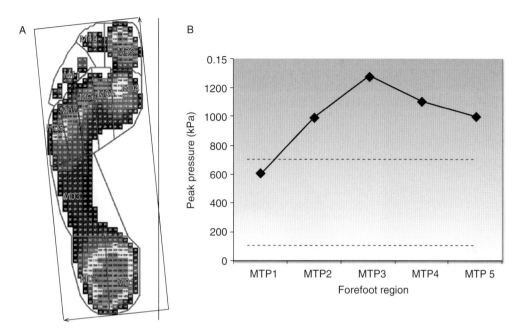

Figure 2.23 (A) masking technique for regional pressure analysis. (B) distribution and magnitude of peak pressure across the MTP joint regions in comparison with normal range (area between dashed lines represent the normal range [mean ±2SD]).

contact is made, but only for 0.18 s in late stance and function is diminished as the peak pressure values are under normal limits for this region. Interestingly, pressure distribution is normal in the 1st metatarsal head region and the hallux.

The utility of these data emerges when we consider the clinical picture (Fig. 2.24). This 59-year-old male patient presented with longstanding bilateral forefoot pain, deformity of his toes and self-reported changes to his walking style (slow, avoidance of uneven surfaces, and careful foot placement). On examination, the MTP and interphalangeal joints were retracted with claw-toe deformity, although range of motion was within normal limits. The fatty-fibro padding was displaced anteriorly and dorsally and moderate callus and adventitious bursae were observed over the 2nd–5th MTP joints (Figure 2.24A and B). He tested positive to the metatarsal squeeze test, and all 5 MTP joints were tender on direct palpation. Radiographically, all 5 MTP joints scored 5 on the Scott modification of the Larsen index, indicating severe erosion and deformity. The tarsus and ankles of both feet were unremarkable. The sites of high pressures are entirely consistent with the pathology and clinical features at the MTP joints (Fig. 2.24C).

The foot pressure distribution pattern in able-bodied persons is variable and Hughes et al. (1991), using a discriminant analysis technique, classified four basic patterns (medial, medial-central, central, lateral). In RA, these basic patterns are influenced by the extent of forefoot pain and deformity, and any compensation strategy to off-load sites and by the transfer of load forward from the heel and midfoot particularly when these sites are deformed and painful. In Figure 2.25, we noticed our patient was uncomfortable when standing and was rolling the foot outwards to off-load the medial forefoot region. The patient, with 2 months of disease, was tender at the medial three MTP joints, the first and second of which had synovitis confirmed by ultrasonography. Early in the disease there were no major foot deformities, but the daylight sign confirmed spreading of the forefoot. She had no plantar pressure lesions, and when the peak pressures were averaged the loading pattern was medial according to the Hughes Classification. However, when individual steps were considered, two other patterns were observed on subsequent steps and we believe this demonstrates a variable off-loading pattern in response to the medial forefoot symptoms.

Clinical utility of plantar pressure measurement has been demonstrated in a number of studies. Sharma et al. (1979) for instance, showed that forefoot loading was associated with lesser toe deformity and increased severity of clinical symptoms and radiographic joint damage. In three cohorts of patients

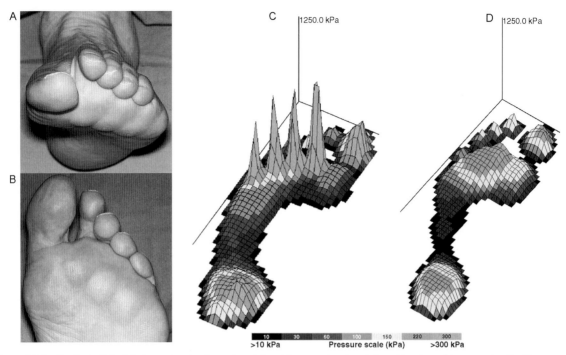

Figure 2.24   Forefoot clinical features showing lesser toe deformities, prominent metatarsal heads, and bursa and callosities overlying the MTP joints (A) and (B). Peak pressure profile in presented case (C) and foot of age and sex matched normal subject (D).

Figure 2.25   Patient with early disease off-loading the medial forefoot region, which was both tender and inflamed. The daylight sign is seen on standing at the 1st and 2nd toe clefts. The pressure distribution pattern is variable ranging from central to medial. The symptoms (RAI: Ritchie Articular Index scores for tenderness ranging in severity from 0 to 3), presence of inflammation (HRUS: high-resolution ultrasound), and peak plantar pressure (PP) values for each MTP joint are presented in the table.

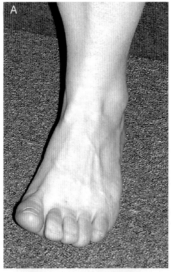

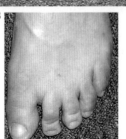

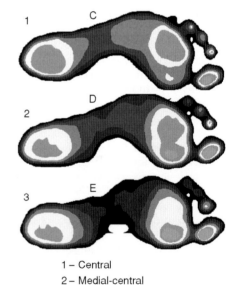

1 – Central
2 – Medial-central
3 – Medial

MTP	RAI	Lesion	HRUS	PP (kPa)
1	2	–	+	445
2	3	–	+	280
3	1	–	–	265
4	0	–	–	205
5	0	–	–	110

presenting with progressively worse radiological damage (not based on any current scoring system), loading on the hallux, second and lateral toes (regional analysis) were markedly reduced in comparison with normal with significantly less loading in the lateral toe regions (Sharma 1979). The area of toe contact and the force generation capacity of the lesser toes appear critical in relation to abnormally high peak pressures in the forefoot (Collis & Jayson 1972, Sharma 1979, Simkin 1981, Minns & Craxford 1984, Soames et al. 1985). In Figure 2.26, a series of six feet are presented with varying severity of forefoot impairment characterized, if viewed from left to right, with increasing loss of toe function. In each case, focal areas of high pressure with a sharp gradient from adjacent sites were observed and consistent with MTP deformity including hallux valgus and claw and hammer toe. These patterns are observed in patients who have predominantly forefoot disease and in all cases a well-defined medial longitudinal arch is present. This serves to decrease the contact area proximal to the metatarsal head region in some cases and this is well demonstrated in the right most foot.

The case series above perfectly illustrates why it is impossible to attempt to define a typical pattern of forefoot loading in patients with RA. In addition to deformity, plantar pressure measurement may be affected by local factors such as skin and soft-tissue thickness, plantar callosities (Sharma 1979, Woodburn & Helliwell 1996) and the extent of bony erosion at the MTP joints (Sharma 1979, Soames et al. 1985, Tuna et al. 2004). Sites of forefoot plantar callus are proxy indicators of localized high pressure and these are useful to detect during clinical examination. In most

instances, the callus has an underlying adventitious bursa and both serve to increase the contact area over which the forces are distributed. Hence the debate as to whether these lesions are protective or harmful (Woodburn et al. 2000, Davys et al. 2005). We do know, however, that elevated focal pressures are associated with the development of ulceration in some feet and three pressure profiles are shown in Figure 2.27. In each case, the peak pressures are in excess of normal values, and are experienced for prolonged periods during stance. Extensive deformity, bone erosion and fatty-fibro padding displacement are important in all three cases and, characteristically, the ulcer sites have steep pressure gradients from the adjacent normal or under-loaded skin sites. Toe function is universally non-existent.

Attention to underlying structure is important and four groups (Sharma et al. 1979, Soames et al. 1985, Tuna et al. 2004, Davys et al. 2005) noted higher pressures in patients with more erosive disease in the MTP joints. These joints are frequently subluxed or dislocated and through erosion have irregular surfaces and sharp spikes. When the fatty-fibro padding is displaced it is of little surprise that these feet have sharp focal pressures, severe symptoms and are at risk from ulceration. The pathomechanics of this process has been well described by Stainsby and others in rheumatoid arthritis (Dixon 1969, Mann & Coughlin 1979, Stainsby 1997, Briggs 2003). Briefly, synovitis and effusion leads to capsular stretching, which results in loss of integrity of the collateral ligaments (hypothetically with greater involvement of the medial collateral ligaments that leads to fibular toe drift) and capsule itself. The plantar plate moves distally around the metatarsal head (see

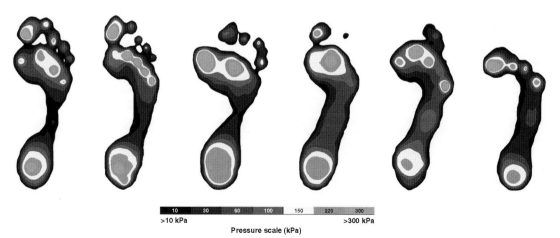

Figure 2.26   Peak pressure distribution profiles for six patients with rheumatoid arthritis with varying severity of foot impairment characterized from left to right with increasing loss of toe function and decreased forefoot contact area.

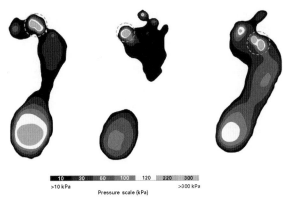

Figure 2.27 Peak pressure distribution profiles for three patients with forefoot ulceration. Ulcer sites are indicated with a red circle.

Fig. 2.28), and in severe deformity as frequently encountered in RA, the metatarsal head dislocates through the proximal joint capsule of the MTP and the two slips of the plantar aponeurosis where attached at the sides of the plantar plate. Dorsiflexion stress leads to subluxation and eventual dislocation at the MTP joints. Erosion may lead to bony spikes and the normal fatty-fibro padding under the metatarsal heads is displaced dorso-anteriorly. Secondary pressure lesions occur in the skin overlying the metatarsal head, often accompanied by an adventitious bursa.

When foot pressures are measured, the duration of pressure experienced at each site must be considered alongside the absolute peak pressure value and this is generally longer in RA patients than normal, so moderate-high pressures may also be experienced for longer in discrete regions such as the forefoot. If plotted as a function of time, the pressure integral or impulse can also be higher (Turner et al. 2003, Otter et al. 2004). This, however, mostly depends on symptoms because those patients with severe forefoot pain at sites of high peak pressure can compensate by delaying load transfer into the forefoot and then rapidly off-loading by eliminating the third rocker function (Simkin 1981, Soames et al. 1985). This can be assessed by measuring the time spent by and the velocity of the COP through the heel, midfoot, forefoot and toe regions of the foot. A typical case is shown in Figure 2.29. In the able-bodied subject, the first rocker function of the foot is shown by the rapid forward progression of the COP in the heel region, followed by forward progression of the COP between 0.3 and 0.5 m/s through the midfoot, forefoot and toe at approximately 22%, 42% and 85% of stance phase respectively. By contrast, the patient has no first rocker function and maintains the COP in the heel region until 70% of stance. The velocity rises sharply through the mid- and forefoot regions, peaking at 2.0 m/s, with the forefoot and toe contact together only making 11% of stance phase contact. The foot is

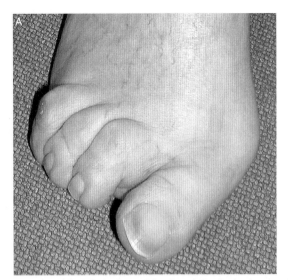

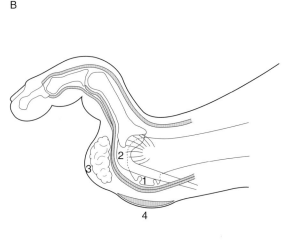

Figure 2.28 (A) typical advanced forefoot deformity in rheumatoid arthritis with clawing of the lesser toes. (B) Schematic showing eroded metatarsal head [1], dorsal and anterior displacement of the plantar plate [2] and forefoot fat pad [3] with overlying metatarsal head callosity [4] (adapted from Briggs 2003).

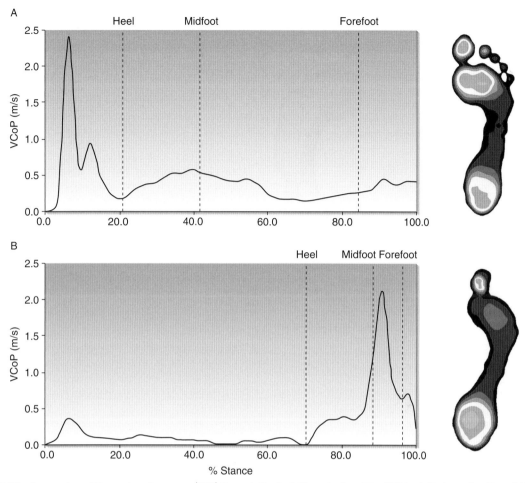

Figure 2.29 Progression of the centre of pressure (COP) through the foot. The velocity of the COP is plotted as a function of time in (A) a typical able-bodied individual and (B) a patient with severe forefoot impairment (pain located to the central MTP joints with overlying callosities and claw toe deformity).

lifted from the ground indicating loss of the second and third rocker functions.

Further work is necessary to elucidate further the compensation strategies adopted by patients to alleviate symptoms. They appear to be highly variable. The case above is predominantly compensating, using a sagittal plane strategy, but contrasts that with two further patients shown in Figure 2.30. These patients both had persistent and severe forefoot symptoms starting early in the course of their disease and had compensated by holding the foot in a stiff varus position to off-load the more painful medial side. The long-term consequence is fixed varus foot deformity with elevated pressures and new symptoms at the lateral forefoot.

The planovalgus foot in RA reveals interesting changes in pressure distribution and these have been described in a number of studies (Stockley et al. 1990, Woodburn & Helliwell 1996, Turner et al. 2003). Stockley's group found an association between valgus heel deformity and elevated medial forefoot pressures in patients who had undergone forefoot arthroplasty (Stockley et al. 1990). Since these patients fared worse surgically than their counterparts with normal heel alignment, they concluded that load transfer from the heel to forefoot was an important factor in foot function. A later study confirmed this showing a similar medial distribution of forefoot peak pressures and callus patterns in patients with valgus heel deformity (Woodburn & Helliwell 1996). More recently, a

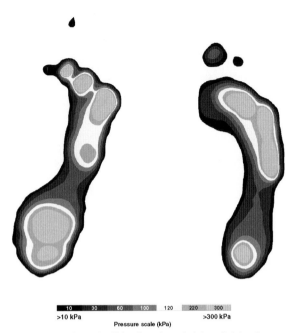

Pressure scale (kPa)
>10 kPa   >300 kPa

Figure 2.30   Lateral off-loading the painful medial forefoot region in two patients with rheumatoid arthritis.

comprehensive study of 23 cases with clinically defined pes planovalgus incorporated spatial-temporal and 3D ankle joint complex kinematics with plantar pressure measurement (Turner et al. 2003). Typical pronatory motion for the ankle joint complex was found with changes to the plantar pressure and force distribution patterns. The patients walked slower and remained in double-support longer and these compensatory mechanisms reduced the amplitude of the pressure and force variables, but may have served to increase the cumulative load because of the longer contact time. This was demonstrated in the heel region and the effect may be beneficial to reduce painful symptoms in the peri-talar region during the loading response. As expected, medial longitudinal arch collapse resulted in a large increase in the contact area in the midfoot and medial forefoot as the soft-tissue and bony architecture changed. Furthermore, higher midfoot peak pressures and pressure-time integrals may be related to tissue viability problems and skin callosities were noted over the talonavicular joint area in several patients with severe deformity. Internal joint loads may be harmful in the midfoot region where peak force, force-time integrals and contact time are increased and this was demonstrated in the patients. In agreement with others, forefoot loading was altered from a central to a medial pattern, peak pressure and pressure- and

force-time integrals were greater, and lateral forefoot off-loading was present in the group with RA (Fig. 2.31). The findings from this study confirm the observation that pes planovalgus may have detrimental effects on the entire structure and function of the foot.

The progression of pes planovalgus has been estimated in radiographic studies, but these techniques are not advisable for routine clinical use. Plantar pressure measurement offers quick assessment of overall foot geometry and loading characteristics. From the Turner et al. study of 2003 six cases are presented in Figure 2.32 to show the progressive features of pes planovalgus. From left to right, progressive off-loading in the lateral heel and forefoot regions with increased loading medially and increased contact area in the midfoot region can be observed. Two extreme cases on the far right are shown with severe midfoot collapse with high focal pressures in the navicular-medial cuneiform region consistent with sites of pain and overlying callus.

Plantar pressure measurement is useful in determining functional changes in our patients who have multiple impairments throughout the foot. Figure 2.33 shows the profile from a female patient in her 60s with over 25 years of disease duration. Although her disease is well controlled on biologic therapy she has persistent forefoot pain. She presented with hallux valgus fixed at ~15° of dorsiflexion, claw toes, which were retracted and non-weightbearing when standing, and a valgus heel deformity with low medial longitudinal arch profile. Her walking speed was slow at 0.78 m/s, cadence 113 steps/min, cycle time 1.06 s and stride length 0.83 m. In the forefoot the normal geometry of the MTP parabola had been disturbed through a combination of disease activity (erosion and deformity) and surgical intervention (arthrodesis and arthroplasty). The sharp distal margins of the eroded 5th MTP and arthrodesed 1st MTP were evident on plain X-ray. The fatty-fibro padding was displaced anteriorly and a callus was present over the 1st MTP joint. The heel fat pad was atrophied and a firm palpable mass consistent with a nodule or bursa present over the medial calcaneal tubercle. From her pressure profile a number of features can be determined. The superimposed COP shows normal progression in the heel region, delay in the midfoot and rapid progression through the forefoot consistent with an off-loading pattern described earlier. The elevated medial heel pressures are located as the site of the plantar nodule or bursa. Although her arch profile is low, it has stiffened in that posture rather than collapse as the pressure profile shows a normal arch distribution.

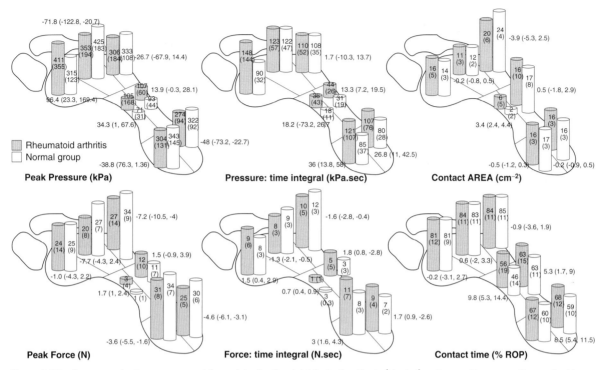

Figure 2.31 Summary plantar pressure and force data for the right foot of patients (shaded) and normative group. The vertical bars are scaled to the absolute mean values with SD in parentheses. The mean group differences are presented with 95% confidence intervals of the difference given in parentheses. The foot is divided into regions of interest including the medial and lateral heel and the midfoot and medial, central and lateral forefoot. Six summary variables are presented (From Turner et al. 2003).

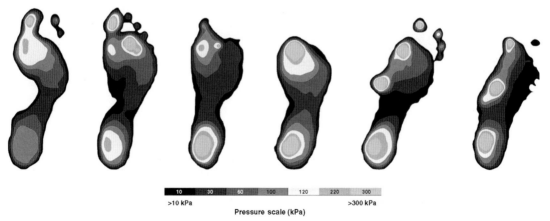

Figure 2.32 Peak pressure distribution profiles for six patients with varying severity of pes planovalgus.

Armed with this information one can go about systematically linking structural and functional impairment with knowledge of the disease pathology, symptoms, compensation strategies and effects of past interventions. In the forefoot, the heel position has resulted in high medial pressures concentrated over the first metatarsal head, which is dorsiflexed and immobile. This is further exacerbated by the fixed dorsiflexed position of the 1st MTP with the hallux undergoing minimal ground contact. Laterally, the eroded 5th

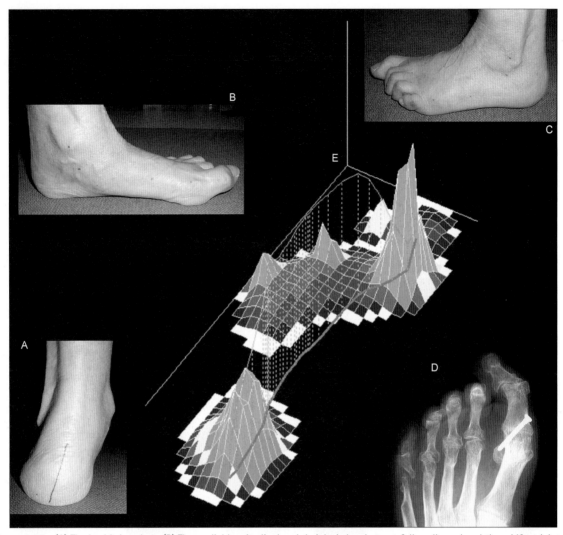

Figure 2.33 (A) The heel is in valgus. (B) The medial longitudinal arch height is low but not fully collapsed and the midfoot joints are stiff. (C) The lesser toes are retracted, deformed and non-weight bearing. (D) The 1st MTP is arthrodesed, the 2nd, 3rd and 4th MTP joints are severely eroded, and the 5th MTP has undergone excision of the metatarsal head and proximal phalanx. (E) Peak pressure profile with vertical ground reaction and centre-of-pressure line superimposed.

metatarsal head may be responsible for the spike of pressure at the MTP joint region. The 3rd metatarsal head was slightly longer and prominent on palpation and the toe made no ground contact explaining the elevated pressure here. Pain is significant enough to slow the walking speed and shorten the stride length.

The pressure information from this case was used to assist surgical planning and it is here that PPM has been used as a functional outcome tool (Betts et al. 1988, Phillipson et al. 1994, Dereymaeker et al. 1997, Bitzan 1997). Findings have been variable and

difficult to compare due to methodological differences with the pressure measurement and variance in the patient cohorts, surgical procedures undertaken and follow-up time. As a rule, detrimental peak pressures can be reduced in the forefoot with arthroplasty procedures and these tend to be associated with clinical improvement in symptoms and function (Betts et al. 1988, Dereymaeker et al. 1997, Bitzan 1997). Betts and colleagues found that pre- and post-operative pressure analysis allowed them to appraise their surgical techniques after encountering good pressure reduction in the central metatarsal heads, but not at the 1st or 5th (Betts et al. 1988). They attributed this to a shallow arc created during the metatarsal head resection thereby transferring load from the central metatarsal heads outwards to the first and fifth. Dereymaeker et al. (1997) detected a reduction of abnormal high pressure areas in just over 50% of cases with increased toe loading and resolution of plantar callosities at 35 months post-surgery. After a similar period, by contrast, Phillipson and colleagues found an increase in both peak pressure and the pressure-time integral in 15 patients, although not all were RA. This was partly attributed to increased walking speed following surgery, although this change was not formally reported and the greatest changes were reported under the first metatarsal head and associated with recurrent callosities. Clearly, more controlled studies with well-defined end points are required to clarify some of the anomalies arising from the current literature.

Elsewhere, in-shoe pressure measurement has been used to assess the off-loading properties of custom and prefabricated orthotic devices. Shrader and Siegel, from the National Institutes of Health, present a very detailed and excellent case history, showing the effective reduction of peak pressure and pressure-time integral in the forefoot using a custom-fabricated orthosis (Shrader & Siegel 2003). The pressure relief was accompanied by improvement to symptoms and ability to perform activities of daily living requiring standing and walking. In more controlled studies, both prefabricated and custom orthoses have been shown to be effective for reducing forefoot pressure and improving symptoms with moderate evidence to suggest custom devices are more effective (Hodge et al. 1999, Li 2000). The Leeds randomized controlled trial of custom orthoses manufactured in carbon-graphite, followed 101 patients with early disease and mobile correctable valgus heel deformity for 30 months (Woodburn 2001). Results showed effective off-loading of the medial forefoot region, increased contact area and force in the midfoot and decreased pressure in the heel region, all favourable changes for the foot type being treated.

Noteworthy is the use of padded hosiery as these too, in the short term, have pressure-relieving function similar to orthotics. In Leeds, the effect of scalpel debridement on forefoot pressures at callus sites has also been studied and showed no significant difference in the change between a real and sham procedure (Davys et al. 2005). Again, these areas will benefit from further studies that are well controlled, adequately powered to detect pressure differences and appropriately disease-staged.

> ## KEY POINTS
>
> - Plantar pressure (P) is defined as the force (F) per unit area (A) (P=F/A).
> - Plantar pressure distribution can be measured using platform or in-shoe systems.
> - The pressure footprint can be used to determine the plantar geometry
> - Peak pressure and the pressure-time integral are frequently higher than normal in the forefoot in RA and are associated with impairment including pain, stiffness and deformity.
> - In pes planovalgus collapse of the medial longitudinal arch is associated with increased contact and force in the midfoot region.
> - Plantar pressure relief, pain reduction and functional improvement have been reported following surgical and non-surgical interventions for symptomatic forefoot disease in RA.

MUSCLE FUNCTION (SEE ALSO CHAPTERS 3 AND 4)

Determining muscle function from electromyography has been rarely studied in RA. Perry (1992) suggested that the loss of muscle strength was a major pathomechanical factor in foot disease in RA. Two mechanisms were postulated: (1) inflammation causes joint and soft-tissue pain that inhibits muscle function, thereby reducing the force transmission at painful joint sites and (2) through the above action motion is decreased, which results in reduced activity and the development of secondary muscle weakness. This was demonstrated in a single RA patient with gastrocnemius and soleus weakness secondary to MTP joint inflammation showing loss of third rocker function as described earlier (Perry 1992). The same group used fine-wire electromyography (EMG) to study extrinsic foot muscle function in patients with RA with and without valgus deformity of the foot (Keenan et al. 1991). This work eloquently showed increased intensity and duration of activity of the tibialis posterior, supposedly in an effort to support the medial longitudinal arch in those patients with valgus heel deformity. This group believed the compensatory action of tibialis posterior was due to primary weakness in calf muscles that, despite increased activity on EMG testing, were weak on manual muscle testing. Combined with motion, structural and clinical data, the integrated approach demonstrated in this work facilitates a better understanding of changes in foot function resulting from primary pathology. Electromyography is one of the more difficult techniques to undertake during routine gait analysis and we have yet to fully integrate this technique to the approaches described above.

ENERGY CONSUMPTION

When patients who have RA walk with painful joints and undertake compensatory strategies we can postulate that the gait is less energy efficient than normal. Measurement of metabolic energy expenditure is a useful global measure of overall gait performance and allows the physiological cost of pathological gait to be estimated. Measurement techniques are not routinely performed since they typically involve collection and analysis of blood gases and heart rate whilst walking or exercising. The physiological cost index (PCI) was previously proposed as an objective measure of disability and as an outcome for intervention studies in RA (Steven et al. 1993, Kavlak et al. 2003). The index is based on the observation that any voluntary increase in walking speed demands an increase in energy expenditure that is relatively disproportionate in disabled persons. Past studies have shown that NSAID therapy leads to a statistically significant improvement in the PCI, but that the improvement was not correlated with conventional clinical measurements such as tender/swollen joints, pain score or ESR (Steven et al. 1983). Kavlak and colleagues (2003) found a significant improvement in foot pain, step and stride length, and the physiological cost index after 3 months of foot orthotic therapy. Beyond these two applications, the PCI has not been widely adopted in clinical research and this is understandable when disability can be easily measured using valid and reliable global and foot-specific questionnaires.

CONCLUSIONS

This chapter has summarized currently available gait analysis techniques that are available to the clinician and researcher. We have appraised the available information and where evidence was lacking appropriate cases were presented to illustrate the use of the various techniques in our own laboratory. Plantar pressure measurement probably represents the extent that most clinical units will invest in gait equipment and we believe this is reasonable given its ease of use and affordability. This technique yields valuable information on foot structure and function in RA. We are steadily refining other techniques and using them for clinical research and practice. 3D joint kinematic and kinetic analyses are more difficult to perform and interpret, but we have shown some valuable uses in patients at various stages of the disease to detect changes associated with impairment and as compensation strategies. We hope that gait analysis will be become more readily available in the future, as it has important uses for determining the structural and functional changes in the foot brought about by inflammation in the joints and soft-tissues of the foot. Moreover, treatment planning and evaluation can be greatly aided by gait information, especially in complex cases undergoing surgical intervention. In terms of clinical research, gait analysis will be used to drive experimental work aimed at further advancing our core knowledge and, in translational studies, inform future development of customized approaches to footwear and orthosis manufacture as well as foot surgery.

References

Betts RP, Stockley I, Getty CJ, Rowley DI, Duckworth T, Franks CI Foot pressure studies in the assessment of forefoot arthroplasty in the rheumatoid foot. Foot and Ankle 1988; 8: 315–326.

Bilney B, Morris M, Webster K Concurrent related validity of the GAITRite walkway system for quantification of the spatial and temporal parameters of gait. Gait Posture 2003; 7: 68–74.

Bitzan P, Giurea A, Wanivenhaus A Plantar pressure distribution after resection of the metatarsal heads in rheumatoid arthritis. Foot and Ankle International 1997; 18: 391–397.

Bouysset M, Tebib J, Tavernier T et al. Posterior tibial tendon and subtalar joint complex in rheumatoid arthritis: magnetic resonance imaging study. Journal of Rheumatology 2003; 30: 1951–1954.

Bouysset M, Tebib JG, Weil G, Lejeune E, Bouvier M Deformation of the adult rheumatoid rearfoot. A radiographic study. Clinical Rheumatology 1987; 6: 539–544.

Briggs PJ Controversies and perils. Reconstruction of the rheumatoid forefoot. The Stainsby operation. Techniques in Orthopaedics 2003; 18: 303–310.

Buczek FL, Kepple TM, Lohmann Siegel K, Stanhope SJ Translational and rotational joint power terms in a six degree-of-freedom model of the normal ankle complex. Journal of Biomechanics 1994; 27: 1447–1457.

Carson MC, Harrington ME, Thompson N, O'Connor JJ and Theologis TN Kinematic analysis of a multi-segment foot model for research and clinical applications: a repeatability analysis. Journal of Biomechanics 2001; 34: 1299–1307.

Coakley FV, Smanta AK, Finlay DB Ultrasonography of the tibialis posterior tendon in rheumatoid arthritis. British Journal of Rheumatology 1994; 33: 273–277.

Collis WJMF, Jayson MIV Measurement of pedal pressures. An illustration of a method. Annals of Rheumatic Diseases 1972; 31: 215–217.

Davys HJ, Turner DE, Helliwell PS, Conaghan PG, Emery P, Woodburn J Debridement of plantar callosities in rheumatoid arthritis: a randomized controlled trial. Rheumatology 2005; 44: 207–210.

Dereymaeker G, Mulier T, Stuer P, Peeraer L, Fabry G Pedodynographic measurements after forefoot reconstruction in rheumatoid arthritis patients. Foot and Ankle International 1997; 18: 270–276.

Dixon A St J The rheumatoid foot. Proceedings of the Royal Society of Medicine 1970; 63: 677–679.

Eng JJ, Winter DA Kinetic analysis of the lower limbs during walking: what information can be gained from a three-dimensional model? Journal of Biomechanics 1995; 28: 753–758.

Fransen M, Edmonds J Off-the-shelf orthopaedic footwear for people with rheumatoid arthritis. Arthritis Care Research 1997; 10: 250–256.

Fransen M, Edmonds J Gait variables: appropriate objective outcome measures in rheumatoid arthritis. Rheumatology 1999; 38: 663–667.

Grace EM, Gerecz EM, Kassam YB, Buchanan HM, Buchanan WW, Tugwell PS 50-foot walking time: a critical assessment of an outcome measure in clinical therapeutic trials of antirheumatic drugs. British Journal of Rheumatology 1988; 27:372–374.

Hamilton J, Brydson G, Fraser S, Grant M Walking ability as a measure of treatment effect in early rheumatoid arthritis. Clinical Rehabilitation 2001; 15: 142–147.

Hodge MC, Bach TM, Carter GM Orthotic management of plantar pressure and pain in rheumatoid arthritis. Clinical Biomechanics 1999; 14: 567–575.

Hughes J, Clark P, Jagoe JR, Gerber C, Klenerman L The pattern of pressure distribution under the weightbearing forefoot. Foot 1991; 1: 117–124.

Hunt GC, Fromherz WA, Gerber LH, Hurwitz SR Hindfoot pain treated by a leg–hindfoot orthosis. Physical Therapy 1987; 67: 1384–1388.

Isacson, J, Brostrom LA Gait in rheumatoid arthritis: an electrogoniometric investigation. Journal of Biomechanics 1988; 21: 451–457.

Jernberg ET, Simkin P, Kravette M, Lowe P, Gardner G The posterior tibial tendon and tarsal sinus in rheumatoid flat foot: magnetic resonance imaging of 40 feet. Journal of Rheumatology 1999; 26: 289–293.

Kavlak Y, Uygur F, Korkmaz C, Bek N Outcome of orthoses intervention in the rheumatoid foot. Foot and Ankle International 2003; 24: 494–499.

Keenan MAE, Peabody TD, Gronley JK, Perry J Valgus deformity of the feet and characteristics of gait in patients who have rheumatoid arthritis. Journal of Bone and Joint Surgery 1991; 73A: 237–247.

Kjaersgaard-Andersen P, Wethelund JO, Helmig P, Soballe K The stabilising effect of the ligamentous structures in the sinus and canalis tarsi on movements in the hindfoot. American Journal of Sports Medicine 1988; 16: 512–516.

Klenerman L The foot and ankle in rheumatoid arthritis. British Journal of Rheumatology 1995: 34: 443–448

Lehtinen A, Paimela L, Kreula J, Leirisalo-Repo M, Taavitsainen M Painful ankle region in rheumatoid arthritis. Acta Radiologica 1996; 37: 572–577.

Li CY, Imaishi K, Shiba N, Tagawa Y, Maeda T, Matsuo S, Goto T, Yamanaka K Biomechanical evaluation of foot pressure and loading force during gait in rheumatoid arthritic patients with and without foot orthosis. Kurume Medical Journal 2000; 47:211–217.

Locke M, Perry J, Campbell J, Thomas L Ankle and subtalar motion during gait in arthritic patients. Physical Therapy 1984; 64: 504–509.

Lundberg A, Svensson OK, Bylund C, Goldie I, Selvik G Kinematics of the ankle/foot complex—Part 2: Pronation and supination. Foot and Ankle 1989; 9: 248–253.

MacSween A, Brydson G, Hamilton J The effects of custom moulded ethyl vinyl acetate foot orthoses on the gait of patients with rheumatoid arthritis. The Foot 1999; 9: 128–133.

Mann RA, Coughlin MJ The rheumatoid foot. Review of the literature and method of treatment. Orthopaedic Review 1979; 13:105–112.

Marshall RN, Myers DB, Palmer DG Disturbance of gait due to rheumatoid disease? Journal of Rheumatology 1980; 7: 617–23.

Masterton E, Mulcahy D, McElwain J, McInerney D The planovalgus rheumatoid foot: is tibialis posterior rupture a factor? British Journal of Rheumatology 1995; 34(645): 645–646.

McDonough AL, Batavia M, Chen FC, Kwon S, Ziai J The validity and reliability of the GAITRite system's measurement: a preliminary evaluation. Archives of Physical Medicine and Rehabilitation 2001; 82: 419–425.

Mejjad O, Vittecoq O, Pouplin S, Grassin–Delyle L, Weber J, Le Loet X Foot orthotics decrease pain but do not improve gait in rheumatoid arthritis patients. Joint, Bone, Spine: Revue du rhumatisme 2004; 71: 542–545.

Minns RJ, Craxford AD. Pressure under the forefoot in rheumatoid arthritis: a comparison of static and dynamic methods of assessment. Clinical Orthopaedics and Related Research 1984; 187: 235–242.

Moriggl B, Kumai T, Milz S, Benjamin M The structure and histopathology of the 'enthesis organ' at the navicular insertion of the tendon of tibialis posterior. Journal of Rheumatology 2003; 30: 508–517.

O'Connell PG, Siegel KL, Kepple TM, Stanhope SJ, Gerber LH Forefoot deformity, pain, and mobility in rheumatoid and nonarthritic subjects. Journal of Rheumatology 1998; 25:1681–1689.

Ottenbacher K, Barrett K Measures of effect size in reporting of rehabilitation research. American Journal of Physical Medicine and Rehabilitation 1989; 68: 52–57.

Otter SJ, Bowen CJ, Young AK Forefoot plantar pressures in rheumatoid arthritis. Journal of American Podiatric Medical Association 2004; 94: 255–260.

Perry J Gait Analysis. Normal and Pathological Function. Slack, Inc., Thorofare, NJ, 1992.

Phillipson A, Dhar S, Linge K, McCabe C, Klenerman L Forefoot arthroplasty and changes in plantar foot pressures. Foot and Ankle International 1994; 15: 595–598.

Platto MJ, O'Connell PG, Hicks JE, Gerber LH The relationship of pain and deformity of the rheumatoid foot to gait and an index of functional limitation. Journal of Rheumatology 1991; 18: 38–43.

Premkumar A, Perry MB, Dwyer AJ, Gerber LH, Johnson D, Venzon D, Shawker TH Sonography and MR imaging of posterior tibial tendinopathy. Am J Roentgen 2002; 178: 223–232.

Sharma M, Dhanendran M, Hutton WC, Corbett M Changes in load bearing in the rheumatoid foot. Annals of Rheumatic Diseases 1979; 38: 549–552.

Shrader JA, Siegel KL Postsurgical hindfoot deformity of a patient with rheumatoid arthritis treated with custom-made foot orthoses and shoe modifications. Physical Therapy 1997; 77: 296–305.

Shrader JA, Siegel KL. Nonoperative management of functional hallux limitus in a patient with rheumatoid arthritis. Physical Therapy 2003; 83: 831–843.

Siegel KL, Kepple TM, O'Connell PG, Gerber LH, Stanhope SJ A technique to evaluate foot function during the stance phase of gait. Foot & Ankle 1995; 16: 764–770.

Simkin A The dynamic vertical force distribution during level walking under normal and rheumatic feet. Rheumatology Rehabilitation 1981; 20: 88–97.

Soames RW, Carter PG, Towle JA The rheumatoid foot during gait. In: Whittle M and Harris D (eds) Biomechanical Measurement in Orthopaedic Practice. Oxford University Press. New York, 1985; pp. 167–178.

Spiegel TM and Spiegel JS Rheumatoid arthritis in the foot and ankle – diagnosis, pathology, and treatment. Foot & Ankle 1982; 2: 318–324.

Stainsby GD Pathological anatomy and the dynamic effect of the displaced plantar plate and the importance of the integrity of the plantar plate–deep transverse metatarsal ligament tie-bar. Annals of the Royal College of Surgery of England 1997; 79: 58–68.

Steven MM, Capell HA, Sturrock RD, MacGregor The Physiological cost index of gait (PCG): a new technique for evaluating nonsteroidal anti-inflammatory drugs in rheumatoid arthritis. British Journal of Rheumatology 1983; 22: 141–145.

Stockley I, Betts RP, Rowley DI, Getty CJM, Duckworth T The importance of valgus hindfoot in forefoot surgery in rheumatoid arthritis. Journal of Bone and Joint Surgery 1990; 72–B: 705–708.

Tuna H, Birtane M, Tastekin N, Kokino S Pedobarography and its relation to radiologic erosion scores in rheumatoid arthritis. Rheumatology International 2005; 26(1): 42–47.

Turner DE, Woodburn J, Helliwell PS, Cornwall ME, Emery P Pes planovalgus in rheumatoid arthritis: a descriptive and analytical study of foot function determined by gait analysis. Musculoskeletal Care 2003; 1: 21–33.

Woodburn J Plantar pressure and footprint analysis in rheumatoid arthritis: a comparison of patients classified by 3D MRI image analysis of the subtalar and midtarsal joints. Proceedings from the VIIIth emed Scientific meeting, Kananaskis, Calgary, Alberta, Canada, August 2002.

Woodburn J Kinematics at the ankle joint complex in rheumatoid arthritis. PhD Thesis. The University of Leeds. 2001.

Woodburn J, Cornwall MW, Soames RW, Helliwell PS Selectively attenuating soft-tissues close to sites of inflammation in the peri-talar region of patients with rheumatoid arthritis leads to the development of pes planovalgus. Journal of Rheumatology 2005; 32: 268–274.

Woodburn J, Helliwell PS. The relationship between valgus heel deformity and the distribution of forefoot plantar pressures and callosities in rheumatoid arthritis. Annals of Rheumatic Diseases 1996; 55: 806–810.

Woodburn J, Helliwell PS, Barker S Three-dimensional kinematics at the ankle joint complex in rheumatoid arthritis patients with painful valgus deformity of the rearfoot. Rheumatology 2002; 41: 1406–1412.

Woodburn J, Helliwell PS, Barker S Changes in three-dimensional joint kinematics supports the continuous use of foot orthoses in the management of painful rearfoot deformity in rheumatoid arthritis. Journal of Rheumatology 2003; 30: 2356–2364.

Woodburn J, Nelson KM, Lohmann Siegel K, Kepple TM, Gerber LH Multisegment foot motion during gait: proof of concept in rheumatoid arthritis. Journal of Rheumatology 2004; 31: 1918–1927.

Woodburn J, Stableford Z, Helliwell PS Preliminary investigation of debridement of plantar callosities in rheumatoid arthritis. Rheumatology 2000; 39: 652–654.

Woodburn J, Turner DE, Helliwell PS Barker S A preliminary study determining the feasibility of electromagnetic tracking for kinematics at the ankle joint complex. Rheumatology 1999; 38: 1260–1268.

Woodburn J, Udupa JK, Hirsch BE et al. The geometrical architecture of the subtalar and midtarsal joints in rheumatoid arthritis based on MR imaging. Arthritis Rheum 2002; 46: 3168–3177.

Yao L, Gentili A, Cracchiolo A MR imaging findings in spring ligament insufficiency. Skeletal Radiology 1999; 28: 245–250.

Further reading

Perry J Gait Analysis. Normal and Pathological Function. Thorofare, NJ: Slack, Inc, 1992.

Robertson G, Caldwell G, Hamill J, Kamen G, Whittlesey S Research Methods in Biomechanics. Champaign, Illinois. Human Kinetics, 2004

Whittle M Gait Analysis. An Introduction. 3rd Edition. Butterworth Heinemann Health, 2001.

Chapter **3**

Clinical features of the foot in rheumatoid arthritis

JOINT DISEASE: UNDERSTANDING HOW SYNOVITIS PRESENTS IN THE FOOT AND CAUSES THE CHANGES SEEN IN RHEUMATOID ARTHRITIS

In the section on the pathogenesis of rheumatoid arthritis (RA) (Chapter 1), the putative triggers and mechanisms behind the development of synovitis, the hallmark of RA, were described. In RA, synovitis can develop in any joint, simultaneously or consecutively. There are no rules that govern which joint or group of joints become involved at any particular time. In fact, it is likely that virtually all synovial joints have some degree of inflammation if we were to look hard enough, by synovial biopsy, for example. Imaging modalities, such as ultrasound (U/S) and magnetic resonance imaging (MRI) have shown that clinical examination is a crude technique for detecting synovial inflammation at an early stage (see Chapter 5).

Given that synovial inflammation is probably widespread, what sort of factors might govern the progression of inflammation and the onset of bone damage and deformity? With respect to the foot, the most important factor must be joint loading. What governs the degree of joint loading in the foot? Body weight is an important variable in this respect, but we don't know how important this is, having no epidemiological data to advise us. Ambulation, both in quantity and quality, is important. There is some evidence that stride length is a significant indicator of joint loading (see section on Gait in Chapter 2) but, all other things being equal, the amount of time spent upright will greatly influence the cumulative loading of the lower limb joints. While we would not advocate a return to the times when patients with early RA were admitted to hospital, there to rest in bed for up to 3 months, methods to reduce joint loading and abnormal forces should be a priority in early disease.

Are any of the joints of the foot and ankle more susceptible to excessive joint loading? There is evidence that the talo-crural joint is rarely involved by osteoarthritis and it has been suggested that this joint in particular has a good surface area to load ratio despite having to withstand forces of up to four times body weight during normal ambulation (Swann & Seedhom 1993). For theoretical reasons, therefore, it might be expected that the ankle joint is involved less frequently and later than other joints in this region. The evidence for this is contradictory, however, as was discussed in the section on the Epidemiology of Foot Disease in Chapter 1. On the whole the evidence points to a lower prevalence of disease in the talo-crural joint, but it must be recognized that many of these figures were obtained by clinical examination. However, figures from radiological surveys (i.e. of deformity and erosion) support the low prevalence and later onset of disease in this joint.

The progression of disease and the appearance of joint deformity will also be influenced by the structure and function of the joint. The subtalar joint, for example, is a complex structure that permits a triplanar movement through which forces are transmitted between the ground and the body during locomotion. Although the anterior and posterior parts of the joint are normally separated, this separation is soon lost in RA as inflammatory changes cause attenuation of joint structures. In fact, the loss of the normal anatomical boundaries between joints is a frequent occurrence in established RA. This is readily apparent when contrast is injected into the joints; a common finding is communication between the anterior and posterior parts of the subtalar joint and communication between these and the talo-crural joint (see Fig. 6.4) and within the mid-tarsal and mid-carpal joints.

The subtalar joint also contains important ligamentous structures that contribute to the stability of the ankle joint complex; the talo-calcaneal and cervical ligaments in particular. Intra-articular ligaments such as these are particularly vulnerable to the advancing rheumatoid pannus. However, another mechanism that contributes to the loss of joint stability is the laxity in joint capsule consequent to tense intra-articular effusions. When a joint first becomes inflamed the intra-articular pressure is high due to the effusion occurring within the normal anatomical confines of the joint capsule. The high pressure may contribute, incidentally, to articular damage due to ischaemic changes (as the pressure of the effusion exceeds that of arterial pressure) (Blake et al. 1989, Jayson & Dixon 1970). With time and persistence, however, the joint

capsule adapts and becomes distended and lax so that the intra-articular pressure falls.

The sub-talar joint is particularly vulnerable to inflammation in RA. There are a number of reasons for this. Firstly, as mentioned above, the sub-talar is a complex joint the stability of which may be readily compromised by inflammation. Secondly, pronation at this joint is not an uncommon finding in 'normal' people, the prevalence being around 25%. Thirdly, abnormal gait patterns resulting from painful forefoot disease may lead to excessive pronation of the foot and the resulting pes planovalgus deformity (see Figs. 1.3, 2.6). Fourthly, inflammation and attenuation of medial juxta-articular structures such as the tibialis posterior tendon and the deltoid ligament will exacerbate and contribute to advancing deformity (see Fig. 2.10).

Compensation mechanisms occurring in neighbouring structures are often adequate for the purpose of minimizing functional limitation imposed by specific, localized pathology. Symptoms will arise, however, if the compensations are inadequate or when the act of compensation itself precipitates other dysfunction. An example of this process is in the development of a *varus* hindfoot deformity in RA. This inverted positional deformity of the calcaneus contrasts with the more usual valgus deformity and is seen in only 3–5% of people with RA. The mechanism for the varus deformity is not well understood, but it is seen in patients with severe and painful forefoot disease on the medial side and so it is thought likely that it is a structural consequence of a functional change brought about by offloading the painful joints.

In the mid-tarsal region one joint in particular seems to be involved early and is often the source of much discomfort in RA; the talo-navicular joint. The reason this joint is so pivotal in this disease is not entirely clear, other than some of the factors adduced to be important in the sub-talar joint will apply here. These include a low joint surface-area-to-load ratio. In addition, increasingly large forces will come to bear on this joint as the medial arch of the foot begins to displace inferiorly with progression of disease in the subtalar joint and as a result of the inflammatory changes in the ligamentous structures of the foot.

In the metatarsophalangeal joints early inflammatory change may cause, through disruption of the joint capsule, widening of adjacent toes (daylight sign: see Fig. 2.15) and pressure on the inter-digital nerve (Morton's 'neuroma' – see below). These clinical pointers are unique to this area, possibly as a result of the anatomy of the metatarsophalangeal joint and the surrounding structures in the web space. Extension of synovial pannus into the contiguous ligamentous structures, such as the deep transverse metatarsal ligament, will cause disruption of this structure and thus widening of the forefoot at this point. The subsequent development of the typical changes seen in RA are a consequence both of synovitis, attenuation of joint capsule and ligaments, altered mechanical forces and unequal pull of the long and intrinsic tendons crossing the joints (see Fig. 2.24).

Morton's 'neuroma' is a misnomer in this situation. Although Morton originally described the syndrome in association with a swelling of the inter-digital nerve adjacent to the metatarsophalangeal joint, it seems likely that in RA it is synovitis in the joint that is causing compression of the nerve (Awerbuch et al. 1982). The presentation is the same: a sharp pain radiating into the ipsilateral digit, worse on weight bearing and reproduced by pressure across the metatarsophalangeal joints.

Understanding the effects of synovitis in the foot in rheumatoid arthritis

- Joint loading is an important factor interacting with synovitis to produce joint deformity. Many factors contribute to this including body weight and stride length.
- Synovial pannus weakens intra-articular and periarticular ligamentous structures. Joint effusions distort the joint capsule.
- Certain joints deform early – the subtalar joint is vulnerable because of its complex anatomical structure, vulnerable supporting structures and pivotal biomechanical role in walking.
- Similarly the talo-navicular joint is frequently involved because of its pivotal position and function in the integrity of the medial lingitudinal arch.
- Forefoot deformity, manifest as widening, occurs early and may manifest as difficulty getting footwear to fit.
- Sesamoiditis in the forefoot may be an important cause of symptoms.

Further manifestations of the inflammatory process are manifest in the sesamoid bones and in the tendons with synovial sheaths. The major sesamoid bones, in particular those associated with the hallux, may develop an associated inflammatory synovitis as their anatomy reveals a synovial sheath around the bone. Rheumatoid synovitis then results in what is essentially 'sesamoiditis', a major consequence of which is pain and altered gait to avoid loading the area.

Tenosynovitis is frequently seen in the major tendons that cross the ankle joint where they are encased in sheaths lined with a synovial membrane. The most frequent areas are the peroneal tendons on the lateral aspect (see Fig. 4.9) and tibialis posterior on the medial aspect, but changes are also often seen anteriorly beneath the extensor retinaculum. The inflammation may arise de novo in these tendon sheaths, but is occasionally seen as an extension of the inflammatory process in adjacent joints: a phenomenon seen occasionally at arthrography. Importantly, sustained inflammation in the tendon sheaths will eventually lead to deterioration of the collagenous substance of the tendon itself with subsequent rupture. The tendon may be functionally inadequate, however, purely in the presence of inflammation as the individual seeks to avoid loading the affected part (see Chapter 7).

In summary, the hallmark changes of RA (inflammatory synovitis) may affect any synovial tissue and, although the pathological processes are common to all joints, the effects of the inflammation will be modified according to local factors, including the joint anatomy, the periarticular structures and the individual's response to the painful pathological processes that are underway in the feet. Finally, as befits our adoption of the ICF model, it is worth considering what effect footwear and walking surfaces have on the processes of synovitis in the foot affected by RA. Dixon has argued that some of the deformities of the foot in RA, particularly the forefoot, are the result of wearing ill-fitting shoes (Dixon 1987). His comments are aimed mainly at the narrow fashion 'court' shoes worn by women in Western society that contribute to the common deformities seen in the hallux. In support of his contention is the common absence of this deformity in developing countries. Whether this is true or not, patients with RA commonly complain of painful feet and an inability to wear comfortable footwear. There is no doubt that once the disease progresses the resulting pain and ensuing deformity make obtaining comfortable footwear that fits a difficult task. On the other hand, many of the patients supplied with footwear designed to accommodate their foot problems do not ultimately wear the new shoes (Williams & Meacher 2001). This remains an important area for further work both from the perspective of our patients, whose mobility is compromised as a result, and from the perspective of the NHS, whose finite resources must be used in the most cost-effective manner.

JOINT SYMPTOMS IN EARLY AND LATE DISEASE

Two of the cardinal symptoms of rheumatoid arthritis (joint pain and stiffness) are manifest early in the foot and ankle. Symptoms change with the duration and stage of disease, and these will be discussed separately in relation to the underlying pathological changes.

At onset RA comes as a completely new set of sensory experiences and frequently results in a level of impairment and disability that both shocks and dismays the sufferer. What were previously regarded as automatic activities, walking and running, are suddenly very difficult and present significant obstacles to mobility. Pain is usually felt under the metatarsophalangeal joints and is worst in the early morning and evening when weight bearing. Patients describe their feet as 'throbbing'. At this stage, and long before there is deformity of the forefoot with callus formation, patients will describe a sensation of walking with pebbles in their shoes. Inflammation of the mid-tarsal and sub-talar joints can be equally disabling and results in an aversion to walking on uneven ground or cobbles. A particular environmental obstacle in this respect is the so called 'tactile pavement' now in widespread use at junctions to help visually disabled pedestrians.

At the early stages patients may prefer to walk barefoot as their usual footwear aggravates their symptoms. Attempts to find more comfortable footwear, which is also cosmetically acceptable, results in the complaint of multiple pairs of discarded shoes, none of which are worn. Many patients find 'trainers' the most comfortable option. As the disease progresses the desire is to find wider fitting shoes to accommodate the broadening forefoot.

Later in the process of the disease the patient may have symptoms that relate to deformity and associated consequences. At this stage patients may only be able to walk with shoes on as their bare feet are no longer able to provide a stable base for ambulation. Hammer toes will rub on the toe box of the shoe and some patients will wear, as a consequence, only sandals. Hard callus under subluxed metatarsal heads will cause discomfort in addition to adventitial bursae associated with these. A mid-foot that is collapsing will cause excessive activity in tibialis posterior (if the tendon is still intact) and consequent medial calf pain. Nodules in the heel pad will cause significant pain and interfere with mobility.

At all stages of disease foot morbidity will impair mobility and cause much anger and frustration. Patients say they feel slowed down and that they slow others down. No longer can they run for a bus, or across the road. Everything must be planned in advance. As the disease progresses patients feel unsafe and can't keep their balance. This is due partly to loss of proprioception from damaged joints (in all lower limb joints), partly weakness and, in some cases,

because of neuropathy. Health professionals are now advocating the use of a stick or a frame, but these walking aids are problematic because of upper-limb involvement. The patient sees the dreaded wheelchair looming, understandably becoming more despondent. Their once dainty feet are now deformed and painful, they can't wear a decent shoe and previous enjoyable activities, such as walking and dancing, are now impossible.

This may seem a negative account of the natural history of foot and ankle symptoms of RA, but many of these symptoms are experienced and patients do entertain thoughts such as those given above. It is important for health professionals to be aware of this when treating patients; *we* know we can do a lot to help and even prevent these symptoms and disability, but we should appreciate that patients may not, initially at least, share these views.

JOINT STIFFNESS AND EARLY-MORNING STIFFNESS

Stiffness, particularly early-morning stiffness, is a symptom eagerly sought by rheumatologists, since it is believed to be a cardinal symptom of inflammation. Indeed, such is the importance attached to this symptom that it was included as one of the original items used for diagnosis of RA and was retained in the 1987 revised diagnostic classification criteria (Arnett et al. 1988, Ropes et al. 1959). Further, the duration of morning stiffness is often used both in the clinic and in research studies as a guide to disease activity. However, other conditions may cause stiffness: osteoarthritis, in particular, can also cause early-morning stiffness and may also be associated with stiffness that comes on after a period of inactivity such as sitting in a chair: the so-called articular gelling. Some authors have suggested that it is difficult to separate osteoarthritis from RA just on the duration of morning stiffness, although the severity of morning stiffness (as measured on a visual analogue scale) seems a better discriminator (Hazes et al. 1993). Of course, it is often difficult for the patient to comply with the request to quantify the timing of stiffness as often it doesn't just disappear; in metrology there is a tendency to quantify even that which cannot be measured, certainly not precisely.

Discussion of the significance of the symptom of stiffness requires some definition of terms. In engineering terms, stiffness is defined as the resistance to movement. Not surprisingly, this may not be the definition used by patients. In fact, when a patient uses the term 'stiffness', or responds to a question about this symptom, they may be referring to a wide spectrum of definitions (Helliwell & Wright 1990). Using an array

Joint stiffness in rheumatoid arthritis

- Prolonged early morning joint stiffness is an important symptom
- It is one of the criteria used for classification of the disease
- Duration of early morning stiffness is often used to reflect disease activity
- Patients confuse the symptoms of joint pain and stiffness but describe a lack of movement and resistance to movement
- Joint stiffness can be quantified and can be used to measure change in inflammation in the joint but it is quicker and easier and, probably more relevant, to measure a serum marker of inflammation such as the C reactive protein

of definitions provided by a broad selection of patients, Helliwell was able to demonstrate that patients using the term 'stiffness' predominantly mean 'resistance to movement' or 'lack of movement', but nevertheless often confuse stiffness with pain (Helliwell 1995).

Given the definition of stiffness as resistance to movement, and given the importance of the symptom in the diagnosis and monitoring of the disease, it was inevitable that engineers would attempt to devise instruments to quantify this symptom. Original devices were cumbersome and tended to cause the patient some discomfort (Wright et al. 1969), but later machines were light and portable and enabled measurement of a large number of patients in the clinic situation (Howe et al. 1985). Unfortunately, using such a device Helliwell was unable to demonstrate any increase in articular stiffness in this disorder (Helliwell et al. 1988b).

Further work made the situation clearer. When measuring stiffness it is generally necessary to move the distal part of the joint with the patient relaxed while at the same time measuring the resistance to movement. The mistake that was made was to assume that the articular structures were the major tissues contributing to stiffness when measured this way. In fact, later experiments revealed that the muscles serving the tendons that cross the joint contribute about 50% to total joint stiffness. It was generally known that muscle wasting is a feature of RA and this was demonstrated using hand dynamometry and, later, by the measurement of forearm circumference (Helliwell et al. 1987, Helliwell & Jackson 1994). Finally, a study of wrist stiffness using an entirely new system of measurement, and correcting for forearm circumference,

found an appropriate increase in articular stiffness in RA (Helliwell et al. 1995). Earlier measurements on the finger were able to be revisited and corrected for muscle wasting, thus revealing the erroneous nature of these original measurements.

It is clear, therefore, that we can quantify the symptom of joint stiffness, but that the effort required probably outweighs the precision and reliability of the result. This comment is particularly true if we are using stiffness as a measure of joint inflammation; it is quicker and easier and, probably more relevant, to measure a serum marker of inflammation such as the C reactive protein. The symptom itself is still worth seeking as it may provide a guide to disease activity and may provide prior information about limited range of movement at the joints. This may be especially relevant at the ankle joint where a limited range of dorsiflexion is readily perceptible and may be identified by the patient as a cause of altered gait. It is doubtful that patients will be aware of reduced movement at other joints as often the functional range is small and even a very restricted range may still permit adequate function (Woodburn et al. 2002).

MODIFYING FACTORS AND ASSOCIATED SYMPTOMS

RA is a disease of remissions and relapses. Although overall involvement of the foot and ankle is common, the degree of involvement is fairly unpredictable and is dependent on a range of intrinsic and extrinsic factors. The foot contributes to limitation in walking ability in some three-quarters of patients with RA, and is the primary or sole cause of walking limitation in about one-quarter (Kerry et al. 1994). The symptoms of RA and their effects in the foot can be modified, either positively or negatively, by a range of mediators, many of which can be influenced by the patient or the rheumatology team (see Fig. 3.1).

Intrinsic factors affecting rheumatoid arthritis symptoms in the foot

Disease activity

The effect of RA on the foot is closely related to disease activity and, by extension, its control (Scott et al. 2000). Increased RA activity is known to lead to greater pain (Covic et al. 2003) and considerable impairment of walking function (O'Connell et al. 1998, Wickman et al. 2004). The most widely used measure of disease activity is the Disease Activity Score (DAS), which is an index derived from counts of tender and swollen joints, erythrocyte sedimentation rate, and global

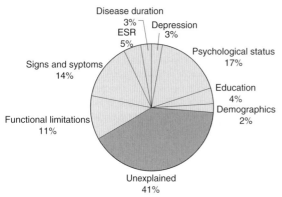

Contribution of factors to disablement in RA

Figure 3.1 Contributors to disability in rheumatoid arthritis.

health measured by a visual analogue scale (van der Heijde et al. 1990). The original DAS score and the truncated 28 joint version (DAS-28) are well validated and are used widely as a measure of disease activity (see Chapter 8).

The variability of the disease process is evidenced by the degree of intra-individual variation in functional scores over time within individuals (Wells et al. 1993). This is especially true in early disease where functional measures such as the Health Assessment Questionnaire (HAQ: see Chapter 8) vary with disease activity. In general, good medical control will generally improve walking ability in patients with RA (Hamilton et al. 2001).

Innate intrinsic factors

Intrinsic factors such as age and gender are also known to affect impairment. These factors are unalterable and so are often dismissed, but warrant recognition. It is known for example that HAQ scores worsen with age (Anderson et al. 1988, Sokka et al. 2003), which reflects the accumulation of joint damage associated with the disease, as well as the functional limitations associated with the natural ageing process (Anderson 1988). Poorer functional scores are also reported by women than men, although it is not clear why (Escalante & Del Rincon 1999, Thompson & Pegley 1991).

Cultural and ethnic factors have been reported to be influential in RA (Griffiths et al. 2000).

A high BMI of >30 is known to be associated with an increased risk of developing RA (OR=3.74) (Symmons et al. 1997) and this may impact on the disease course, as indicated above. Patients with RA are prone to becoming more obese over time, possibly

through decreased physical activities (Morgan et al. 1997). Change in BMI is not thought to be associated with disease activity however (Morgan et al. 1997) and, perhaps surprisingly, patients with lower BMI in one study demonstrated more substantial change in Larsen scores over 2 years than those with higher BMI (Kaufmann et al. 2003).

In the early stages of the disease, the best predictor of the severity of functional impairment appears to be disease activity, but as the disease progresses joint damage is more important. Forty percent of maximal joint damage occurs in the first 20 years of disease, although the earliest degeneration is most aggressive and results in some 16% of damage occurring in the first 5 years (Scott et al. 2000).

Soft-tissue involvement may contribute to symptoms. Bursitis, tenosynovitis and enthesopathy may complicate the presentation of the articular disease. In later disease callus formation and the presence of adventitious bursae may make a significant contribution to symptom presentation.

Extra-articular features such as vasculitis, ulceration and neuropathy (see below) may also add to the symptom complex, usually in the latter stages of disease.

Inability to maintain own foot care

There are no formal data on the capacity of people with RA to maintain their own foot care, but anecdotal reports suggest that limitations in manual dexterity and in spinal flexibility, coupled with joint restriction, all combine to lead to difficulties with maintaining foot care. Hygiene may become problematic, although it has been suggested that this is more a concern to clinicians than to patients (Macran et al. 2003), but inability to continue with nail care and control of callosities has the potential to contribute to symptoms. Inability to moisturize the skin of the feet can increase the rate of callus re-growth, and fissures may lead to opportunistic infection.

Extrinsic factors affecting rheumatoid arthritis symptoms in the foot (environmental factors of the ICF)

Psycho-social, socio-cultural and lifestyle demands

The impact of living, long-term, with a chronic and painful disease has profound effects on the patients' perceptions of themselves, their surroundings, and the disease itself. It is has been proposed recently that psychosocial factors, such as psychological status, learned helplessness, and self-efficacy explain nearly one-fifth of the disability associated in rheumatoid arthritis and, as such, have been significantly undervalued previously (Escalante & Del Rincon 1999). People with RA have a chronic pain condition and all the psycho-social consequences associated with this. Over time, pain pathways become increasingly sensitized, and the threshold for generating and passing pain messages lowers leading to increased severity of symptoms (Gaston-Johansson & Gustafsson 1990). Depression and hopelessness will adversely affect motivation and coping (Whalley et al. 1997). In the longer term, negative stress-vulnerability factors and poor social support are also known to be detrimental to overall function, although the short-term influence of these factors appears less significant (Evers et al. 2003).

Reduced capacity to undertake valued leisure or home-role activities can result in higher indices of depression, but conflicts between functional capacity and demands of work also result in high levels of work instability and lost productivity (Puolakka et al. 2004). It is known that the impairment secondary to RA results in some one-third of patients retiring from work within 5 years, and one-half retiring within 10 years due to decline in physical function (Yelin et al. 1987, Yelin et al. 1980), although the varying demands of specific work roles mean that the misfit between functional status and continued employment can be variable (Escalante & Del Rincon 2002).

More subtle socio-cultural factors include cultural background and ethnicity, level of education and occupation/income as well as marital status and social support (Escalante & Del Rincon 2002, Gaston-Johansson & Gustafsson 1990, Hewlett et al. 2002), although the effects of these are not well understood, particularly in relation to the foot.

Environmental factors can influence symptoms and function, with factors such as walking surface, presence of uneven terrain, steps and stairs, contributing to the misfit between capacity and functional demands (Escalante & Del Rincon 2002).

Footwear

Footwear can be either detrimental to symptoms in the foot or can be used therapeutically to improve an existing disease state. Patients will often report problems with their footwear, as standard retail footwear is often poorly suited to the altered structure of the rheumatoid foot. Problems can occur with fitting due to deformity, or with accommodation of insoles or orthoses. Off-the-shelf orthopaedic footwear has been shown to result in immediate improvement in walking function (Fransen & Edmonds 1997), and its bespoke nature should result in improved comfort levels. The role of footwear is discussed in more detail in Chapter 6.

FUNCTIONAL STATUS

An understanding of functional status is important to those managing patients with RA because functional status represents, for many patients, the bottom-line as far as the impact of their disease is concerned. Type and severity of pain, and the local effects of inflammatory joint disease have already been discussed and these factors are important in their own right. They do, however, represent only part of the picture, as it is changes in functional status that will influence patients ability to participate fully in their activities of work, social roles and leisure. A patient's functional status will of course be affected by the severity and type of symptoms, although function will in turn also affect symptoms (Anderson et al. 1988, Chen et al. 2003, Escalante & Del Rincon 1999). A detailed discussion of the various measures of patient functional status is presented in Chapter 8.

Joint pain presents both a physical and psychological barrier to normal function. Tasks generally take longer, and physically demanding tasks may appear especially daunting. In addition, patients with RA often report increased levels of fatigue and weakness, which makes a range of activities of daily living more draining.

Even in early disease, the effect on functional status causes a threat to continued employment, and this link is continued into established disease (Barrett et al. 2000). Functional status will worsen steadily over the course of the disease in most people (Hazes 2003), but variations in disease activity are highly influential. Patients experiencing a flare in their arthritis may find, therefore, that their symptoms are worse, and their functional capacity temporarily reduced during a flare, even in longstanding disease (Drossaers-Bakker et al. 1999, Hazes 2003). During a flare, patients will typically find the duration of morning stiffness increased, as is the severity of the stiffness. Morning stiffness is problematic to working people as it reduces functional capacity during a busy period of the day, although for all sufferers it necessitates prioritization of activities. Increased disease activity affecting the upper limbs will make it more difficult for patients to undertake basic activities of daily living that require manual dexterity or the capacity to stretch or to lift, such as dressing, washing and cooking. Increased disease activity in the lower limb likewise brings its own problems, as foot pain is known to impact on functional status even in the general population (Benvenuti et al. 1995, Chen et al. 2003, Leveille et al. 1998). Damage to the large joints accumulating over time affects function significantly in its own right and is often further compounded by associated damage in small joints such as those in the foot (Drossaers-Bakker et al. 2000). Activities requiring standing for any period of time may become problematic, posing problems for people whose work requires standing, or for undertaking domestic duties such as dish washing or ironing. Discomfort associated with dynamic activities such as walking will limit the distances that can be covered, will increase the time taken to undertake tasks requiring walking (O'Connell et al. 1998, Platto et al. 1991) and contribute to increased fatigue (Chen et al. 2003).

Other factors affecting functional status are less explicitly related to the physical manifestations of the disease. Psychological factors have been shown to be important, with poorer functional status associated with depression (Anderson et al. 1988, Hazes 2003), while those with stress-vulnerability profiles better suited to coping, show less disability (Evers et al. 2003). Equally interesting is the relationship between socio-economic factors and functional status, as it has been demonstrated that patients with a poorer socio-economic background show greater functional impairment and a poorer disease course generally than those with less deprivation (ERAS-Study-Group 2000). The reason for this is again unclear but does reflect the increased morbidity from other disorders in this group.

Foot involvement generally is a significant predictor of impaired functional status (Wickman et al. 2004). Progressive structural change in the hindfoot leads to permanent diminishment of functional ability and may, in turn, contribute to structural changes in neighbouring joints, which exacerbate the loss of function. Inflammation of the midfoot region can be particularly disabling because of its coupling with the hindfoot (Astion et al. 1997). Patients find it difficult to compensate for functional loss in the mid-foot region. In the forefoot, in early disease, involvement of the metatarsophalangeal joints leads to pain in the forefoot and difficulties for the patient in loading this part of the foot (Turner 2003). Patients often complain of a feeling of pebbles in the shoes. If the symptoms are confined to one or two joints then the patient may be able to retain function by compensation mechanisms such as offloading on the other, less painful joints (O'Connell et al. 1998). While this may have other undesirable consequences, such as the development of structural changes in the foot (see above), it minimizes the impact on global function.

ENTHESOPATHY

The enthesis is the point of attachment of ligament or tendon to bone. There are, therefore, literally hundreds of entheses in the foot and many more elsewhere in the skeleton. Additionally, Benjamin has introduced the concept of 'functional' entheses. Functional entheses occur where tendinous and ligamentous structures, while not actually attaching to bone, are adjacent and in a close relationship to the underlying bone. Forces, both shear and direct, occurring as a result of this juxtaposition effectively result in an enthesis at this point (Benjamin & McGonagle 2001). Often there is a bursa between the tendon and the bone: an example would be the gluteal tendon as it passes round the greater trochanter of the femur. Examples in the foot are the tendons of the peroneals and tibialis posterior as they pass around the lateral and medial malleoli respectively.

Traditionally, enthesitis has been one of the hallmarks of the seronegative spondyloarthropathies: ankylosing spondylitis, psoriatic arthritis and reactive arthritis (Wright & Moll 1976). The traditional sites for enthesopathy in this group of disorders have been the heel (the insertion of the plantar fascia into the medial tubercle of the calcaneum and the insertion of the Achilles tendon into the posterior aspect of the calcaneum), around the pelvis, the sacroiliac joints and the inter-vertebral ligaments. However, to reflect the widespread distribution of enthuses, an index of enthesitis has been developed that takes in palpable entheses from a number of other locations (Mander et al. 1987). The Mander index scores the degree of tenderness at 18 possible locations in the spine and upper and lower limbs. In clinical practice, however, many patients with ankylosing spondylitis have an enthesis score of zero and there are problems with inter-rater reliability. As a result of these limitations, a much reduced version has been introduced (Heuft-Dorenbosch et al. 2003).

Clinically, it is still believed that the two enthesitis sites at the heel are important and readily accessible and that involvement of these sites is a good differentiating feature between seronegative spondyloarthropathies and other inflammatory arthritides. McGonagle and colleagues have been at the forefront of rekindling interest in this topic. They have subsequently studied calcaneal enthesopathy using MRI in 17 cases of early spondyloarthropathy (including four cases of psoriatic arthritis, three cases of reactive arthritis and three cases of ankylosing spondylitis) and 11 cases of non-inflammatory heel pain (McGonagle et al. 2002). Bone oedema at entheseal insertions was seen in both inflammatory and non-inflammatory conditions, but was found to be more severe in the spondyloarthropathy cases. Calcaneal spurs occurred with equal frequency between the two classes of disorder.

Calcaneal enthesopathy has also been studied using ultrasonography by an Italian group (Falsetti P et al. 2003). Spur formation, both posteriorly and inferiorly was common in erosive osteoarthritis, nodal osteoarthritis, psoriatic arthritis, and rheumatoid arthritis, but was less frequently found in a non-arthritic control group. However, erosive changes at the enthesis were only found in psoriatic arthritis (5% posterior, 1% inferior) and RA (12% posterior, 6% inferior), a surprising result in view of the enthesitis hypothesis (McGonagle et al. 1998).

It would appear, therefore, that calcaneal spurs and erosions occur reasonably frequently in RA, an observation made clinically in the original large series by Vainio (Vainio 1991). It is also worth remembering that the retrocalcaneal bursa is a synovial lined structure and so will be vulnerable to the inflammatory process of RA per se, independent of any associated problems in the adjacent enthesis. The many other anatomical and functional entheses in the foot may also be involved and contribute to symptoms in this disorder.

BURSAE, SKIN AND NAIL DISEASE

A bursa is an enclosed space or sac that may contain fluid and may be lined by synovial-like tissue. Anatomical bursae are common around synovial joints and may communicate with them. Bursae may also develop in response to repeated trauma and, as such, are named adventitious bursae. Adventitious bursae are commonly seen in the foot in people with RA. They may become periodically inflamed and painful and they may develop secondary infection. Bursae are often seen under the MTP joints (Boutry et al. 2003), where the plantar fat pad is displaced and pressures are high, or, less commonly, over other sites of increased pressure, such as the posterior aspect of the calcaneus (Stiskal et al. 1997). It has also been demonstrated that local pressures are elevated under metatarsophalangeal joints with greater joint degeneration (Davys et al. 2004).

Bursae may be relatively symptom free most of the time, but may become inflamed periodically leading to intense discomfort on weight bearing. The treatments discussed in Chapter 6 include strategies to offload the area and aspiration; the latter relieves symptoms and permits infection to be excluded.

Compressive and shearing forces acting on the skin can lead to corn and callus formation, and the presence of scarring from surgical interventions will also increase the chances of the person with RA developing symptomatic callus (Fig. 3.2). Calluses usually become problematic only when the thickness of the callused plaque limits skin elasticity. Where cornified nuclei are involved in a callus, local areas of high pressure lead to more significant symptoms. Periodic reduction of

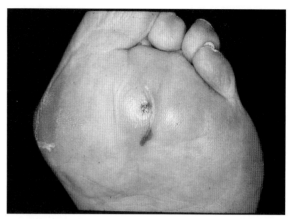

Figure 3.2   Callus formation under the metatarsophalangeal joints with deep haemorrhage, indicating incipient ulceration.

the callus is usually carried out, but the callus can be expected to re-grow within 1–6 weeks, creating a need for ongoing care. Offloading of the area may be helpful in limiting callus regrowth and can be achieved through the use of a rigid functional foot orthosis to redistribute forces to the mid foot or simple forefoot padding (see Chapter 6).

Abnormalities of the nails are frequently seen in clinical practice, although there has been no systematic study of these in RA. Difficulty with hand function due to arthritis of the small joints of the hand, coupled with involvement of large joints of the upper and lower limb, may also make it difficult for the patient to reach and cut the toe nails. This may lead to infection around the nail bed manifest as paronychia and ingrowing toe nail. Long-term immunosuppression of the disease may also play a part in the pathogenesis of infection around the nail and within the nail by fungi and yeasts.

EXTRA-ARTICULAR DISEASE

RA is a systemic inflammatory connective tissue disease. Occasionally, the disease will present with systemic features, such as vasculitis or pulmonary nodules, with the joint inflammation developing as a late and often minor feature. Extra-articular features are, as the name implies, clinical and pathological manifestations of the disease outside the synovial joints.

A number of general observations can be made:

- They are often associated with inflammation in the blood vessels, called vasculitis.
- The presence of extra-articular features is associated with a worse prognosis in terms of mortality, although modern aggressive treatment with

immunosuppressive regimes has made an impact on this.

- People with extra-articular features are usually older, male, have rheumatoid nodules and are seropositive.

Extra-articular features in rheumatoid arthritis

- Rheumatoid arthritis can affect any organ in the body
- Extra-articular features are generally caused by vasculitis
- Patients with extra-articular features are usually male, seropositive and nodular
- Extra-articular features are associated with a worse prognosis and higher mortality

Can we predict which patients will develop extra-articular features? The risk factors for severity discussed in Chapter 1 (homozygosity for the shared epitope, rheumatoid factor, age, smoking, and social deprivation) are a guide only. We still have no clear evidence that targeting this group for more aggressive treatment reduces the complications or improves the mortality. The problems with extended longitudinal observational studies, let alone randomized controlled trials, have been noted in Chapter 1.

Vasculitis and leg ulceration

Clinically, vasculitis is an uncommon finding, but like its counterpart, neuropathy, much of the disease is probably sub-clinical. Post-mortem studies have found evidence of vasculitis in up to 14% of cases of RA, but clinically the prevalence is much less. Turesson and colleagues found a prevalence of extra-articular features of 1.8% annually, with approximately one-third of these cases manifesting as cutaneous vasculitis (Turesson et al. 1999). In fact, vasculitis, neuropathy, and nodules are all part of the same pathological process with inflammation of blood vessels being the underlying lesion. (However, if nodularity is a defining feature of vasculitis, then it is clinically more common than generally believed.)

Vasculitis may present clinically in one of three ways (for a full discussion see Breedveld (Breedveld FC 2003):

- Small vessel digital arteritis manifest as tiny nail fold infarcts (Fig. 3.3)

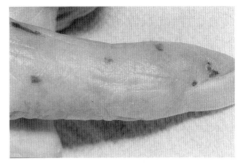

Figure 3.3   Small vessel digital arteries manifesting as nail fold infarcts.

- Inflammation of venules and small arteries usually manifest as a purpuric rash (Fig. 3.4)
- Necrotizing arteritis of small- and medium-sized arteries, which causes major organ damage and may lead to digital gangrene (Fig. 3.5)

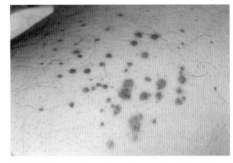

Figure 3.4   Inflammation of venules and small arteries usually manifests as a purpuric rash.

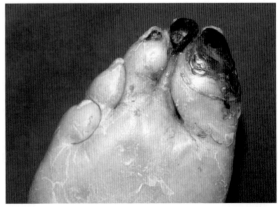

Figure 3.5   Necrotizing arteritis of small- and medium-sized arteries can lead to digital gangrene.

It is important to note that each of these manifestations is not mutually exclusive and all three types may occur in the same patient, although this is uncommon. The first type, manifest as nail-fold infarcts, is most commonly seen with an overall clinical prevalence of about 10%. Many patients develop nail-fold infarcts and little other evidence of vasculitis and appear to come to no harm from these. Both of the other two types of vasculitis may be associated with systemic disease and carry a graver prognosis. For example, necrotizing arteritis is a bad sign and is associated with a high mortality rate (25% to 45% mortality over 2 years).

Clinically, there are features often shared by those who develop vasculitis and other extra-articular features of disease. These include a high titre of rheumatoid factor, the presence of rheumatoid nodules, the older age groups, a higher percentage of males, frequent treatment with corticosteroids, and those with extremely destructive disease. Clinical features suggesting vasculitis include the following (Voskuyl et al. 2003):

- Systemic features, such as weight loss, fever, malaise
- Cutaneous features, such as a purpuric rash, nail-fold infarcts, leg ulcers (often multiple with a sharply demarcated punched out edge and often associated with extreme pain see Fig. 3.6), and rheumatoid nodules
- Eye signs: scleritis and episcleritis
- Major organ damage:
  - heart: pericarditis, heart valve lesions
  - lungs: pulmonary fibrosis, pleurisy, pulmonary nodules
  - kidney: glomerulonephritis
  - bowel: mesenteric infarcts
  - nervous system: peripheral neuropathy (thought by some authors to be the prime sign of an underlying vasculitis. Schmid et al. found 59% of their cases of biopsy proven vasculitis had a neuropathy (Schmid et al. 1961).

Leg ulceration in RA is not uncommon and merits a separate paragraph. It is estimated that 9% of rheumatology out-patients have a leg ulcer at any one time, the figure for in-patients being 0.6–8% (McRorie et al. 1994). Leg ulceration in this situation is thought to be multifactorial, but the relative weights of the individual factors are unknown. Certainly, in many cases there appears to be a vasculitic element and such patients often share the same features as those with vasculitis elsewhere: older age, severe deforming disease, seropositive and nodular. Treatment for vasculitis will frequently result in healing of the ulcer. However, other factors are likely to be contributing (McRorie et al. 1994):

- Venous insufficiency. There are good theoretical reasons why venous insufficiency is present, including immobility, decreased ankle movement due to arthritis (thus impairing the venous pump action of the calf muscles). McRorie and colleagues have argued that 50–80% of patients with leg ulcers have venous drainage problems (McRorie et al. 1998).
- Macrovascular arterial disease. Using the ankle-brachial index 41% of patients with ulcers had an index of less than 0.9, the threshold for arterial insufficiency.
- Some ulcers may start as pyoderma gangrenosum, the basis of which is probably vasculitic. These lesions can be seen in a number of diseases: they often start as a painful nodule that quickly breaks down to produce a deep sloughy ulcer with undermined edges.

It is not known how chronic leg ulceration in RA relates to chronic ulceration on the foot, but it is possible that similar factors are operative. However, with foot ulcers, there may be other important factors, foot deformity, areas of high pressure and neuropathy, for example, which are more akin to the risk factors for ulceration in diabetes mellitus.

Macrovascular disease

In addition to the distinctive features caused by inflammation of the blood vessels in RA it is important to note that morbidity and mortality from macrovascular arterial disease (atherosclerosis leading to cardiovascular, cerebrovascular and peripheral

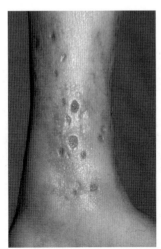

Figure 3.6 Vasulitic ulcers are often multiple with sharply demarcated punched out edges.

vascular morbidity) is increased in RA (Symmons et al. 1998, Doran et al. 2002, Mitchell et al. 1986).

There appear to be a number of reasons for this. Firstly, conventional risk factors for atherosclerosis are increased in RA; these include hypercholesterolaemia, smoking, lack of exercise and use of corticosteroids. However, Alkaabi and colleagues have shown abnormalities independent of traditional risk factors (Alkaabi et al. 2003). Alkaabi et al. measured intimal wall thickness by ultrasound, the ankle-brachial pressure index and an index of cardiovascular risk (the QT dispersion time from the electrocardiograph) finding all three abnormal compared to age and sex matched controls.

Secondly, the pathological mechanisms underlying atherosclerosis are very similar to RA with, in this case, the arterial wall being the target organ. Thus, there is an inflammatory cell infiltrate, and cellular proliferation with production of cytokines similar to those produced in RA (Kaplan & McClune 2003). Conversely, treatment with disease-modifying drugs such as methotrexate may have an anti-inflammatory and anti-atherosclerosis effect beyond their effect on the rheumatoid disease (Choi et al. 2002).

Thirdly, serum levels of homocysteine, high levels of which have been associated with accelerated atherosclerosis, are abnormally elevated in RA. Treatment with methotrexate may exacerbate this, although folic acid, which is often used as a co-treatment with methotrexate, suppresses homocysteine levels.

For these reasons, all patients with RA should have an assessment of their risk factors for atherosclerosis at regular intervals and appropriate interventions made to reduce these factors where possible.

Neuropathy

From a clinical point of view neuropathy is uncommon but if looked for (by biopsy and targeted clinical examination) appears to be present in up to half the cases (Lanzillo et al. 1998). Lanzillo and colleagues examined 40 consecutive cases where clinical symptoms of peripheral neuropathy were absent. Of these, 43% had absent vibration perception in the legs and fully 58% had a sensorimotor peripheral neuropathy on electrophysiological testing. As with vasculitis, which underlies these two pathologies, there is an appreciable sub-clinical spectrum of disease.

It is important to note that clinical detection of peripheral neuropathy may not be straightforward in RA. Firstly, pain may arise from a number of different tissues and from a number of different mechanisms: it is sometimes hard for the patient and the clinician to distinguish a new onset neuropathic pain from an existing articular pain. Secondly, articular pain will prevent an accurate assessment of muscle strength. Thirdly, articular disease may mask neurological sensory signs: joint damage will affect joint proprioception and inflammatory oedema may prevent an accurate assessment of vibration loss.

Another important point is that early studies were pre-occupied with the association of vasculitis and neuropathy with the use of therapeutic steroids (Hart & Golding 1960). It now seems likely that this association was not causal but resulted from the more frequent use of steroids in cases more likely to develop extra-articular features: that is the more severe cases. At that time steroids had only been in use for about 10 years and their benefit and side-effect profile was still emerging. Observational studies had noted the association of steroid use with the systemic complications of RA and authors quite rightly discussed the possible aetiological role of these drugs.

A suggested scheme for classifying neuropathy in RA is as follows (Chamberlain & Bruckner 1970):

- Compression neuropathies
- Distal sensory neuropathy
- Severe fulminating sensorimotor polyneuropathy
- Mononeuritis and mononeuritis multiplex.

The first two are much more common; the latter two, while less commonly seen, carry a worse prognosis. As already mentioned, Lanzillo and colleagues found 23/40 subjects without clinical symptoms of peripheral neuropathy had electrophysiological evidence of a mild sensorimotor peripheral neuropathy (Lanzillo et al. 1998). Lanzillo et al. also found a fairly high prevalence of asymptomatic compression neuropathy with 5/40 subjects having carpal tunnel syndrome. Other studies looking at compression neuropathies in the foot have found a high prevalence of asymptomatic tarsal tunnel syndrome in RA (Baylan et al. 1981). While these results remain unconfirmed they are consistent and indicate that many patients have asymptomatic neurological abnormalities associated with their disease.

Compression neuropathies

Clinically, the commonest compression neuropathy in RA is carpal tunnel syndrome, due to compression of the median nerve at the wrist as it passes, along with the long flexor tendons and their sheaths, under the relatively tight retinaculum. Other compression neuropathies in the upper limb are, in decreasing order of frequency, lesions of the ulnar nerve, as it courses through the cubital tunnel at the elbow and the posterior interosseous nerve, as it pierces the fascia of the supinator muscle just distal to the lateral epicondyle of the elbow.

In the lower limb, more importantly for this book, the following entrapment syndromes are of importance:

- Entrapment of the tibial nerve as it passes through the tarsal tunnel at the ankle
- Lesions of the common peroneal nerve at the knee which may result in foot drop
- Compression of the deep peroneal nerve under the extensor retinaculum at the ankle
- Mortons' interdigital 'neuroma'.

Five sensory nerves innervate the foot: the sural, the superficial peroneal, the deep peroneal, the lateral and medial plantar (both arising from the tibial nerve). Potential causes of entrapment include compression from proliferative synovitis or tenosynovitis, rheumatoid nodules or bony deformity. In practice, the only significant problems occur due to tarsal tunnel syndrome and Morton's neuroma as the other nerves are seldom in a position to be compromised by the above factors.

By far the most important of these is the so-called 'tarsal tunnel syndrome'. The tarsal tunnel lies on the medial side of the ankle and is bounded by the calcaneus, the flexor retinaculum (ligamentum lacinatum) and the tendinous arch of abductor hallucis (Pecina et al. 2001). Also found passing through the 'tunnel' are the posterior tibial artery and the tendons of tibialis posterior and flexor hallucis longus. Tenosynovitis in the sheaths of the latter is the most likely cause of this problem in RA. As already noted, the syndrome may be more common than clinically indicated, if electrophysiological studies are used as the 'gold standard'. McGuigan and colleagues found a relatively high point prevalence of 13% (McGuigan et al. 1983), while a prevalence of 25% was found by Baylan et al. (1981). Of importance in the latter study was the lack of relationship between several other variables (including symptoms, duration of disease, severity of disease, treatment, and age) and the presence of tarsal tunnel syndrome, a similar finding to that of Chamberlain (Chamberlain & Bruckner 1970). It could be argued from these studies that the syndrome is of no clinical significance, but without a systematic study comparing those with and without the syndrome and following cases prospectively this statement cannot be justified. Clinical symptoms include pain and paraesthesiae on the plantar aspect of the foot, more so on the medial side. The pain may be confused with that arising from the joints and the paraesthesiae as coming from a more proximal location (such as the back). Like carpal tunnel syndrome, symptoms may be worse at night. Usually there is little to find objec-tively and if this syndrome is suspected clinically the patient should be referred for nerve conduction tests.

Lesions of the common peroneal nerve, while not strictly relating to the foot and ankle, are mentioned here because they may result in foot drop. The common peroneal nerve is vulnerable to entrapment as it winds around the head of the fibula at the knee. The commonest cause is trauma: plaster casts, operations and pressure from the other leg, giving rise to the other name for this condition ('crossed legs' palsy). In RA it may be compressed by a ganglion, rheumatoid nodule, an extension of synovial hypertrophy from the knee or even a large knee osteophyte.

Compression of the deep peroneal nerve is unusual clinically, but there are no systematic studies of this problem using electrophysiology, so the actual prevalence in rheumatoid arthritis is unknown. The nerve is vulnerable to compression as it passes under the extensor retinaculum and, certainly, hypertrophic tenosynovitis in this location is frequently seen. The clinical effects are painful hyperaesthesiae in the space between the first and second toes and weakness of extensor hallucis brevis (the strength of this muscle must be tested with the ankle in full dorsiflexion to negate the effects of the long extensor tendon to the great toe).

A Morton's 'neuroma' is a common early presentation of RA. As mentioned in the section on 'Synovitis and the foot' in this chapter, the pathology is not of a neuroma of the inter-digital nerve, but more often is a synovitis and bulging of the capsule of the adjacent metatarsophalangeal joint or, in later stages, a rheumatoid nodule (Awerbuch et al. 1982). The name has stuck and the clinical manifestation is similar, but it is unfortunate that the original pathology described by Morton is not seen in these other conditions.

Distal sensory neuropathy

Like the entrapment neuropathies distal sensory neuropathy is found more frequently on electrophysiological testing than it is clinically. When it is clinically evident it often presents with an unpleasant burning sensation in the feet. It is often symmetrical and affects the feet more than the hands. There is a higher proportion of male patients. Clinical findings include loss of vibration sense and light touch at the foot and sometimes loss of ankle reflexes. Biopsy of peripheral nerves and/or muscle biopsy may reveal vasculitis (Chamberlain & Bruckner 1970, Hart & Golding 1960). There is a poor prognosis generally; in one series survival was 57% at 5 years (Peuchal et al. 1995). Voskuyl reported that a peripheral neuropathy was one of the main distinguishing features for rheumatoid vasculitis (Voskuyl et al. 2003).

Severe fulminating sensorimotor polyneuropathy
This is the less common variety of peripheral neuropathy usually carrying a worse prognosis. It is often associated with severe pre-existing disability, male predominance, erosive seropositive disease, and often presenting dramatically with palsy, such as a foot drop, and carrying a poor prognosis (Chamberlain & Bruckner 1970). In one series of selected patients, all those with a distal sensorimotor peripheral neuropathy died with visceral ischaemia (Pallis & Scott 1965).

Mononeuritis and mononeuritis multiplex
In terms of severity a mononeuropathy or a mononeuritis multiplex are of grave prognostic importance, mainly because they signal arteritis of medium-sized arteries and usually major organ involvement. Clinically, there is often a sudden onset of nerve palsy. Typically, the patient will present with a foot drop, sometimes unnoticed, or a wrist drop (radial nerve palsy). There will be a preceding history of weight loss and the other typical features of extra-articular disease will be found. Digital gangrene may occur. In fact Voskuyl found that the more the extra-articular features the more likely the patient had a systemic vasculitis, including major organ involvement (Voskuyl et al. 2003). The feared complication of medium-vessel arteritis is mesenteric artery obstruction and necrosis of a segment of bowel. It is feared, because it may present late, after the bowel has perforated, with the patient septicaemic and in shock. Unfortunately, as most of these patients are already on systemic steroids the classical symptoms and signs are often masked until the problem is well advanced.

Along with the medium-vessel arteritis, a small-vessel vasculitis results in the other major organ damage: pericardial and cardiac involvement, renal and pulmonary involvement. Slowly progressive pulmonary fibrosis unresponsive to the usual treatments is also a grave prognostic sign. The patient already severely disabled by RA deformities who develops progressive pulmonary fibrosis and who, at each clinic appointment, is more and more breathless, is a distressing sight in the face of our therapeutic impotence.

In the series of Peuchal fully 23 of 32 cases with biopsy proven vasculitis had evidence of a major nerve involvement, and 38% of patients had cutaneous lesions: these included purpura, ulcers, nailfold infarcts, livedo reticularis and gangrene. Factors predicting decreased survival were a cutaneous feature, a multifocal neuropathy or a decreased serum complement (Peuchal et al. 1995).

Sub-cutaneous nodules

Rheumatoid nodules have been found to affect between 17 and 34% of patients with RA (Turesson et al. 1999). When present they are an important clinical marker of rheumatoid disease, helping differentiate RA from other causes of inflammatory arthritis. They may, on occasions, occur before the development of arthritis, both in a subcutaneous distribution and in the lungs. Nodules on the feet are a possible risk factor for ulceration as they have the potential to increase pressure and friction from footwear as well as affecting local tissue viability.

The initial event in the formation of a rheumatoid nodule is vasculitis. Possibly trauma has a part to play, as the traditional sites for rheumatoid nodules are over bony prominences and areas of repeated abrasion such as the elbow, knuckles or heel pad. Histologically, rheumatoid nodules initially comprise vascular granulation tissue that undergoes involution until it forms a central area of necrosis, bordered by a palisade of radially arranged elongated cells and encapsulated in scar tissue. In keeping with other extra-articular manifestations of disease, nodules are associated with more severe, seropositive disease in males and are, therefore, considered to be a poor prognostic marker.

Nodules tend to occur over bony prominences where the skin and subcutaneous tissues are already under increased stress. They vary in size and number and may persist indefinitely or can regress at the time. Common sites in the foot include the Achilles tendon (Fig. 3.7), over the first and fifth metatarsal heads and the heel pad, where they can be particularly troublesome to the patient. Treatment with methotrexate can, paradoxically, make nodulosis worse increasing the number and the prominence of the nodules. On occasions this is a reason for treatment discontinuation.

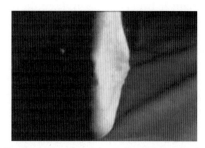

Figure 3.7 Rheumatoid nodules in the Achilles tendon.

Hyperviscosity syndrome

The viscosity of whole blood is a function of the plasma viscosity and the cellular content, the red and white blood cells and the platelets. The viscosity of plasma is largely influenced by the protein content: the quantity and the quality of protein in terms of the size of the molecules and their shape. In conditions where excess protein is produced the serum viscosity may rise to the point where this hyperviscosity produces clinical and pathological effects. This syndrome usually occurs in situations where large amounts of immunoglobulin are produced, such as Waldenstroms macroglobulinaemia or multiple myeloma where excess light and heavy chain proteins occur (Pruzanski & Watt 1972). The plasma viscosity can rise from a normal value of under 2 to over 10. The plasma viscosity is sometimes used as an indicator of inflammation as it is influenced by acute-phase proteins. It can, therefore, be markedly elevated in RA, usually in association with the production of large amounts of rheumatoid factor. The clinical syndrome does not usually occur unless the plasma viscosity is 4 or over.

Clinically, this syndrome may manifest in the following way:

- Neurological symptoms and signs. Dizziness, headaches, lethargy, confusion and weakness. Enlarged, 'sausage like' veins may be visible in the retina, sometimes with haemorrhages and exudates
- Haematological. Patients may present with abnormal bleeding, purpura, bruising on the legs and feet, and epistaxis.
- The bleeding disorder may also be manifest in the gastro-intestinal tract with bleeding gums and rectal bleeding.

Treatment to reduce the production of excess protein, in RA, is aimed at the immune cells producing immunoglobulin, the B lymphocytes. Treatment of this condition is, therefore, with immunosuppressive drugs. Sometimes, in severe cases, the excess protein is removed by plasmapheresis.

Muscle disease

Although pain and stiffness are the main symptoms of RA, they are closely followed by weakness, particularly of grip strength. There are several reasons for this.

Firstly, patients often complain that their limbs seem to have lost bulk since the beginning of their disease. It has, however, been remarkably difficult to demonstrate this with appropriately matched control subjects. Using a validated method for measuring anatomical cross-sectional area, Helliwell found a significant reduction in RA: forearm muscle cross-sectional area in RA 25.9 cm^2 and in normals 29.7cm^2 (Helliwell & Jackson 1994). Although this difference appears minimal in terms of force generation by the forearm muscles it is a considerable reduction.

Secondly, the inflammatory process of RA may affect the muscles directly thereby reducing the effective force generation. The likely mechanism for this is vasculitis, although drugs used in RA (in particular steroids) may contribute. Steinberg and Wynn-Parry found electromyographic evidence of muscle inflammation in 85% of their subjects (Steinberg & Wynn-Parry 1961).

Thirdly, joint inflammation and deformity may contribute to weakness as a result of afferent impulses from joint mechanoreceptors and nociceptors; a phenomenon known as arthrogenous muscle inhibition. The same mechanism is responsible for the sudden giving way of the knee and ankle when someone treads on a sharp nail. People with inflamed foot and ankle joints must fight to overcome this reflex with every step. A further electromyographic study found surface abnormalities of the EMG signal, consistent with this mechanism, in 65% of cases with RA (Lenman & Potter 1966).

Fourthly, deformity of joints may disrupt the normal mechanical architecture that allows purposeful movement at the joint. Inflammation and attrition of tendons will also contribute to these 'biomechanical' factors. These mechanisms are readily observable in the ankle of someone with longstanding RA, particularly if a prominent pes plano-valgus deformity is present.

There is no doubt that people with RA are weaker than their non-affected counterparts and fatigue more easily (Helliwell et al. 1988a). Significant muscle wasting occurs, but there are also doubts about the quality of the muscle itself and the contribution of arthrogenous muscle inhibition. In the study by Helliwell a multiple regression model incorporating an index of joint pain and deformity found that both these variables, in addition to muscle wasting, contributed significantly to the weakness but the model as a whole only accounted for 38% of the variation in grip strength (Helliwell & Jackson 1994). Muscle biopsy studies in selected subjects have confirmed a relatively high prevalence of myositis, but have found, in addition, evidence of neuropathy in 26% of cases (Haslock et al. 1970). The problem is, therefore, clearly multifactorial and in rehabilitation terms must be addressed as a multidisciplinary problem if improvements are to be made.

References

Alkaabi JK, Ho M, Levison R, Pullar T and Belch JJF
Rheumatoid arthritis and macrovascular disease.
Rheumatology 2003; 42: 292–297

Anderson KO, Keefe FJ, Bradley LA et al. Prediction of pain
behavior and functional status of rheumatoid arthritis
patients using medical status and psychological
variables. Pain 1988; 33(1): 25–32

Arnett FC, Edworthy SM and Bloch DA The American
Rheumatism Association 1987 revised criteria for the
classification of rheumatoid arthritis. Arthritis and
Rheumatism 1988; 31(3): 315–324

Astion DJ, Deland JT, Otis JC and Kenneally S Motion of the
hindfoot after simulated arthrodesis. Journal of Bone &
Joint Surgery – American Volume 1997; 79(2): 241–246.

Awerbuch MS, Shephard E and Vernon-Roberts B Mortons
metatarsalgia due to intermetatarsophalangeal bursitis as
an early manifestation of rheumatoid arthritis. Clinical
Orthopaedics & Related Research 1982; 167: 214–221.

Barrett EM, Scott DG, Wiles NJ and Symmons DP The
impact of rheumatoid arthritis on employment status in
the early years of disease: a UK community-based study.
Rheumatology 2000; 39(12): 1403–1409.

Baylan SP, Paik SW, Barnert AL, Ko KH, Yu J and Persellin
RH Prevalence of the tarsal tunnel syndrome in
rheumatoid arthritis. Rheumatology & Rehabilitation
1981; 20(3): 148–150.

Benjamin M and McGonagle D The anatomical basis for
disease localisation in seronegative spondyloarthropathy
at entheses and related sites. Journal of Anatomy 2001;
199(5): 5–26.

Benvenuti F, Ferrucci L, Guralnik JM, Gangemi S and
Baroni A Foot pain and disability in older persons: an
epidemiologic survey. Journal of the American Geriatrics
Society 1995; 43(5): 479–484.

Blake DR, Merry P, Unsworth J et al. Hypoxic–reperfusion
injury in the inflamed human joint. Lancet 1989; 1: 289.

Boutry N, Larde A, Lapegue F, Solau-Gervais E, Flipo RM
and Cotten A Magnetic resonance imaging appearance of
the hands and feet in patients with early rheumatoid
arthritis. Journal of Rheumatology 2003; 30(4): 671–679.

Breedveld FC Vasculitis associated with connective tissue
disease. Baillières Clinical Rheumatology 2003; 11(2):
315–334.

Chamberlain MA and Bruckner FE Rheumatoid neuropathy:
clinical and electrophysiological features. Annals of
Rheumatic Diseases 1970; 29: 609–616.

Chen J, Devine A, Dick IM, Dhaliwal SS and Prince RL
Prevalence of lower extremity pain and its association
with functionality and quality of life in elderly women in
Australia. Journal of Rheumatology 2003; 30(12):
2689–2693.

Choi HK, Hernan MA, Seeger JD, Ropes MW and Wolfe F
Methotrexate and mortality in patients with rheumatoid
arthritis: a prospective study. Lancet 2002; 359:
1173–1177.

Covic T, Adamson B, Spencer D and Howe G
A biopsychosocial model of pain and depression in
rheumatoid arthritis: A 12-month longitudinal study.
Rheumatology 2003; 42(11): 1287–1294.

Davys HJ, Turner DE, Emery PE and Woodburn J
A comparison of scalpel debridement versus sham
procedure for painful forefoot callosities in rheumatoid
arthritis. Annals of the Rheumatic Diseases 2004;
63(Suppl 1): 427.

Dixon A J The anterior tarsus and forefoot. Baillières Clinical
Rheumatology 1987; 1(2): 261–274.

Doran MF, Pond GR, Crowson CS, OFallon WM and Gabriel
SE Trends in incidence and mortality in rheumatoid
arthritis in Rochester, Minnesota over a forty year
period. Arthritis and Rheumatism 2002; 46: 625–631.

Drossaers-Bakker KW, de Buck M, van Zeben D,
Zwinderman AH, Breedveld FC and Hazes JM Long-
term course and outcome of functional capacity in
rheumatoid arthritis: the effect of disease activity and
radiologic damage over time. Arthritis & Rheumatism
1999; 42(9): 1854–1860.

Drossaers-Bakker KW, Kroon HM, Zwinderman AH,
Breedveld FC and Hazes JM Radiographic damage of
large joints in long-term rheumatoid arthritis and its
relation to function. Rheumatology 2000; 39(9): 998–1003.

ERAS Study Group Socioeconomic deprivation and
rheumatoid disease: what lessons for the health service?
Annals of the Rheumatic Diseases 2000; 59(10): 794–799.

Escalante A and Del Rincon I How much disability in
rheumatoid arthritis is explained by rheumatoid
arthritis? Arthritis & Rheumatism 1999; 42(8): 1712–1721.

Escalante A and Del Rincon I The disablement process in
rheumatoid arthritis. Arthritis & Rheumatism 2002; 47(3):
333–342.

Evers AW, Kraaimaat FW, Geenen R, Jacobs JW and Bijlsma
JW Stress-vulnerability factors as long-term predictors of
disease activity in early rheumatoid arthritis. Journal of
Psychosomatic Research 2003; 55(4): 293–302.

Falsetti P, Frediani B, Fioravanti A, Acciai C, Baldi F, Filippou
G and Marcolongo R Sonographic study of calcaneal
entheses in erosive osteoarthritis, nodal osteoarthritis,
rheumatoid arthritis and psoriatic arthritis. Scandinavian
Journal of Rheumatology 2003; 32: 229–234.

Fransen M and Edmonds J Off-the-shelf orthopedic
footwear for people with rheumatoid arthritis. Arthritis
Care & Research 1997; 10(4): 250–256.

Gaston-Johansson F and Gustafsson M Rheumatoid arthritis:
determination of pain characteristics and comparison of
RAI and VAS in its measurement. Pain 1990; 41(1): 35–40.

Griffiths B, Situnayake RD, Clark B, Tennant A, Salmon M
and Emery P Racial origin and its effect on disease
expression and HLA-DRB1 types in patients with
rheumatoid arthritis: a matched cross-sectional study.
Rheumatology 2000; 39(8): 857–864.

Hamilton J, Brydson G, Fraser S and Grant M Walking ability
as a measure of treatment effect in early rheumatoid
arthritis. Clinical Rehabilitation 2001; 15(2): 142–147.

Hart FD and Golding JR Rheumatoid neuropathy. British
Medical Journal 1960; 1: 1594–1600.

Haslock DI, Wright V and Harriman DGF Neuromuscular disorder in rheumatoid arthritis. Quarterly Journal of Medicine 1970; 39: 335–358.

Hazes J, Hayton R and Silman AJ A re-evaluation of the symptom of morning stiffness. Journal of Rheumatology 1993; 20: 1138–1142.

Hazes JM Determinants of physical function in rheumatoid arthritis: association with the disease process. Rheumatology 2003; 42(Suppl 2): ii17–21.

Helliwell PS The semeiology of arthritis: discriminating between patients on the basis of their symptoms. Annals of the Rheumatic Diseases 1995; 54(11): 924–926.

Helliwell P, Howe A and Wright V Functional assessment of the hand: reproducibility, and utility of a new system for measuring strength. Annals of the Rheumatic Diseases 1987; 46: 203–208.

Helliwell PS, Howe A and Wright V An evaluation of the dynamic qualities of isometric grip strength. Annals of the Rheumatic Diseases 1988a; 47(11): 934–939.

Helliwell PS, Howe A and Wright V Lack of objective evidence of stiffness in rheumatoid arthritis. Annals of the Rheumatic Diseases 1988b; 47(9): 754–758.

Helliwell PS and Jackson S Relationship between weakness and muscle wasting in rheumatoid-arthritis. Annals of the Rheumatic Diseases 1994; 53(11): 726–728.

Helliwell PS, Smeathers JE and Wright V The contribution of different tissues to stiffness in the joint. Proceedings of the Institution of Mechanical Engineers: Part H. Engineering in Medicine 1995; 208: 223–228.

Helliwell PS and Wright V Stiffness – a useful symptom but an elusive quantity. RSM Current Medical Literature. Rheumatology 1990: 9: 95–99.

Heuft-Dorenbosch L, Spoorenberg A, van Tubergen A, Landewe R, van ver T H, Mielants H, Dougados M and van der HD Assessment of enthesitis in ankylosing spondylitis. Annals of the Rheumatic Diseases 2003; 62(2): 127–132.

Hewlett S, Smith AP and Kirwan JR Measuring the meaning of disability in rheumatoid arthritis: The personal impact Health Assessment Questionnaire (PI HAQ). Annals of the Rheumatic Diseases 2002; 61(11): 986–993.

Howe A, Thompson D and Wright V Microprocessor-mediated measurement of mcp joint stiffness. British Journal of Rheumatology 985; 24: 220.

Jayson MIV and Dixon A St J Intra-articular pressure in rheumatoid arthritis of the knee. I Pressure changes during passive joint distension. Annals of the Rheumatic Diseases 1970; 29: 261–265.

Kaplan MJ and McClune WJ New evidence for vascular disease in patients with early rheumatoid arthritis. Lancet 2003; 361: 1068–1069.

Kaufmann J, Kielstein V, Kilian S, Stein G and Hein G Relation between body mass index and radiological progression in patients with rheumatoid arthritis. Journal of Rheumatology 2003; 30(11): 2350–2355.

Kerry RM, Holt GM and Stockley I The foot in chronic rheumatoid arthritis: A continuing problem. Foot 1994; 4(4): 201–203.

Lanzillo B, Pappone N, Crisci C, Di Girolamo R, Massini R and Caruso G Subclinical peripheral nerve involvement in patients with rheumatoid arthritis. Arthritis and Rheumatism 1998; 41(7): 1196–1202.

Lenman JAR and Potter JL Electromyographic measurement of fatigue in rheumatoid arthritis and neuromuscular disease. Annals of the Rheumatic Diseases 1966; 25: 76–84.

Leveille SG, Guralnik JM, Ferrucci L, Hirsch R, Simonsick E and Hochberg MC Foot pain and disability in older women. American Journal of Epidemiology 1998; 148(7): 657–665.

Macran S, Kind P, Collingwood J, Hull R, McDonald I and Parkinson L Evaluating podiatry services: testing a treatment specific measure of health status. Quality of Life Research 2003; 12(2): 177–188.

Mander M, Simpson JM, McLellan A, Walker D, Goodacre JA and Dick WC Studies with an enthesis index as a method of clinical assessment in ankylosing spondylitis. Annals of the Rheumatic Diseases 1987; 46: 197–202.

McGonagle D, Gibbon W and Emery P Classification of inflammatory arthritis by enthesitis. Lancet 1998; 352: 1137–1140.

McGonagle D, Marzo-Ortega H, OConnor P, Gibbon W, Pease C, Reece R and Emery P The role of biomechanical factors and HLA-B27 in magnetic resonance imaging-determined bone changes in plantar fascia enthesopathy. Arthritis & Rheumatism 2002; 46(2): 489–493.

McGuigan L, Burke D and Fleming A Tarsal tunnel syndrome and peripheral neuropathy in rheumatoid disease. Annals of the Rheumatic Diseases 1983; 42(2): 128–131.

McRorie ER, Jobanputra P, Ruckley CV and Nuki G Leg ulceration in rheumatoid arthritis. British Journal of Rheumatology 1994; 33: 1078–1084.

McRorie ER, Ruckley CV and Nuki G The relevance of large-vessel vascular disease and restricted ankle movement to the aetiology of leg ulceration in rheumatoid arthritis. British Journal of Rheumatology 1998; 37(12): 1295–1298.

Mitchell DM, Spitz PW, Young DY, Block DA, McShane DJ and Fries JF Survival, prognosis, and causes of death in rheumatoid arthritis. Arthritis and Rheumatism 1986; 29: 706–714.

Morgan SL, Anderson AM, Hood SM, Matthews PA, Lee JY and Alarcon GS Nutrient intake patterns, body mass index, and vitamin levels in patients with rheumatoid arthritis. Arthritis Care & Research 1997; 10(1): 9–17.

OConnell PG, Lohmann Siegel K, Kepple TM, Stanhope SJ and Gerber LH Forefoot deformity, pain, and mobility in rheumatoid and nonarthritic subjects. Journal of Rheumatology 1998; 25(9): 1681–1686.

Pallis CA and Scott JT Peripheral neuropathy in rheumatoid arthritis. British Medical Journal 1965; 1: 1141–1147.

Pecina MM, Krmpotic-Nemanic J and Markiewitz AD Tunnel Syndromes, 3rd ed, CRC Press, Boca Raton, 2001.

Platto MJ, OConnell PG, Hicks JE and Gerber LH The relationship of pain and deformity of the rheumatoid foot to gait and an index of functional ambulation. Journal of Rheumatology 1991; 18(1): 38–43.

Pruzanski W and Watt JG Serum viscosity and hyperviscosity syndromes. Annals of Internal Medicine 1972; 7: 853–860.

Puechal X, Said G, Hilliquin P, Coste J, Job-Deslandre C, Lacroix C and Menkes CJ Peripheral neuropathy with necrotising vasculitis in rheumatoid arthritis. Arthritis and Rheumatism 1995; 38(11): 1618–1629.

Puolakka K, Kautiainen H, Mottonen T et al. Impact of initial aggressive drug treatment with a combination of disease-modifying antirheumatic drugs on the development of work disability in early rheumatoid arthritis: a five-year randomized followup trial. Arthritis & Rheumatism 2004; 50(1): 55–62.

Ropes MW, Bennett GA, Cobb S, Jacob T and Jessar RA 1958 revision of diagnostic criteria for rheumatoid arthritis. Arthritis and Rheumatism 1959; 2: 16–20.

Schmid FR, Cooper NS, Ziff M and McEwen C Arteritis in rheumatoid arthritis. American Journal of Medicine 1961; 30: 56–83.

Scott DL, Pugner K, Kaarela K, Doyle DV, Woolf A, Holmes J and Hieke K The links between joint damage and disability in rheumatoid arthritis. Rheumatology 2000; 39(2): 122–132.

Sokka T, Krishnan E, Hakkinen A and Hannonen P Functional disability in rheumatoid arthritis patients compared with a community population in Finland. Arthritis & Rheumatism 2003; 48(1): 59–63.

Steinberg VL and Wynn-Parry CB Electromyographic changes in rheumatoid arthritis. British Medical Journal 1961; 1: 630–632.

Stiskal M, Szolar DH, Stenzel I, Steiner E, Mesaric P, Czembirek H and Preidler KW Magnetic resonance imaging of Achilles tendon in patients with rheumatoid arthritis. Investigative Radiology 1997; 32(10): 602–608.

Swann AC and Seedhom BB The stiffness of normal articular cartilage and the predominant acting stress levels: implications for the aetiology of osteoarthrosis. British Journal of Rheumatology 1993; 32: 16–25.

Symmons DP, Bankhead CR, Harrison BJ, Brennan P, Barrett EM, Scott DG and Silman AJ Blood transfusion, smoking, and obesity as risk factors for the development of rheumatoid arthritis: results from a primary care-based incident case–control study in Norfolk, England. Arthritis & Rheumatism 1997; 40(11): 1955–1961.

Symmons DPM, Jones MA, Scott DL and Prior P Long term mortality outcome in patients with rheumatoid arthritis: early presenters continue to do well. Journal of Rheumatology 1998; S25(6): 1072–1077.

Thompson PW and Pegley FS A comparison of disability measured by the Stanford Health Assessment Questionnaire disability scales (HAQ) in male and female rheumatoid outpatients. British Journal of Rheumatology 1991; 30(4): 298–300.

Turesson C, Jacobsson L and Bergstrom U Extra–articular rheumatoid arthritis: prevalence and mortality. Rheumatology 1999; 38: 668–674.

Turner DWJ, Woodburn J, Helliwell PS, Cornwall MW, Emery P Pes planovalgus in RA: a descriptive and analytical study of foot function determined by gait analysis. Musculoskeletal Care 2003; 1(1): 21–33.

Vainio K The rheumatoid foot. A clinical study with pathological and roentgenological comments. Clinical Orthopaedics & Related Research 1991; 265: 4–8.

van der Heijde DM, van t Hof MA, van Riel PL et al. Judging disease activity in clinical practice in rheumatoid arthritis: first step in the development of a disease activity score. Annals of the Rheumatic Diseases 1990; 49(11): 916–920.

Voskuyl AE, Hazes JMW, Zwinderman AH, Paleolog EM, van der Meer FJM, Daha MR and Breedveld FC Diagnostic strategy for the assessment of rheumatoid vasculitis. Annals of the Rheumatic Diseases 2003; 62(5): 407–413.

Wells GA, Tugwell P, Kraag GR, Baker PR, Groh J and Redelmeier DA Minimum important difference between patients with rheumatoid arthritis: the patients perspective. Journal of Rheumatology 1993; 20(3): 557–560.

Whalley D, McKenna SP, de Jong Z and van der Heijde D Quality of life in rheumatoid arthritis. British Journal of Rheumatology 1997; 36(8): 884–888.

Wickman AM, Pinzur MS, Kadanoff R and Juknelis D Health-related quality of life for patients with rheumatoid arthritis foot involvement. Foot & Ankle International 2004; 25(1): 19–26.

Williams A and Meacher K Shoes in the cupboard: the fate of prescribed footwear? Prosthetics and Orthotics International 2001; 25: 53–59.

Woodburn J, Helliwell PS and Barker S Three dimensional kinematics at the ankle joint complex in rheumatoid arthritis patients with a painful valgus deformity of the rearfoot. Rheumatology 2002; 41(12): 1406–1412.

Wright V, Dowson D and Longfield MD Joint stiffness – its characterisation and significance. Biomedical Engineering 1969; 4: 8–14.

Wright V and Moll JMH Seronegative Polyarthritis. North Holland Publishing Co, Amsterdam, 1976.

Yelin E, Henke C and Epstein W The work dynamics of the person with rheumatoid arthritis. Arthritis & Rheumatism 1987; 30(5): 507–512.

Yelin E, Meenan R, Nevitt M and Epstein W Work disability in rheumatoid arthritis: effects of disease, social, and work factors. Annals of Internal Medicine 1980; 93(4): 551–556.

Chapter 4

Clinical assessment

SCREENING TOOLS

There is no standardized method by which to assess the musculoskeletal system. Assessment of this nature is often perceived to be very difficult and time consuming by students and health professionals and there is evidence of neglect of musculoskeletal examination in clinical practice (Doherty et al. 1990). In an attempt to overcome lack of standardization, a simple screening tool (GALS – Gait, Arms, Legs and Spine) was developed and has found widespread acceptance (http//www.arc.org.uk) (Doherty & Doherty 1992). The screening consists of asking the patient three questions: (1) Do you have any pain or stiffness in your muscles, joints or back? (2) Can you dress yourself completely without any help? (3) Can you walk up and down the stairs without any help? This is followed by a brief structured examination of the patient's gait, arms, legs and spine (Table 4.1). GALS is a short, simple, standardized history and examination of the locomotor system, which has been shown to be useful for the detection of joint abnormalities. However, it is not a substitute for a more detailed examination. GALS allows identification of abnormality to a specific region, which should then be subject to a more detailed regional examination.

Recently, a set of core regional examination skills for medical students has been developed (Regional Examination of the Musculoskeletal System [REMS]). These core skills have been developed by national consensus (Coady et al. 2004). Initially, focus groups of rheumatologists, orthopaedic surgeons, geriatricians and general practitioners were used to inform the content of a national questionnaire. Questionnaires were sent to 3373 doctors, in which they were asked to assign a value to each regional musculoskeletal clinical skill using a five-point Likert scale ranging from 'definitely

Table 4.1   Summary of GALS (Doherty et al. 1992).

Gait	Symmetry and smoothness of movement Normal stride length Ability to turn normally
Arms Hands	Assess wrist/finger swelling deformity Squeeze across 2nd to 5th metacarpals Inspect hands for muscle wasting Assess normal pronation/supination of forearm
Grip strength	Assess power grip (make a tight fist) Assess precision grip (put fingers on thumb)
Elbows	Can patient fully extend at the elbow (arms out straight)
Shoulders	Can patient place their hands behind their head
Legs Knees	Assess for knee swelling and deformity Assess for quadriceps muscle bulk Assess for knee effusion Assess for crepitus during knee flexion
Hips	Assess internal and external rotation
Feet	Squeeze across metatarsal for tenderness Check for callosities
Spine Assess from behind for	Scoliosis Symmetrical muscle bulk Level iliac crests No popliteal swelling Normal hindfoot alignment
Palpate for	Tenderness over mid-supraspinatus
Assess from the side for	Kyphosis Flexion (can you touch your toes)

Assess from
    the front
	Assess lateral flexion at the neck
	    (can you touch your shoulder with
	    your ear)

The core set of musculoskeletal examination skills for the feet identified by REMS

Examine sole of patient's feet
Recognize hallux valgus, claw and hammer toes
Assess a patient's feet with them standing
Assess for flat feet (including patient standing on tiptoe)
Recognize hind foot/heel pathologies
Assess plantar and dorsi-flexion of the ankle
Assess movements of inversion and eversion of the foot
Assess the sub-talar joint
Perform a lateral squeeze across the metatarso-phalangeal joints
Assess flexion/extension of the big toe
Examine a patient's footwear.

individual clinical tests did not appear to influence the decision of clinicians in accepting it as 'core' for students. It is also not surprising that the survey also showed consistently that examination of the feet was one of the least popular techniques. This finding is not exclusive to musculoskeletal examinations and is consistent with evidence of low rates of foot examination in other disciplines such as diabetes mellitus. Examination of the foot has been shown to be one of the most effective mechanisms for preventing diabetic foot complications. However, it remains the most neglected part of the diabetic assessment (Levin 2001). Low rates of foot examination have been reported during out-patient and in-patient consultations (Wylie-Rosett et al. 1995).

Whilst GALS and REMS are a useful starting point for examination of the foot in a patient with RA, the assessment is aimed at a broad group of patients and is not specific to patients with RA. As RA is a heterogeneous disease, it is not possible to develop a gold standard for assessment. However, given the likely sites of involvement (outlined in Chapter 3) it is possible to examine these sites using a structured and systematic approach. Generally, there is a lack of 'gold jstandard' diagnostic tests. Despite the poor sensitivity and specificity of many of the examination tests, they are included for the purposes of completeness. It is hoped that future research will address this issue.

As with any assessment of a patient, taking a patient history is essential. Full descriptions of successful strategies used in gathering patient history

not required' to 'essential'. Findings from the focus groups and national survey were assessed using a group nominative technique with national representation from the above-listed specialties. This resulted in the identification of 50 core regional musculoskeletal examination skills deemed to be appropriate for medical students. The results are available in handbook and DVD format through the ARC (http//www.arc.org.uk).

It is interesting to note that the national questionnaire showed that the sensitivity and specificity of (non-verbal communication, environmental factors, etc.) have been described in detail elsewhere (Bickley & Szilagyi 2003). It is important to determine what has brought the patient to the consultation, the pattern of distribution and chronological development of symptoms, the impact of the problem and the patient's concerns and expectations. Our clinical experience at Leeds suggests that many patients do not know why they have been referred to the podiatrists and generally have a low expectation for treatment. For the purposes of this chapter, some suggestions of prompts, which are particularly useful when taking a history in a patient with RA foot problems, are outlined below.

Useful prompts for history taking—cont'd

FOOT HISTORY
1. How does your arthritis affect your feet?
2. Has it always affected your feet?
3. As your arthritis progressed, tell me how it has affected your feet over time?
4. Using your hands, can you show me exactly where you get the problems you have described?
5. In what way does the arthritis in your feet impact on your life?
6. How are your feet in comparison to other joints, such as your knees or hand joints?

Useful prompts for history taking

HISTORY
1. When did your arthritis first start?
2. How did it start?
3. What made you seek help?
4. How was the diagnosis made?
5. You have had your arthritis now for ___ years, tell me how it has developed over that time?
6. How has your arthritis been this week (is it active or quiet?)
7. How is your arthritis today (in comparison with when it's at its best and when it's at its worst)?

TREATMENT HISTORY
1. What treatment are you currently receiving for your arthritis (in terms of medicines, tablets, pills or injections)?
2. How do you take these treatments (self or at clinic)?
3. What treatments have you had in the past?
4. What do you feel has been the most effective treatment and why?

OTHER HISTORY
1. Some people with your type of arthritis have other problems, for example chest problems. Do you know if you have any of these?
2. Do you go to see any other medical person because of problems with your arthritis (for example some people go to the chest clinic, others to the eye clinic)
3. Have you had any special investigations for your arthritis?

Continued

MONITORING PROGRESSION OF THE DISEASE

Assessing functional limitation and participation restriction are addressed in the Chapter on Outcome Evaluation (Chapter 8).

The core set of data collected in RA comprises of: tender and swollen joint counts, pain assessment, patient and physician global assessment and an acute phase marker such as the ESR or CRP. The assessment is completed by the patient to ascertain functional limitation. These items will be discussed in more detail in Chapter 8.

Assessment of pain

By far the most common reason for referral to rheumatology departments is pain. Foot pain is the most common reason for referral to podiatry. Pain is a complex, subjective sensation and difficulties arise when one attempts to define, explain or measure it. There has been some suggestion in the literature that there are gender and disease differences in pain thresholds and that patients with RA may have lower pain thresholds than, for example, ankylosing spondylitis (Buskila et al. 1992, Gerecz-Simon et al. 1989, Huskisson & Dudley Hart 1972, Walker & Carmody 1998).

Discordance of pain with tender and swollen joint counts is often apparent during clinical examination and is highlighted in the summary of clinical data shown in Figure 4.1. The number of tender, swollen and patient reported painful joints in the feet was recorded in 40 consecutive patients with RA with varying disease duration and disease activity. Most patients reported far less painful joints than actually were found to be either tender or swollen during examination.

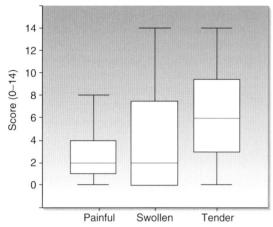

Figure 4.1   Painful, swollen and tender joint counts.

There are many outcome tools that can be used in clinical practice to establish the extent of foot pain and the resultant functional limitation and activity restriction. Some are specifically validated for the use in RA and others aimed at community-based populations. These are described in detail in Chapter 8. A useful strategy, which helps to determine nature and sites of involvement, is to ask the patient to complete a lower limb map. This helps the patient focus on their symptoms and can provide useful clues as to the possible aetiology of the underlying problem (see Fig. 4.2). Pain in small joints tends to be more accurately localized by patients than pain in larger joints. The character of

pain is often helpful in determining the structures involved (for example, aching suggests pain within the joint, whereas, burning, tingling, stabling, radiating suggests neurological elements). The presence or absence of pain during different activities can also be helpful.

ASSESSING DISEASE ACTIVITY IN THE FOOT

It is essential to be able to distinguish if lower limb pain and functional limitation is related primarily to biomechanical dysfunction or related to increased disease activity, or a combination of the two. Objective measurements should be taken during routine clinical practice, to determine the activity level of the RA. It is important to take measures of disease activity as part of routine practice to:

- monitor the patient over time
- predict further outcome
- assess change over time as an effect of systemic and local treatments
- make decisions on treatment change.

Studies have shown that patients attending early inflammatory arthritis clinics may have evidence of bone erosions (Harrison & Symmons 2000, Machold et al. 2002). This suggests that damage related to disease activity can occur in a relatively short time frame. Therefore, it is important that practitioners assess patients on every visit for indicators of increased disease activity and take appropriate action.

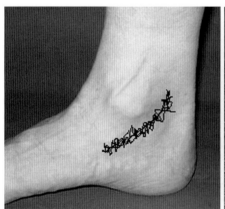
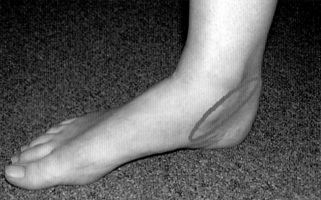

Figure 4.2   This patient was referred to the podiatry department with persistent medial ankle pain. She had been diagnosed with rheumatoid arthritis for 18 months and her disease activity was generally low. A copy of her completed foot map can be seen above. The photograph shows obvious swelling along the muscle tendon of tibialis posterior. The area was painful and felt warm and 'boggy' on palpation. The patient has a low medial arch profile and failure of the calcaneus to invert when standing on tiptoe. High-resolution ultrasound scanning showed tibialis posterior tenosynovitis. Provision of functional orthoses along with an ultrasound guided corticosteroid injection fully resolved the tenosynovitis.

Determining the number of tender and swollen joints is a key component in the clinical assessment of RA to monitor disease status and to assess treatment response. There is a strong relationship between disease activity, structural damage and functional disability.

A number of different joint scoring systems are available and there is not complete agreement on which joints should be evaluated. Two methods (the 66/68 and the 28 joint counts) are widely used in clinical practice. The 28 joint count is simpler to perform and takes less time and is reported to be comparable with the 66/68 joint count in terms of the value of the information it provides and reproducibility (Smolen et al. 1995). The main difference between the two scoring methods is that the 28 joint count excludes the joints of the feet and ankles so that potentially relevant clinical information about the feet is not recorded.

Considerable variation between observers in the assessment of tender and swollen joint counts has been highlighted in the literature. Scott et al. (1996) investigated the extent of variation between different examiners (medical and nursing practitioners) in the measurement of joint swelling and tenderness, based on the 28 joint count. A high coefficient of variation between examiners performing the 28 joint count was reported (up to a maximum of 204%). The study also highlighted the importance of training and standardization. After training, the mean coefficient of variation for tender and swollen joints had improved, but was still high, at 65% and 59% respectively (Scott et al. 1996).

DAS (Disease Activity Score) 28 can be determined with the number of tender and swollen joints (based on the 28 joint score), with a measure of patient's global assessment (on a 100 mm visual analogue scale) and with an acute phase reactant, usually the ESR or CRP (Fig. 4.3). Values have been established and can determine if a patient is in a flare or not. A full description can be found in Chapter 8. The DAS 28 is endorsed by EULAR and has been used more widely to direct decisions on systemic management.

Allied health practitioners working in primary care teams or distant sites may not easily have access to laboratory reports that include details on acute-phase reactants. If it is not possible to access blood results, the number of tender, swollen and painful joints can act as a reflective marker of disease activity (greater number of swollen, tender and painful joints relate to increased disease activity). The number of tender, swollen and painful joints can be serially plotted over time to monitor disease progression as can the number of joints with deformity. The number of tender,

swollen and painful foot joints can be recorded; a suggested format is shown in Figure 4.4.

Painful joints

Patient self-reported joint pain, and perceived disease activity can be helpful in clinical assessment; however, there is debate whether these measures are reliable and valid (Houssien et al. 1999, Stewart et al. 1993, Stucki et al. 1995). Agreement between physician and patient derived scores of disease activity are sufficient to allow patients' derived scores to be used in clinical research, although physician and patient scoring systems are not directly interchangeable (Houssien et al. 1999).

Asking patients to describe the character of pain is helpful in understanding the underlying cause. The presence or absence of pain during specific activities can also provide useful clues. Many common lower limb pathologies have common patterns of foot pain. It is important to recognize these patterns; for example, plantar heel pain on first weight bearing, which is relieved initially by walking and then is made worse by standing and walking is the classical feature of plantar fasciitis.

Swelling

Joint swelling can be either due to soft tissues or bony proliferation. When performing swollen joint counts, only swelling of the soft tissues should be included; swelling associated with osteophytic proliferation or deformity is not included. Swelling is usually detectable along the joint margins and is usually confined to a discrete area and conforms to an underlying anatomical structure. It is often hard to distinguish between swelling due to joint effusion, synovitis or inflammation of periarticular structures. There is evidence of greater sensitivity of imaging modalities in the detection of synovitis, tenosynovitis and tendon tears: synovitis in the foot, in particular, is detected at the MTP joints more often with ultrasound than by clinical examination (Karim et al. 2001).

Tenderness

Joint tenderness is pain in a joint under defined circumstances. These include pain at rest with pressure (for example, at the metatarsophalangeal (MTP) joints) or pain on movement of the joint. The pressure used to elicit joint tenderness should be exerted by the examiner's thumb and index finger, which is sufficient to cause 'whitening' of the examiner's nail bed. Different techniques can be used to elicit joint tenderness, either a two- or four-finger technique.

DAS 28

Tender joint count

The number of swollen joints are counted as follows:
0 = not tender
1 = tender

Tenderness will be assessed for 28 joints on both right and left side. The following joints will be evaluated: 10 proximal interphalangeal joints and 10 metacarpophalangeal joints, 2 wrists, 2 elbows, 2 shoulders and 2 knees.
Tenderness will be elicited by firm pressure over the joint margin

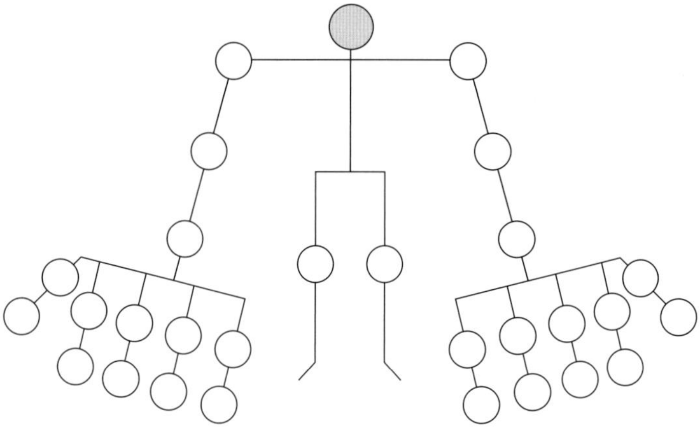

Number

Swollen joint count

The number of swollen joints are counted as follows:
0 = not swollen
1 = swollen

Swelling will be evaluated by palpation, only soft tissue swelling will be accounted for. The same 28 joints as for tenderness will be assessed for swelling.

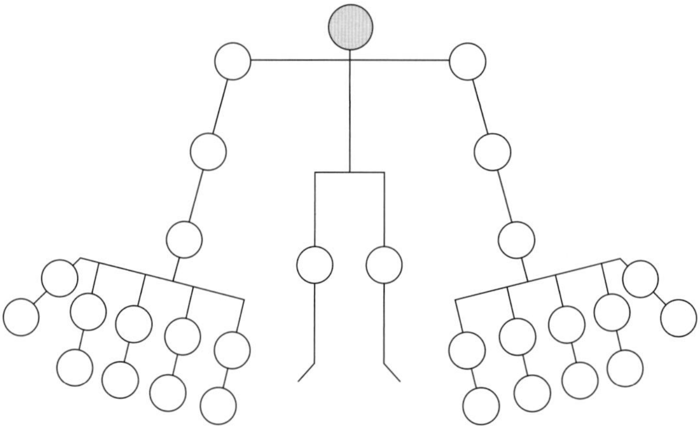

Number

ESR (mm/hr)

Patient General Health

Please mark on the line with a cross the response which best describes your general health in the last week

Best possible health ├───────────────────┤ Worst possible health

Score mm

Figure 4.3 A proforma used for recording tender and swollen joint counts that may also be used for calculating the DAS28 score.

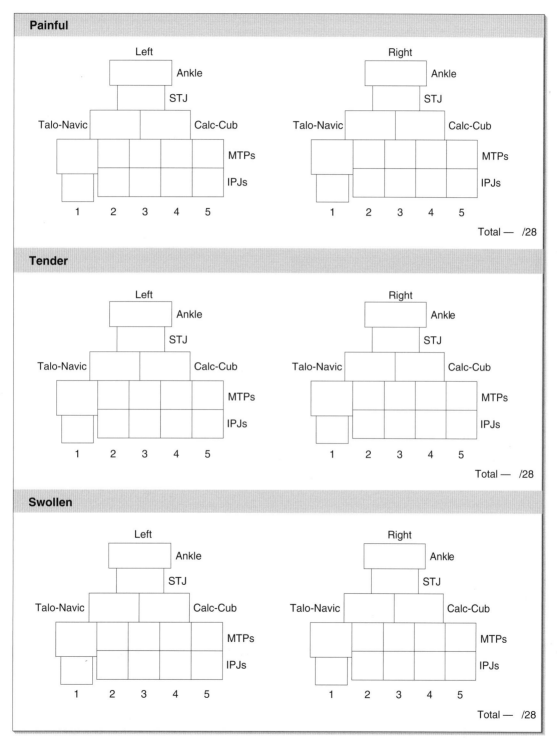

Figure 4.4 Suggested tender and swollen joint count.

A full description of joint counts can be found in the EULAR handbook (http//www.eular.org). As considerable variation exists between examiners and techniques it is recommended that the methods are standardized and, where possible, performed by the same person.

Joint stiffness

Joint stiffness is a complex sensation defined mechanically as increased resistance to movement of the joint. A fuller description can be found in Chapter 3. Joint stiffness is usually more pronounced following periods of inactivity or rest. Many clinicians will use the number of minutes of early morning stiffness, severity and number of joints affected as an objective measure of joint stiffness.

KEY POINTS

- Tender and swollen joint counts are useful in clinical practice to monitor disease activity.
- Considerable variation exists between different examiners. However, standardization of methods and training greatly improve reliability.
- In the absence of acute-phase reactants, serial recording of tender and swollen joint counts, pain and functional limitation can provide useful information on disease progression.
- EULAR standards provide full instructions on how to perform tender and swollen joint counts (Copies can be obtained by contacting the publisher, Van Zuiden Communications, ISBN 90-751-41-90-4.) It is best to have training from someone experienced in performing joint counts.

GENERAL PRINCIPLES OF ASSESSMENT OF IMPAIRMENT IN THE FOOT

The key elements of a foot examination are look, feel and move. It is essential to have an appreciation of the normal surface anatomy, muscle bulk, joint movements and muscle power. Careful inspection should be performed to identify abnormalities and inspection undertaken in both weight bearing and non-weight bearing conditions from all aspects. A structured, systematic approach reduces the possibility of omitting any structures. It is convenient to assess the foot as three units – the rearfoot, midfoot and forefoot. Assessment procedures will be outlined around these three functional units. Table 4.2 summarizes the examination schedule.

Table 4.2   Outline for foot examination.

Examination of skin	Look for: Necrosis Ulceration Nodules Scarring (previous ulceration/trauma/surgical) Corns/callus Haemorrhage into callus Skin infection (bacterial/fungal) Blisters Adventitious bursa formation (inflamed) Interdigital maceration/ulceration/corns Colour changes, venous, ischaemic, vasospastic (pallor/rubor/cyanotic) Oedema Thinning of the skin/bruising (associated with long-term steroid use) Evidence of poor foot hygiene Feel for: Temperature changes Swelling
Examination of the nail	Look for: Fungal nail infections Ingrowing toe nails Splinter haemorrhages/nail fold infarcts Evidence of poor self care/neglect
Examination of the foot	Look for: Muscle bulk/posture Rearfoot deformity/swelling Midfoot deformity/swelling Collapse of medial longitudinal arch Forefoot deformity Daylight sign Prominent metatarsal heads Hallux valgus Lesser toe deformity Bursitis/tendonitis Feel for: Prominent metatarsal heads Tender, painful and swollen joints Assess muscle tendons for swelling and tenderness Assess joints for range of movement Assess muscle strength
Examination of footwear	Look for: Assess fit of the shoe Assess appropriateness of shoe for function Excessive wear patterns Bulging of medial counter Fastenings Feel for: Midsole flexibility Forefoot cushioning

Look

Joint deformity

Joint deformity should be documented to allow assessment of progression of disease over time. An estimation of the degree of deformity, whether the deformity is fixed or mobile and if it is correctable or non-correctable should also be included. Several scoring systems to document foot deformity are available (generic and specific to RA), although they have failed to be investigated thoroughly in terms of reliability.

The American Orthopedic Foot and Ankle Society developed clinical rating score systems for the hindfoot, midfoot and forefoot (the AOFAS clinical rating scores) (American Orthopedic Foot & Ankle Society 1994). These scoring systems have been utilized widely in the orthopaedic literature mainly as outcome measures following surgical interventions. There are four scoring systems for the Ankle-Hindfoot (AH), midfoot (M), Hallux Metatarsophalangeal-Inter-Phalangeal (HMTP-IP) and the Lesser Metatarsophalangeal-Inter-Phalangeal (LMTP-IP). The AH and HMTP-IP scales have been used to evaluate ankle arthrodesis, total ankle replacement, forefoot athrodesis or 1st MTP resection in patients with RA (de Palmer et al. 2000, Mulcahy et al. 2003, Nishikawa et al. 2004). The AH scale has been criticized for its inherent limited precision, which is associated with the small number of response intervals available (Guyton 2001).

Platto and colleagues developed the Structural Index (SI) to quantify structural deformity in patients with RA (Platto et al. 1991). They defined an index of structural deformity for the forefoot, hindfoot and total foot. In the forefoot, scoring is based on the presence or absence of claw, hammer or cock toes; presence of bunion or hallux valgus, exostosis at the 5th MTP joint, and subluxation at the MTP joints. The hindfoot score is dependent on the valgus or varus position of the hindfoot, total passive range of motion at the ankle (dorsi/plantarflexion) and presence or absence of pes planus or pes cavus deformity (Table 4.3).

In the absence of a validated foot deformity scoring system specifically developed for patients with RA, the SI proposed by Platto is the preferred method to quickly quantify extent of foot deformity. However, it must be recognized the SI has not been thoroughly investigated in terms of reliability, and the dichotomous nature of scoring deformity, while improving inter-examiner reliability, will limit its ability to monitor subtle changes in foot posture/deformity over time.

Root and colleagues arbitrarily assigned stages (1–4) to the progression of hallux abductovalgus (HAV) deformity (Root et al. 1977). In stage 1, lateral subluxation of the base of the proximal phalanx of the hallux in relation to the 1st metatarsal head occurs. This is not detectable by clinical examination and is only evident on X-ray. Stage 2 HAV is characterized by abduction deformity of the hallux. The hallux is seen to press against the second toe. In stage 3 there is development of metatarsus primus varus

Table 4.3   Structural index as described by Platto et al. 1991.

Structural indices for fore and hindfeet deformity (after Platto et al. 1991)					
Forefoot score			Hindfoot score		
Deformity	Right	Left	Deformity	Right	Left
Hallux valgus (Yes=1, No=0)			Calcaneal valgus/varus degrees (0–5=0; 6–10 = 1; 11–15 = 2; >15=3)		
5th MTP Exostosis (Yes=1, No=0)			Ankle total ROM (46–60° = 0; 31–45° = 1; 15–30° = 2; <15° = 3)		
Cock/hammer/claw toes present (Number 0–5) MTP subluxed (Number 0–5) Total Score (from 12)			Pes planus/pes cavus (Yes = 1, No = 0) Total score (from 7)		
SI forefoot = right + left ____/24 Score [as ratio from 200] ____/200 Total foot deformity (forefoot + hindfoot) ____/38 Score [as ratio from 200] ____/200			SI hindfoot = right + left ____/14 Score [as ratio from 200] ____/200		

(an abnormally large transverse plane angle between the 1st and 2nd metatarsals, which is detectable on visual inspection of the foot). Stage 4 is the most advanced stage in the progression of HAV, where dislocation or subluxation of the hallux occurs. The hallux most frequently underrides the 2nd toe but in some cases can override the 2nd toe.

Traditional classifications of lesser toe deformity (clawed, hammer, mallet) become increasing difficult to ascertain in patients with the complex types of foot deformities seen with RA. The clinical approach at Leeds uses a functional classification based on whether the lesser toes are weight bearing or non-weight bearing during gait. Anecdotal evidence suggests this classification relates better to the presence/absence of metatarsal head pain, callus and high plantar pressures.

When assessing the forefoot it is also important to check for splaying of the forefoot. Many patients report they have to 'go up a size' in shoes to accommodate increased foot width. Daylight sign (when daylight can be observed between the toes, Fig. 3.4) is a clinical indicator of synovitis or inter-metatarsal mass at the relevant MTP joint. However, sensitivity and specificity data for this clinical sign is lacking.

Foot posture

There are a number of different mechanisms by which to classify foot posture ranging from visual inspection through to measurements of foot anthropometrics and radiographic evaluations. Each method has particular merits and limitations that have been critically reviewed elsewhere (Menz 1998, Razeghi & Batt 2002). There is no general consensus on which measurements to use. Many reliability studies have been performed for various parameters in healthy control subjects and one cannot assume equipoise in patients with RA. It is important to assess foot shape both non-weight bearing, standing and during gait. Although there is an assumption that foot morphology dictates function, literature suggests there is a poor relationship between measures of foot structure and foot function in asymptomatic individuals (Hamill et al. 1989, McPoil & Cornwall 1994, McPoil & Cornwall 1996). It is likely that strategies for pain avoidance used in RA patients (for example minimally loading tender MTP joints) will further complicate the relationship foot structure and function.

Foot postural changes to screen for during visual inspection should include:

- alignment of the rearfoot (valgus or varus position)
- medial longitudinal arch profile (high, normal, low)

- hallux (hallux valgus deformity, non-weight bearing)
- lesser toes (presence of deformity, non-weight bearing).

Muscle

Muscle may be involved as part of the process of RA (see Chapter 3). Joint pain and associated functional limitation may also contribute to disuse muscle atrophy. Pain avoidance strategies adopted by patients may result in weakness and wasting of specific muscle groups. For example, weakness in the gastrocnemius and soleus muscles can develop in patients who fail to create the normal plantarflexion moment at the ankle joint in terminal stance in an attempt to avoid pain across painful MTP joints. A visual inspection of the lower leg for normal muscle bulk should be performed making note of any apparent loss in muscle bulk, hypertrophy or flexion contractures. A summary of muscle testing in the foot is given in Figure 4.5.

Assessment of the skin

Inspection of the foot from all aspects should be undertaken for any pressure induced lesions (hyperkeratotic lesions, adventitious bursae), ulceration, scarring or extra articular features of RA (including nodules and nail fold infarcts). At the posterior aspect of the calcanueus, check the tendo Achilles, retrocalcaneus and subcutaneous bursae for evidence of inflammation and for evidence of skin irritation or hyperkeratotic tissue from a rigid heel counter. On the plantar surface of the mid and forefoot check for any pressure induced lesions. Inspect the dorsal toes for evidence of irritation from footwear and the interdigital areas for maceration, infection, or any lesions.

Footwear

No examination of the foot in RA is complete without an inspection of the footwear. A high proportion of patients wear ill-fitting footwear. One study found that 24% of patients attending general medical outpatient appointments wore shoes that were the wrong size (Reddy et al. 1989). In the elderly, the proportion of people wearing ill-fitting shoes is higher. Burns and colleagues (2002) found 72% of patients on an elderly general rehabilitation ward were wearing ill-fitting shoes (a discrepancy in length of more than half a British shoe size or more than one British width fitting, 7 mm). The study found a significant association between incorrect shoe length and ulceration and self-reported foot pain. Patients with foot deformity find it increasingly difficult to buy footwear that can accommodate their foot shape as deformity progresses.

| Region | Muscle & innervation | Technique | | | Picture |
		Patient position	Stabilization	Resistance	Movement	
Posterior						
	Triceps surae (L5,S1,S2)	Supine	Lower third of leg	Under plantar surface of the foot	Patient has to plantarflex at the ankle against resistance	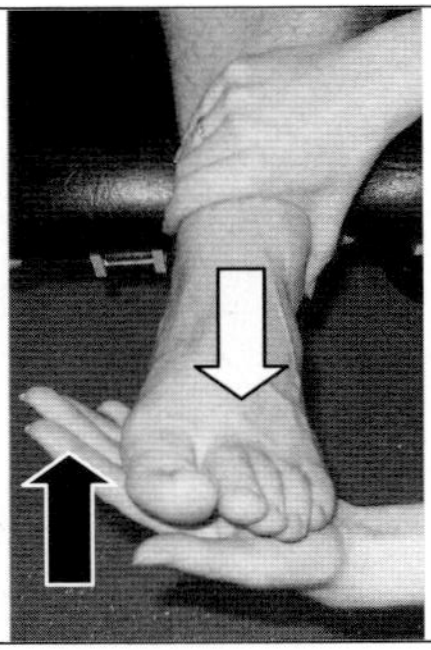
Lateral						
	Peroneus brevis (L4,L5,S1)	Supine	Lower third of leg, above malleolus	Hand over the dorsal, lateral border of the forefoot.	Start position – foot in neutral position. Patient has to evert the foot against resistance (demonstration of desired movement probably needed)	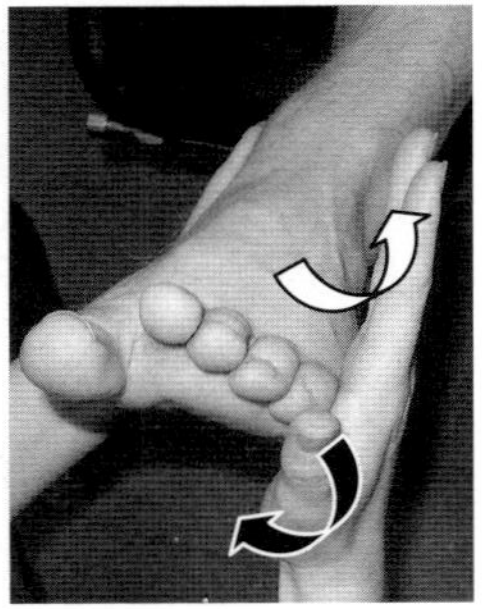
	Peroneus longus (L4,L5,S1)	Supine	Lower third of leg, above malleolus	Hand over the dorsal, lateral border of the forefoot.	Start position – foot in dorsiflexed position. Patient has to evert the foot against resistance.	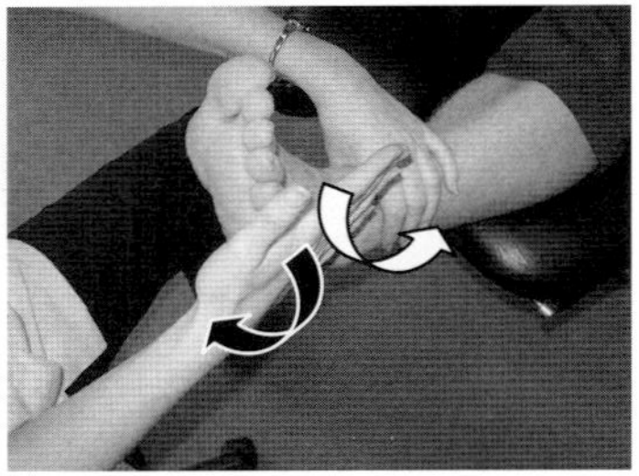

Figure 4.5 Summary of muscle testing.

| Region | Muscle & innervation | Technique | | | Picture |
		Patient position	Stabilization	Resistance	Movement
Anterior	Tibialis anterior (L4,L5,S1)	Supine	Lower third of leg	On dorsal surface of the foot	Patient has to dorsiflex at the ankle against resistance	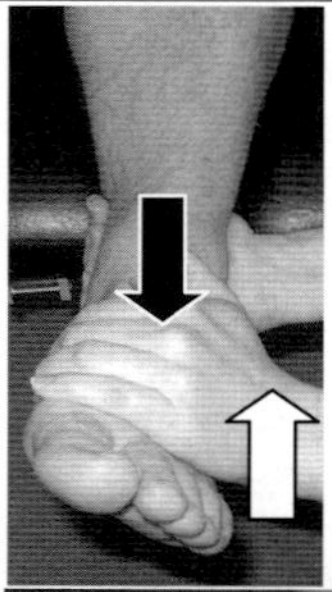
	Extensor hallucis longus (L4,L5,S1)	Supine	Metatarsus	On dorsal aspect of the proximal and distal phalanx of the hallux	Patient has to dorsiflex the hallux against resistance	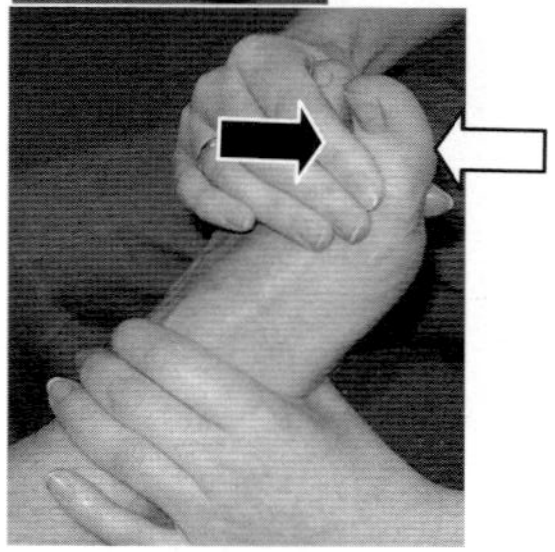
	Extensor digitorum brevis & extensor digitorum longus (L4,L5,S1)	Supine	Metatarsus	On the sides of the proximal phalanges	Patient has to extend the lesser toes against resistance	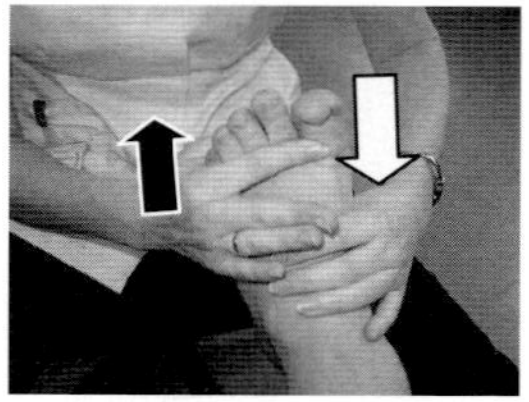

Figure 4.5   Cont'd

| Region | Muscle & innervation | Technique | | | | Picture |
		Patient position	Stabilization	Resistance	Movement	
Medial	Tibialis posterior (L4,L5,S1)	Supine	Lower third of leg just above the malleolus	Hand over the dorsal, medial surface of the foot at the level of the metatarsal heads	Start position – foot is slightly plantarflexed. Patient has to invert the foot against resistance (demonstration of desired movement probably needed)	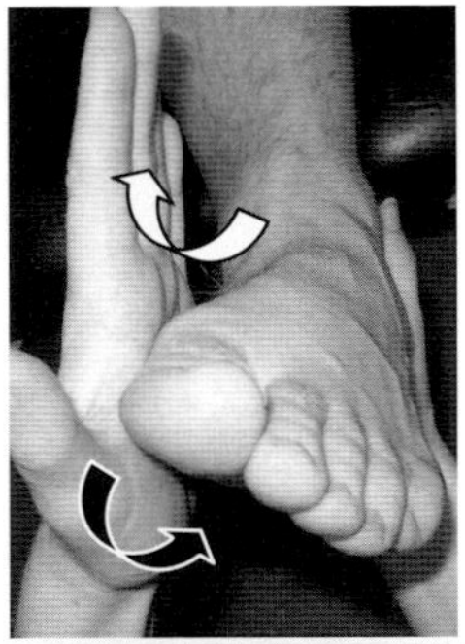
	Flexor hallucis longus (L5,S1,S2)	Supine	Sides of the proximal phalanx of hallux	Plantar surface of distal phalanx of hallux	Patient has to plantar-flex at the 1st interphalangeal joint against resistance	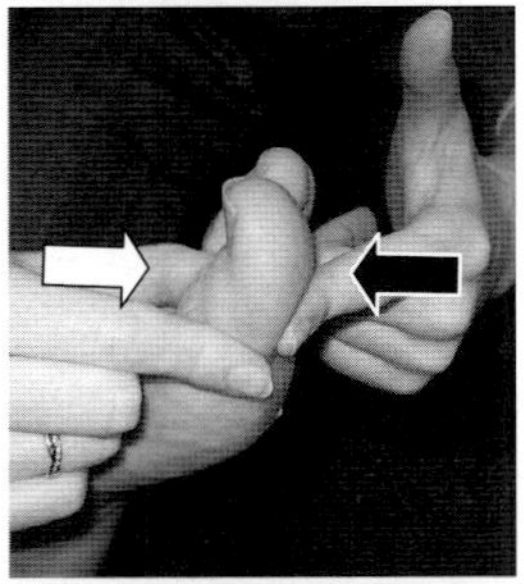
	Flexor digitorum longus (L5,S1)	Supine	Sides of the intermediate phalanx of second toe	Plantar surface of distal phalanx of second toe	Patient has to plantar-flex at the distal interphalangeal joint against resistance	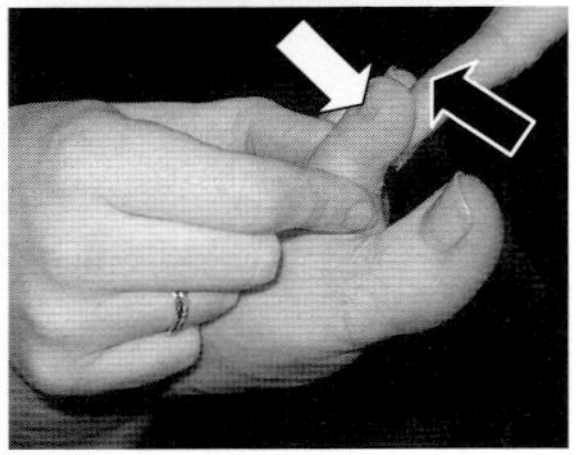

Figure 4.5   Cont'd

Visual analogue scales have been proposed as a reliable measure for subjective footwear comfort (Gramling & Elliot 1992), but the relationship between comfort and fit has not yet been established.

When making an assessment of footwear it is essential to ask the patient about their usual footwear, very often patients will come to hospital appointments in their best/smart shoes or will wear shoes that are easy to remove and put on and it is not necessarily a true reflection of their usual attire. It is important to assess the suitability of footwear for the intended function. Some patients will wear open toe sandals to accommodate forefoot deformities. However, whilst this may be suitable in summer it will not protect the foot in winter.

When assessing footwear fit, attention should be directed to overall length, the forefoot width and toe box depth. Wear marks on the upper, outer sole and insole can provide information on footwear fit and some clues about foot function (Fig. 4.6).

Feel

When there is underlying synovitis at a joint or tenosynovitis, temperature at the site may be elevated. Infrared thermography has been shown to detect

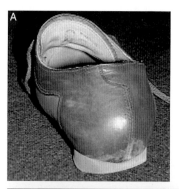

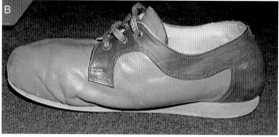

Figure 4.6 Footwear. (A) Note the excessive lateral heel wear. (B) Note the medial bulging of the upper and collapse in the arch area. The medial aspect of the shoe is reinforced with a metal plate. This provides an insight into the magnitude of deforming forces around the mid foot area.

increased heat over an inflamed joint or soft tissue. However, sophisticated objective measures of warmth like this are rarely taken in clinical practice. In the absence of instrumentation to accurately quantify temperature, the backs of the fingers are reported to be sensitive and used to detect temperature changes and, therefore, are recommended for ascertaining 'hot spots'. Assessment of temperature should be taken over sites where inflammation is suspected, making comparison with a reference site on the same limb. Erythema is occasionally visible over superficial joints in acute inflammation due to an increased blood flow to the area. It is always useful to question the patient about recent use of topical rubefacients, counter-irritants or direct heat to exclude this as possible cause of increased skin temperature. When palpating for tenderness, as a general guide pressure should be exerted until either tenderness is elicited or blanching of the examiner's nail bed is apparent. When examining for swelling, one digit should be used to exert pressure on the site and the other as a sensor to detect any fluctuation associated with swelling.

Rearfoot

Anterior   Synovial swelling at the ankle is most likely to be detectable over the anterior or anterior lateral aspect of the joint, because the capsule is more lax in this area. Many tendons cross the ankle joint and it is important to differentiate between the swelling associated with tendon sheaths and the diffuse swelling due to involvement of the ankle. The extensor hallucis longus and extensor digitorum longus tendons should be palpated along their length for tenderness whilst the patient dorsiflexes at the MTP joints against resistance.

Posterior   In the posterior calcaneal region particular attention should be directed to the Achilles tendon and associated bursae. Palpate along the length of the Achilles tendon noting any tenderness or thickening. The key sites to examine are the enthesis, 2–6 cm proximal from the insertion, and the muscle tendon belly junction as these are common sites for injury (Balint 2003). Examine the retrocalcaneal and subcalcaneal tissues for any tenderness, using one digit as a sensor and another as the pressor to detect fluctuation of fluid around the Achilles tendon (Fig. 4.7).

Plantar heel   Palpate the plantar heel area to locate the point of maximum tenderness; a common site of tenderness is the medial tubercle of the calcaneus where the plantar fascia inserts into the calcaneus (Fig. 4.8), tensioning the plantar fascia (with dorsiflexion of the toes) generally accentuates tenderness

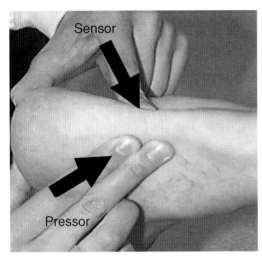

Figure 4.7   Palpating for retrocalcaneal bursitis.

on palpation. Generalized tenderness over the plantar heel may be associated with fat pad atrophy. It is important to examine the subcalcaneal bursa for swelling and tenderness. Nodules develop in pressure areas and can occur in the plantar heel region.

Medial   Palpate along the length of the posterior tibial tendon that runs proximal to the medial malleolus distally to its insertion at the navicular for tenderness or swelling. Asking the patient to invert the foot

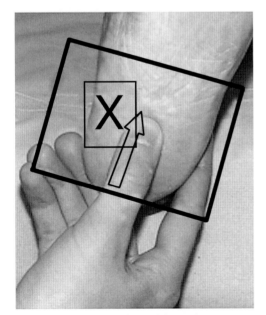

Figure 4.8   Palpation of plantar heel for tenderness.

against resistance whilst palpating the tendon may accentuate tenderness. It is hard to differentiate between inflammation of flexor hallucis longus, flexor digitorum longus and tibialis posterior tendons. From antero-medial to postero-lateral side pass the tendons of tibialis posterior and flexor digitorum longus, the posterior tibial artery with its venae comitantes, the tibial nerve and finally flexor hallucis longus. Asking the patient to activate the appropriate muscle whilst palpating may help to determine which tendon or tendons are involved.

Percussion of the tibial nerve around the medial malleous for Tinel's sign should be performed. Data for the sensitivity and specificity of Tinel's sign for the diagnosis of tarsal tunnel syndrome are lacking. The diagnosis of tarsal tunnel relies primarily on clinical examination with further electrodiagnostic investigations (see Chapter 3).

Lateral   When examining around the lateral rearfoot attention should be directed towards palpation of the sinus tarsi and the peroneal muscle tendons. In sinus tarsi syndrome, clinical presentation typically includes tenderness on palpation of the sinus tarsi, which may be exacerbated by varus tilting of the calcaneus along with a perceived lack of rearfoot stability during gait. This can be confirmed by injection of local anaesthetic into the sinus tarsi, which should alleviate pain and the sensation of instability.

The peroneal muscles make up the lateral compartment of the leg. The tendon of peroneus brevis courses anterior to the peroneus longus tendon at the ankle. It courses over the peroneal tubercle on the calcaneus and inserts into the base of the 5th metatarsal. The tendon of peroneus longus courses behind the peroneus brevis tendon at the level of the ankle and then, usually, courses below the peroneal tubercle; it then deviates sharply in a medial direction to insert into the medial cuneiform and plantar 1st metatarsal. The peroneal tendons share a common tendon sheath proximal to the distal tip of the fibula. More distally, each tendon is housed within its own sheath. The tendons may be separated at the peroneal tubercle with brevis anterior to the tubercle and longus inferior; however, both tendons may pass anterior to the tubercle and separate more distally.

Frequent involvement of both peroneal tendons has been reported in patients with RA (Bouysett et al. 1995). Tenosynovitis can occur in either tendons alone, or both may be involved (Fig. 4.9). Single or multiple longitudinal tears are the most common problem seen with the peroneus brevis tendon. The clinical manifestation is pain; with time, loss of eversion strength may also occur.

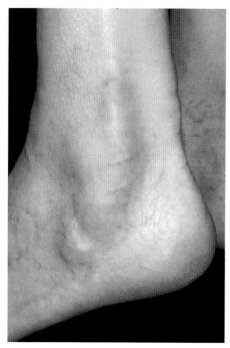

Figure 4.9   Peroneal tenosynovitis.
➤ Note the linear swelling proximal to the lateral malleolus, following the length of the common peroneal sheath.
➤ Note the localized swelling around the malleolus (which could possibly be inflammation of the common bursa of peroneus longus and brevis which lies just behind the lateral malleolus).
➤ Swelling is apparent inferior and distal to the malleolus around the peroneal tubercle where the tendons are likely to separate into individual sheaths.

Midfoot

Synovitis of the intertarsal joints may be difficult to observe, but swelling, erythema and heat may be observed. Each joint should be individually assessed for tenderness.

On the plantar aspect palpate along the length of the plantar fascia for nodules or plantar fibromatosis (a mass of fibrous tissue in the plantar fascia that may or may not be tender on palpation). Dorsiflexion at the ankle, MTP joints and IP joints tightens up the plantar fascia thus facilitating this manoeuvre.

Forefoot

When synovitis in the forefoot is present a lateral squeeze of all the MTP joints causes pain. This clinical test is used as a screen but provides little information on the nature and site of inflammation. Palpation of each individual MTP joint (concurrently above and below the joint) and each inter-metatarsal head space helps to differentiate between MTP joint synovitis, and inter-metatarsal bursitis. Palpation of each MTP joint also provides an opportunity to subjectively assess the thickness and quality of plantar metatarsal head soft tissue and the metatarsal parabola.

Move

Joint movement

When assessing joint movement some appreciation of normal and abnormal ranges and quality of motion is needed. There must also be recognition of the normal age-related reduction in motion and the influence of other factors such as guarding (a protective mechanism commonly used by patients to protect a painful joint). The procedure for assessing joint motion usually involves assessment of the active range (patient moves the joint) and the passive range (examiner moves the joint). The active range is usually less than the passive range. The reliability of measuring joint movement with goniometers is poor, particularly in the foot (where the range of motion is small when compared to the hip and knee) and, therefore has limited value in clinical assessment (Boone et al. 1978, Buckley & Hunt 1997, Ekstrand et al. 1982). A summary of expected values for range of motion at the ankle, subtalar and 1st MTP and description of technique is presented in Figure 4.10.

Whilst assessment of range of motion is important, quality of motion and pain on movement can provide invaluable clues as to the nature of the problem. Crepitation is an audible or palpable grating on movement of a joint. Fine crepitus is audible with stethoscope and may accompany inflammation of bursa, tendon sheath or synovium, whereas coarse crepitus is palpable and reflects cartilage or bone damage (Doherty & Doherty 1992). Patients often will report 'joints cracking'; this is a normal finding due to intraarticular gas bubble formation.

When assessing pain on movement it is useful to examine the patient's face for signs of discomfort and to ask the patient to report the site and nature of any pain as the joint is moved through its passive range. When pain is minimal in mid range but increases towards end of range in all directions this is referred to as 'stress pain'. Universal stress pain is when pain is present throughout most of the range in all directions and can be a sign of synovitis. When pain is present in only one direction this is characteristic of a localized intra- or periarticular lesion (Doherty & Doherty 1992).

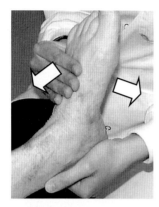

Joint movement – Ankle joint
Plane of motion – Predominantly sagittal plane
Direction of motion – Dorsiflexion / plantarflexion
Expected range of motion – 10° dorsiflexion with knee extended
40 – 70° plantarflexion with knee extended
Description of technique – The knee should be in a fully extended position during the examination. The subtalar joint is placed in the neutral position (neither pronated or supinated) and holding the calcaneus maintains this position. A loading force is applied to the forefoot to allow the ankle joint to dorsiflex and plantarflex to its end ranges of motion. The total range of motion is estimated from visualization.

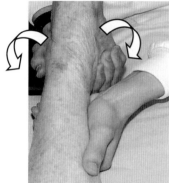

Joint movement – Subtalar joint
Plane of motion – Predominantly frontal plane
Direction of motion – Inversion / eversion
Expected range of motion – 20° inversion
10° eversion
Description of technique – one hand stabilizes the lower third of the leg. The other hand holds the calcaneus and moves the subtalar joint through its range of motion from an inverted to an everted position.

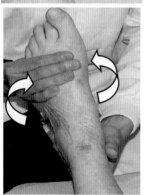

Joint movement – Midtarsal joint (longitudinal axis)
Plane of motion – Predominantly frontal plane
Direction of motion – Inversion / eversion
Expected range of motion – Difficulties and imprecision associated with measurement technique make estimations of range of motion problematic.
Description of technique – The knee should be in a fully extended position during the examination. The subtalar joint is placed in the neutral position (neither pronated or supinated) and holding the calcaneus maintains this position. The other hand holds the forefoot at the level of the base of the metatarsals and moves the midtarsal joint through its range of motion.

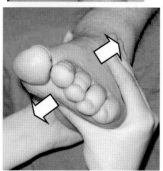

Joint movement – Midtarsal joint (oblique axis)
Plane of motion – Predominantly sagittal plane
Expected range of motion – Difficulties and imprecision associated with measurement technique make estimations of range of motion problematic.
Description of technique – The knee should be in a fully extended position during the examination. The subtalar joint is placed in the neutral position (neither pronated or supinated) and the calcaneus is held to maintain this position. The other hand holds the forefoot at the level of the base of the metatarsals and moves the midtarsal joint through its range of motion, in the direction of dorsiflexion with eversion and plantarflexion with inversion.

Figure 4.10 Summary of joint ranges.

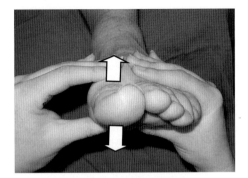

Joint movement – First ray
Plane of motion – Predominantly sagittal plane
Direction of motion – Dorsiflexion / plantarflexion
Expected range of motion – 10 mm dorsal excursion
                                        10 mm plantar excursion
Description of technique – The knee should be fully extended. The subtalar joint is placed in the neutral position. With one hand the examiner holds the second through to fifth metatarsal heads between the thumb and index finger.In a similar manner the other hand holds the first metatarsal head. The first metatarsal is moved dorsally and plantarly and total motion visualized and recorded.

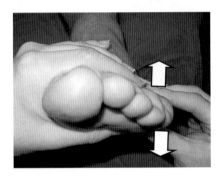

Joint movement – Fifth ray
Plane of motion – Predominantly sagittal plane
Expected range of motion – could not find published reported values
Description of technique – The knee should be fully extended. The subtalar joint is placed in the neutral position. With one hand the examiner holds the first through to fourth metatarsal heads between the thumb and index finger. In a similar manner the other hand holds the fifth metatarsal head. The fifth metatarsal is moved dorsally and plantarly and total motion visualized and recorded.

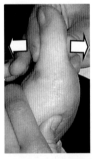

Joint movement – First metatarsophalangeal joint
Plane of motion – Predominantly sagittal plane
Direction of motion – Dorsiflexion / plantarflexion
Expected range of motion – 65–75° dorsiflexion
                                        45° plantarflexion
Description of technique – The first metatarsal shaft is stabilized with one hand. The other hand holds the proximal phalanx of the hallux and moves the first metatarsophalangeal joint through plantarflexion and dorsiflexion.

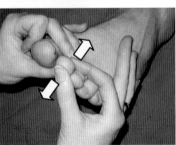

Joint movement – Interphalangeal (IP) joints
Plane of motion – Predominantly sagittal plane
Expected range of motion – 35° flexion
Description of technique – One hand stabilizes the shaft of the proximal phalanx, the other hand holds the intermediate phalanx and moves the proximal IP joint through plantarflexion and dorsiflexion. The range of motion is estimated. The same technique is used to assess the distal IP joint.

Figure 4.10   Cont'd

Assessing muscle weakness

There is a lack of standardized clinical procedure for assessing muscle strength in the lower limb for patients with RA. Although hand-held dynamometers can be used to assess muscle strength (Helliwell et al. 1987), the most common method is the MRC grading system (Medical Research Council/Guarantors of Brain 1986).

MRC muscle strength grading (see text for reference)

0 – No contraction
1 – Flicker
2 – Muscle contraction possible with gravity eliminated
3 – Muscle contraction possible against gravity
4 – Decreased power but muscle contraction possible against resistance
5 – Normal muscle power against resistance.

Functional limitation is often used as a surrogate for weakness. A limitation of this approach is that patient's perceptions of his/her functional capacity do not always correspond to what they are actually able to do. In preference, studies use functional performance tests such as time taken to walk a specified distance or ability to climb stairs. However, these measures are not purely related to muscle strength and can be influenced by other factors such as presence of vascular or neurological disease.

Muscle size decreases with ageing and this quantitative loss of muscle (referred to as sarcopenia) (Evans 1995) has been documented using ultrasound and other imaging modalities. Young and colleagues measured a 25% and 33% smaller cross-sectional area of the quadriceps in older males and females respectively (aged 70–81 years) when compared to younger individuals (aged 20–29 years) using ultrasound (Young et al. 1984, Young et al. 1985). Muscle strength is reported to reach its peak between the second and third decades, gradually decreasing until about 50 years of age and then begins to decline at a rate of about 15% per decade with more rapid losses above the age of 65 years (Lindle et al. 1997). However there is large overlap and individual variation (Helliwell et al. 1987). When assessing muscle bulk and strength it is important to have an appreciation of the normal age-related changes.

Loss of muscle bulk and strength associated with disuse can occur relatively quickly. There have been a number of studies, which have investigated the extent to which muscle function is affected by short-term unloading (mainly bed rest). Milesi et al. (2000) found that short-term bed rest significantly impaired the isometric and isokinetic function of the ankle plantar flexors and this effect continued during the initial 10 days of recovery. Prolonged bed rest (10 days) also significantly decreased the maximal isometric torque of the quadriceps muscles. However, recovery of the proximal muscles to pre-bedrest control values occurred after 4 days of free walking activity (Berg & Tesch 1996).

There are a number of textbooks that provide detailed descriptions of techniques for testing each muscle in the ankle and foot region. In clinical practice, with time constraints, it is not possible, nor is it necessary, to assess each muscle. Furthermore, there is a lack of evidence to demonstrate the ability to isolate individual muscles. At Leeds, assessment directed towards the major muscle groups that have been shown to have an impact of foot function during gait is summarized in Figure 4.5. In the figure white arrows denote the direction of active movement of a body part by the patient. Black arrows denote the direction of resistance exerted by the examiner. All the plantar flexor muscles are active in all positions of plantar flexion testing so that it is not possible to truly isolate gastrocnemius and soleus.

In most movements of the foot, more than one muscle assists the prime mover to achieve movement. For example, foot inversion is predominantly achieved by tibialis posterior but other muscles include tibialis anterior, flexor digitorum longus, flexor hallucis longus, soleus and extensor hallucis longus. In cases of weakness of tibialis posterior substitution by flexor digitorum longus and flexor hallucis longus can occur, so it is important to make sure the toes remain relaxed as the foot inverts. With posterior tibial tendon dysfunction, the hindfoot does not invert on heel raise and resisted inversion of the fully plantarflexed foot is weakened. The patient will have difficulty or will be unable to perform a single heel rise. Although this procedure is widely described in the literature, no evidence regarding sensitivity or specificity could be found. When performing this examination it must also be noted that pain across the MTP joints may prevent the patient from attempting this test or provide an erroneous result.

VASCULAR ASSESSMENT

Vascular disease is evaluated by a combination of clinical signs and symptoms plus results of non-invasive vascular tests. Signs and symptoms of vascular disease are cold feet, blue toes, intermittent claudication, rest pain, night cramps, poor healing, sparse hair growth on lower limb, skin atrophy, muscle wasting and thickened nails. Simple clinical evaluation of the lower limb provides useful information on the arterial circulation. Cold extremities, absent pulses, pallor on elevation and rubor on dependency are all indicative of significant peripheral vascular disease (Levin 2001). The picture can become complicated in the assessment of a patient with RA due to the following factors:

- Joint deformity and pain associated with RA may greatly decrease a patient's activity level and, as a consequence, they may not walk far enough to bring on symptoms of intermittent claudication.
- Patients may also fail to mention symptoms of rest pain and night cramps because they assume they are related to their arthritis.
- Cold feet and peripheral cyanosis may be related to vasospastic disorders and not arterosclerotic changes within the artery.
- Finally, thinning of the skin and nail changes could be related to medication and muscle wasting related to disuse atrophy.

Palpation of pulses is susceptible to variation between observers and the pulses may be masked by the presence of oedema. Non-invasive measurement of blood pressure in peripheral arteries using Doppler ultrasound provides an objective measurement of vascular status. The most commonly used measurement is the Ankle Brachial Pressure Index (ABPI). The ABPI is calculated by dividing the ankle systolic pressure by the brachial systolic pressure. An ABPI is determined for the left and right legs separately and it provides a measure of severity of arteriosclerosis.

A full description of the procedure along with discussion of the limitations is provided elsewhere (Grasty 1999, Marshall 2004). In brief, the patient should be supine and rested for at least 15 minutes prior to measurement. An appropriately sized sphygmomanometer cuff (ensuring the inflation bladder will fully encircle the limb) is placed around the arm. Ultrasound gel is placed over the approximate location of the brachial pulse. A Doppler with an appropriate probe (usually an 8 MHz probe is sufficient but may need to be changed in the presence of severe oedema) is used to locate the brachial artery. Once a clear audible pulsatile signal is found the sphygmomanometer cuff is inflated until the pulsatile signal disappears and then inflated a further 20 mmHg higher. The cuff is deflated at an approximate rate of 2 mmHg per second until the first Doppler signal returns; this value is the systolic pressure and is recorded. This procedure is repeated in the other arm and at both ankles using both the dorsalis pedis and posterior tibial arteries. The details for calculating the ABPI and guidelines for interpretation can be found below.

The ankle/brachial pressure index

$$\frac{\text{Highest ankle systolic pressure (A)}}{\text{Highest brachial systolic pressure (B)}} = \text{ABPI}$$

The ABPI should be calculated for each leg separately:

(A) – The highest systolic ankle pressure, measurements should be taken at both the dosalis pedis and posterior tibial arteries in each foot.
(B) – The highest brachial artery systolic pressure recorded in both arms. A discrepancy greater than 20 mmHg between arms suggests vascular disease of the upper extremity.

Interpretation of results:

ABPI > 1.3	Suggests calcification
ABPI > 1.0–1.3	Normal
ABPI > 0.8–1.0	Indicative of mild arterial disease
ABPI > 0.5–0.8	Indicative of significant arterial disease
ABPI < 0.5	Indicative of severe arterial disease.

Non-invasive tests probably underestimate the severity of arterial insufficiency. Doppler pressures have been noted to correlate poorly with symptoms and angiographic findings (Caputo et al. 1994). The most reliable non-invasive investigation is analysis of the Doppler waveform, often available from handheld Doppler units (Mercer & Berridge 2000, Caputo et al. 1994, Mercer & Berridge 2000). Vascular testing equipment is not always readily available in outpatient settings. Initial screening is based on palpation of pulses, appearance of limb and patient symptoms. If an abnormality in vascular status is suspected, further investigation is performed.

NEUROLOGICAL ASSESSMENT

As noted in Chapter 3 (extra-articular features) significant neurological involvement may be asymptomatic. Neurophysiological testing may reveal abnormalities in the absence of symptoms. Nevertheless, neurological testing is worthwhile as patients may not find it easy to distinguish neurogenic pain from articular pain and articular deformity may result in abnormalities of sensation.

Directed histories and physical examination of the sensory, motor and autonomic systems show a strong correlation with physiological and morphological abnormalities (Kahn 1992). Clinical measures are relatively subjective and are dependent on the aptitude of the examiner. Limited reliability and reproducibility of clinical measures and the lack of sensitivity to change restrict their use as primary outcome measures.

Neurological evaluations attempt to assess the distribution and severity of motor, sensory and autonomic deficits. The traditional methods include evaluation of pain (pin prick), touch pressure (cotton wool, monofilaments), vibration (tuning fork), temperature, reflexes, proprioception and muscle power and tone. The testing is performed at multiple defined sites on the lower limb, with reference testing on other sites of the body (trunk, face) and comparison between limbs. The examination should be systematic and include nerve root and nerve trunk.

Results of sensory tests are more reproducible if classified as normal or abnormal. However, a limitation of assessing deficits in this way is the lack of sensitivity to change once they have become abnormal. These tests are easily applied to the clinical outpatient setting for screening large numbers of patients. Pinprick, light touch sense, vibration sense and ankle reflex, are validated and shown to be adequate for use in daily practice in screening patients with diabetes (Valk et al. 1992, Valk et al. 2000, Valk et al. 1997). Detailed description of neurological examination is beyond the scope of this chapter and can be found elsewhere (Cavanagh & Ulbrecht 1991, Tanenberg et al. 2001).

There is a general lack of published material on neurological assessment in patients with RA. The rationale and clinical evidence to support many of the tests used to screen and quantify neurological deficits in the lower limb are based on findings from patients with diabetic sensory polyneuropathy and are briefly summarized.

Pain assessment

The sensation of superficial pain can be tested by pinprick using a sterile sharp pin or Neurotip (sharp and dull side). Limitations associated with this type of test include difficulty in standardizing the amount of force applied to the skin. The Neuropen (http//www.mortonmedical.co.uk) has been developed in an attempt to allow the examiner to standardize the amount of force used when applying a Neurotip to the skin. However, data to support superiority of the Neuropen over the standard Neurotip in terms of improved reliability are lacking. The superficial pain test has been shown to have comparable sensitivity and specificity with 5.07 monofilament and vibration perception testing in patients with diabetes (Perkins et al. 2001). Valk and associates compared bedside clinical examination with neurophysiological examination and concluded that impairment of pin prick sense was an early indicator of neurological dysfunction and was an important parameter in the clinical diagnosis of diabetic polyneuropathy (Valk et al. 1992).

Touch pressure

Semmes-Weinstein filaments are used for evaluating touch-pressure sensation. The system consists of a series of graded, pressure sensitive nylon filaments of increasing calibre that buckle at a reproducible stress and can measure patient's cutaneous pressure perception threshold. The filaments are pressed perpendicularly onto the skin until buckling occurs. The thicker the filament the greater the force required for buckling. The Semmes-Weinstein filaments are a simple, inexpensive and effective screening method for the detection of loss of sensation. The vibration perception threshold and Semmes-Weinstein filaments have been shown to be the most effective methods of measuring sensory deficits in the hand and foot (Perkins et al. 2001). Birke and Sims found the 4.17 filament represented the approximate lower limit of normal sensation. To characterize the insensate foot, they recommended the use of the 4.17, 5.07 and 6.10 filaments, bending with 1, 10, and 75 g of force respectively (Birke & Sims 1986). There is no standardized methodology for the use of monofilaments (McGill et al. 1998)

Vibration

Measurement of vibration perception threshold is widely used as a sensitive and reproducible test for assessing peripheral large myelinated fibres. In diabetes mellitus, deficit in this function tends to correlate with, but often precedes abnormality in tendon reflexes, light touch and position sense (American Diabetes Association & American Academy of Neurology 1988). A number of instruments are commonly used for detection of vibration perception thresholds (VPTs), including the Biothesiometer (http//www.biothesiometer.com), neurothesiometer and, less technical but commonly used, tuning fork (C_{128}). It has been shown that VPTs correlate significantly with peripheral nerve function, demonstrated by nerve conduction parameters from the sural nerve and clinical scoring systems of neuropathy status (Franklin et al. 1990, Bowditch et al. 1996, Dyck et al. 1995, Smieja et al. 1999, McNeely et al. 1995).

Temperature

There are a number of commercial systems available to test temperature perception; however, they are not widely adopted in clinical practice. Temperature perception is usually tested in the clinical situation by using test tubes filled with hot and cold water. The patient is instructed to close their eyes and asked to identify the temperature as hot and cold test tubes are placed in a random order in contact with their skin. This method is not standardized and there is a lack of evidence to support this as a method to screen for sensory neuropathy (Bowditch et al. 1996, Dyck et al. 1995, Smieja et al. 1999).

Proprioception

Joint position sense is usually assessed first at the inter-phalangeal joint of the hallux. If the patient is unable to detect changes in joint position at this joint, more proximal joints are tested (the 1st metatarsophalangeal joint and the ankle joint). There is no standardized procedure to test joint position sense. Most clinicians will demonstrate moving the hallux joint up, down and a reference position (neither up nor down). The patient is asked to close their eyes and report if they think the position of the hallux is up, down or in the reference position. It has been noted that joint position sense is preserved until late stages of neuropathy. Valk and associates found that joint position sense was normal in 96.4% of patients who had impaired sural nerve function and found discordance between proprioception and other sensory assessment measures (Valk et al. 1992).

Reflexes

The prevalence of absent ankle reflexes in the normal adult population is uncertain, but there is no doubt that they are harder to elicit with increasing age (Bowditch et al. 1996). The frequency of decreased or absent ankle reflexes exceeds 5% in healthy subjects older than 50 years (Dyck et al. 1995). The reflexes at the ankle and knee are usually tested for screening people with diabetes and are usually classified as present, present with reinforcement or absent. The ankle reflex has been shown to be reproducible and has moderate agreement with the Semmes–Weinstein monofilament (Smieja et al. 1999). McNeely and associates found absence of the Achilles tendon reflexes to be a significant independent predictor for foot ulceration in diabetes (McNeely et al. 1995). Similar figures for a population of people with RA are not yet available.

SUMMARY

Clinical assessment of the foot and ankle in people with rheumatoid arthritis should be systematic and thorough and, preferably, follow standard protocols. Joint deformity and associated soft-tissue contracture can make assessment of muscle tone, power and reflexes difficult. In cases where history and brief examination suggests some neurological deficit, further assessment is undertaken. It is recommended that the 10 g Semmes–Weinstein filament is used to screen for sensory loss.

References

American Diabetes Association & American Academy of Neurology Report and recommendations of the San Antonio conference on diabetic neuropathy (Consensus statement). Diabetes Care 1988; 11: 592–597.

American Orthopaedic Foot & Ankle Society AOFAS Clinical rating system. Foot & Ankle International 1994; 15(7).

Balint GP Foot and ankle disorders. Best Practice & Research Clinical Rheumatology 2003; 17(1): 87–111.

Berg HE and Tesch PA Changes in muscle function in response to 10 days of lower limb unloading in humans. Acta Physiologica Scandinavica 1996; 157: 63–70.

Bickley LS and Szilagyi PG Bates' Guide to Clinical Examination and History Taking, 8th edn, Lippincott Williams & Wilkins, Philadelphia, 2003.

Birke JA and Sims DS Plantar sensory threshold in the ulcerative foot. Leprosy Review 1986; 57(3): 261–267.

Boone DC., Azen SP, Lin CM., Spence C., Baron C and Lee L Reliability of goniometric measurements. Physical Therapy 1978; 58(11): 1355–1390.

Bouysett M., Tavernier T, Tebib J, Noel E, Tillman K, Eulry F and Bouvier M CT and MRI evaluation of tenosynovitis of the rheumatoid hindfoot. Clinical Rheumatology 1995; 14(3): 303–307.

Bowditch MG, Sanderson P and Livesey JP The significance of an absent ankle reflex. Journal of Bone and Joint Surgery (B) 1996; 78B(2): 276–279.

Buckley RE and Hunt DV Reliability of clinical measurement of subtalar joint movement. Foot & Ankle International 1997; 18(4): 229–232.

Burns SL, Leese GP and McMurdo MET Older people and ill fitting shoes. Postgraduate Medical Journal 2002; (78): 344–346.

Buskila D, Langevitz P, Gladman DD, Urowitz S and Smythe HA Patients with rheumatoid arthritis are more tender than those with psoriatic arthritis. Journal of Rheumatology 1992; 19(7): 1115–1119.

Caputo GM, Cavanagh PR, Ulbrecht JS, Gibbons GW and Karchmer AW Assessment and management of foot disease in patients with diabetes. New England Journal of Medicine 1994; 331(13): 854–860.

Cavanagh PR and Ulbrecht JS Biomechanics of the diabetic foot: a quantitative approach to the assessment of neuropathy, deformity and plantar pressure. In: Jahss MH (ed.) Disorders of the Foot and Ankle: Medical and Surgical Management, 2nd edn. WB Saunders Company, Philadelphia, 1991; 1864–1907.

Coady D, Walker DJ and Kay L Regional examination of the musculoskeletal system (REMS). Rheumatology 2004; 43: 633–639.

de Palmer L, Santucci A, Verdenelli A, Paladini P and Ventura A Arthroscopic arthrodesis of the ankle in rheumatoid patients. Foot & Ankle Surgery 2000; 6(4): 261.

Doherty M, Abawi J and Pattrick M Audit of medical inpatient examination: a cry from the joint. Journal of Royal College of Physicians 1990; 24: 115–118.

Doherty M and Doherty J Clinical Examination in Rheumatology. Wolfe Publishing Ltd, Aylesbury, 1992.

Dyck PJ, Litchy WJ, Lehman KA, Hokanson JL, Low PA and O'Brien PC Variables influencing neuropathic endpoints: the Rochester Diabetic Neuropathy Study of Healthy Subjects. Neurology 1995; 45(6): 1115–1121.

Ekstrand J, Wiktorsson M, Oberg B and Gillquist J Lower extremity goniometric measurements: a study to determine their reliability. Archives of Physical Medicine and Rehabilitation 1982; 63(4): 171–175.

Evans WJ What is sarcopenia? Journal of Gerontology 1995; 55A(Spec No): 5–8.

Franklin GM, Kahn LB, Bacter J, Marshall JA and Hamman RF Sensory neuropathy in non-insulin dependent diabetes mellitus. The San Luis study. American Journal of Epidemiology 1990; 131: 633–643.

Gerecz–Simon EM., Tunks ER, Heale JA, Kean WF and Buchanan WW Measurement of pain threshold in patients with rheumatoid arthritis, osteoarthritis, ankylosing spondylitis, and healthy controls. Clinical Rheumatology 1989; 8(4): 467–474.

Gramling SE and Elliot TR Efficient pain assessment in clinical settings. Behaviour Research and Therapy 1992; 30: 71–73.

Grasty MS Use of hand held Doppler to detect peripheral vascular disease. The Diabetic Foot 1999; 2(1): 18–22.

Guyton GP Theoretical limitations of the AOFAS scoring systems: An analysis using Monte Carlo modeling. Foot & Ankle International 2001; 22(10): 779–787.

Hamill J, Bates BT, Knutzen KM and Kirkpatrick GM Relationship between selected static and dynamic lower exremity measures Clinical Biomechanics 1989; 4(4): 217–225.

Harrison BJ and Symmons DP Early inflammatory polyarthritis: results from the Norfolk Arthritis Register with a review of the literature II. Outcome at three years. Rheumatology 2000; 39: 939–949.

Helliwell P, Howe A and Wright V Functional assessment of the hand: reproducibility, and utility of a new system for measuring strength. Annals of the Rheumatic Diseases 1987; 46: 203–208.

Houssien DA., Stucki G and Scott DL A patient-derived disease activity score can substitute for a physician-derived disease activity score in clinical research. Rheumatology 1999; 38: 48–52.

Huskisson EC and Dudley Hart F Pain threshold in arthritis. British Medical Journal 1972; 28: 193–195.

Kahn R Proceedings of a conference on standardized measures in diabetic neuropathy. Clinical measures. Diabetes Care 1992; 15(Suppl 3): 1081–1083.

Karim Z, Wakefield RJ, Conaghan PG et al. The impact of ultrasonography on diagnosis and management of patients with musculoskeletal conditions. Arthritis and Rheumatism 2001; 44: 2932–2933.

Levin ME Pathogenesis and general management of foot lesions in the diabetic patient. In: Bowker JH, Pfeifer MA (eds) Levin and O'Neals The Diabetic Foot, 6th edn. Mosby, St Louis 1992; 219–260.

Lindle RS, Metter EJ, Lynch NA, Fleg JL, Fozard JL, Tobin J, Roy TA and Hurley BF Age and gender comparisons of muscle strength in 654 women and men aged 20–93 yr. Journal of Applied Physiology 1997; 83: 1581–1587.

Machold KP, Stamm TA and Elberg GJM Very recent onset arthritis – clinical, laboratory and radiological findings during the first year of disease. Journal of Rheumatology 2002; 29: 2278–2287.

Marshall C The ankle:brachial pressure index. A critical appraisal. British Journal of Podiatry 2004; 7(4): 93–95.

McGill M, Molyneaux L and Yue DK Use of the Semmes–Weinstein 5.07/10 gram monofilament: the long and short of it. Diabetic Medicine 1998; 15: 615–617.

McNeely MJ, Boyko EJ, Ahroni JH, Stensel VL, Reiber GE, Smith DG and Pecoraro RF The independent contributions of diabetic neuropathy and vasculopathy in foot ulceration. How great are the risks? Diabetes Care 1995; 18(2): 216–219.

McPoil TG and Cornwall MW Relationship between neutral subtalar joint position and pattern of rearfoot motion during walking. Foot & Ankle 1994; 15(3):141–145.

McPoil TG and Cornwall MW Relationship between three static angles of the rearfoot and the pattern of rearfoot motion during walking. Journal of Orthopaedics Sports Physical Therapy 1996; 23(6): 370–375.

Medical Research Council/Guarantors of Brain Aids to the examination of the peripheral nervous system Baillière Tindall, London, 1996.

Menz HB Alternative techniques for the clinical assessment of foot pronation. Journal of the American Podiatric Medical Association 1998; 88(3): 119–129.

Mercer KG and Berridge DC Peripheral vascular disease and vascular reconstruction. In: Boulton AJM, Connor H, Cavanagh PR (eds). The foot in diabetes, 3rd edn. John Wiley & Sons Ltd, Chichester, 2000; 215–233.

Milesi S, Capelli C, Denoth J, Hutchinson T and Stussi E Effect of 17 days bedrest on the maximal voluntary isometric torque and neuromuscular activation of the plantar and dorsal flexors of the ankle. European Journal of Applied Physiology 2000; 82: 197–205.

Mulcahy D, Daniels TR, Lau JT, Boyle E and Bogoch E Rheumatoid forefoot deformity: a comparison study of 2 functional methods of reconstruction. Journal of Rheumatology 2003; 30(7): 1440–1450.

Nishikawa M, Tomita T, Fujii M et al. Total ankle replacement in rheumatoid arthritis. International Orthopaedics 2004; 28(2): 123–126.

Perkins BA, Olaleye D, Zinman B and Bril V Simple screening tests for peripheral neuropathy in the diabetes clinic. Diabetes Care 2000; 24(2): 250–256.

Platto MJ, O'Connell PG, Hicks JE and Gerber LH The relationship of pain and deformity of the rheumatoid foot to gait and an index of functional ambulation. Journal of Rheumatology 1991; 18(1): 38–43.

Razeghi M and Batt ME Foot type classification: a critical review of current methods. Gait & Posture 2002; 15: 282–291.

Reddy PV, Vaid MA and Child DF Diabetes and incorrectly fitting shoes. Practical Diabetes 1989; 6: 16–18.

Root ML, Orien WP and Weed JH Normal and abnormal function of the foot, clinical biomechanics. Clinical Biomechanical Corporation, Los Angeles, 1977.

Scott DL, Choy EH, Greeves A, Isenberg D, Kassinor D and Rankin E Standardising joint assessment in rheumatoid arthritis. Clinical Rheumatology 1996; 15(6): 579–582.

Smieja M., Hunt DL, Edelman D, Etchells E, Cornuz J and Simel DL Clinical examination for the detection of protective sensation in feet of diabetic patients. International Cooperative Group for Clinical Examination Research. Journal of General Internal Medicine 1996; 14(7): 418–424.

Smolen JS, Breedveld FC and Ebrel G Validity and reliability of the twenty-eight-joint count for the assessment of rheumatoid arthritis activity. Arthritis & Rheumatism 1995; 38: 38–43.

Stewart MW, Palmer DG, Knight RG and Ilighton J A self-report articular index: relationship to variations in mood and disease activity measures. British Journal of Rheumatology 1993; 32: 631–632.

Stucki G, Stucki, S, Bruhlmann P, Maus, S and Michel BA Comparison of the validity and reliability of self-reported articular indices. British Journal of Rheumatology 1995; 34: 760–766.

Tanenberg RJ, Schumer MP, Greene DA and Pfeifer MA Neuropathic problems of the lower extremity in diabetic patients. In: Bowker JH, Pfeifer MA (eds). Levin and O'Neals The Diabetic Foot, 6th edn. Mosby, St Louis, 2001; 33–64.

Valk GD, de Sonnaville J and van Houtum WH The assessment of diabetic polyneuropathy in daily clinical practice: reproducibility and validity of Semmes – Weinstein monofilaments examination and clinical neurological examination. Muscle & Nerve 1997; 20: 116–118.

Valk GD, Grootenhuis PA, van Eijk JThM, Bouter LM and Bertelsmann FW Methods for assessing diabetic polyneuropathy: validity and reproducibility of the measurement of sensory symptom severity and nerve function tests. Diabetes Research and Clinical Practice 2000; 47: 87–95.

Valk GD, Nauta JJP, Strijers RLM and Bertelsmann FW Clinical examination versus neurophysiological examination in the diagnosis of diabetic polyneuropathy. Diabetic Medicine 1992; 9: 717–721.

Walker JS and Carmody JJ Experimental pain in healthy human subjects: gender differences in nociception and in response to ibuprofen. Anesthesia and Analgesia 1998; 86: 1257–1262.

Wylie-Rosett JF, Walker EA, Shamoon H, Engel S, Basch C and Zybert P Assessment of documented foot examinations for patients with diabetes in inner-city primary care clinics. Archives of Family Medicine 1995; 4(1): 46–50.

Young A, Stokes M and Crowe M Size and strength of the quadriceps muscles of old and young women. European Journal of Clinical Investment 1984; 14: 282–287.

Young A, Stokes M and Crowe M The size and strength of the quadriceps muscle of young and old men. Clinical Physiology 1985; 5: 145–154.

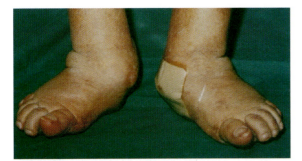

Color Plate 1.3 Typical rear-foot deformity in established rheumatoid arthritis. Note the valgus heel position, loss of longitudinal arch and prominence of navicular bone.

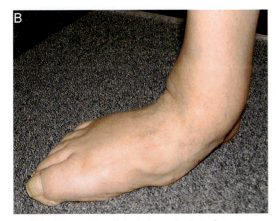

Color Plate 2.12 The clinical picture is that of severe pes planovalgus (B).

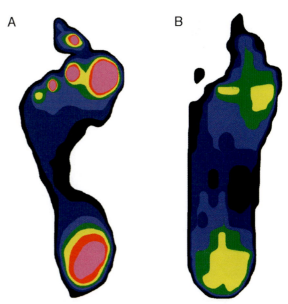

Color Plate 2.20 Plantar pressure distribution pattern from a typical patient with rheumatoid arthritis recorded from (A) platform device and (B) in-shoe device. Both techniques capture the lack of lesser toe contact, Pressure distribution is similar over the metatarsal head region, but the superior spatial resolution of the platform device captures the sharp focal pressure in the middle three metatarsal heads. Furthermore, the in-shoe system is measured at the interface of the foot and contoured custom orthosis, hence, the reduced forefoot pressures and the increased contact are in the midfoot region in comparison with the platform-based technique.

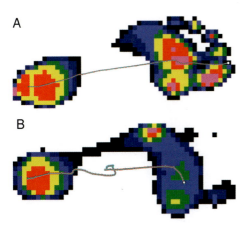

Color Plate 2.16 Sagittal plane ankle joint net muscular moments, power profiles and pressure distribution pattern with COP overlaid in (A) able-bodied adult matched with (B) rheumatoid arthritis case (as presented in Figure 2.15).

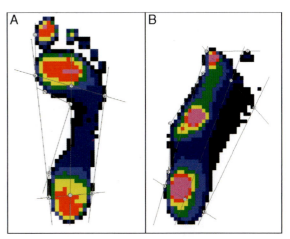

Color Plate 2.21 Foot geometry parameters taken from the footprint of (A) able-bodied subject and (B) patient with severe pes planovalgus. A standard algorithm defines each parameter as a distance or angle measurements taken from anatomically relevant reference lines overlaid on the pressure pattern.

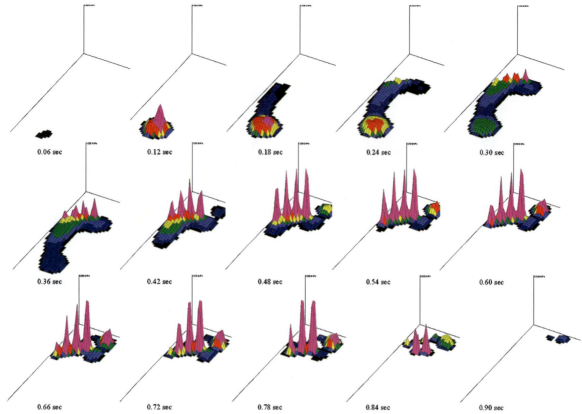

Color Plate 2.22 Plantar pressure distribution pattern in a patient with rheumatoid arthritis. The first frame in the upper left corner is recorded shortly after heel-strike (0.06 s) and then presented every 0.06 s until toe-off in the lower right frame (0.09 s).

A

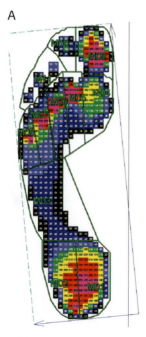

Color Plate 2.23 (A) masking technique for regional pressure analysis.

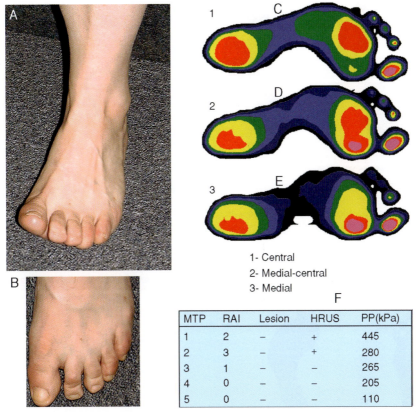

1- Central
2- Medial-central
3- Medial

MTP	RAI	Lesion	HRUS	PP(kPa)
1	2	–	+	445
2	3	–	+	280
3	1	–	–	265
4	0	–	–	205
5	0	–	–	110

Color Plate 2.25 Patient with early disease off-loading the medial forefoot region, which was both tender and inflamed. The daylight sign is seen on standing at the 1st and 2nd toe clefts. The pressure distribution pattern is variable ranging from central to medial. The symptoms (RAI: Ritchie Articular Index scores for tenderness ranging in severity from 0 to 3), presence of inflammation (HRUS: high-resolution ultrasound), and peak plantar pressure (PP) values for each MTP joint are presented in the table.

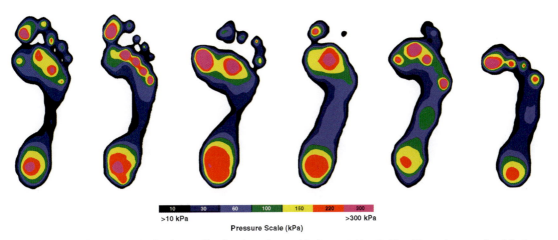

Color Plate 2.26 Peak pressure distribution profiles for six patients with rheumatoid arthritis with varying severity of foot impairment characterized from left to right with increasing loss of toe function and decreased forefoot contact area.

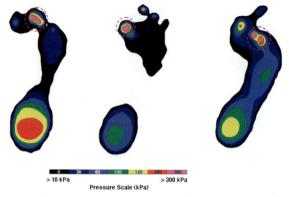

> 10 kPa   > 300 kPa

Pressure Scale (kPa)

Color Plate 2.27 Peak pressure distribution profiles for three patients with forefoot ulceration. Ulcer sites are indicated with a red circle.

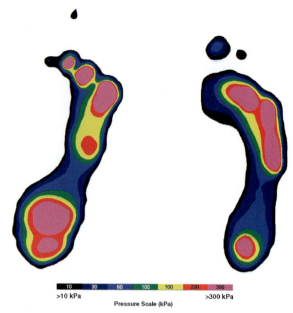

>10 kPa   >300 kPa

Pressure Scale (kPa)

Color Plate 2.30 Lateral off-loading the painful medial forefoot region in two patients with rheumatoid arthritis.

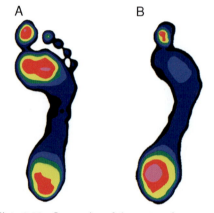

A   B

Color Plate 2.29 Progression of the centre of pressure (COP) through the foot. The velocity of the COP is plotted as a function of time in (A) a typical able-bodied individual and (B) a patient with severe forefoot impairment (pain located to the central MTP joints with overlying callosities and claw toe deformity).

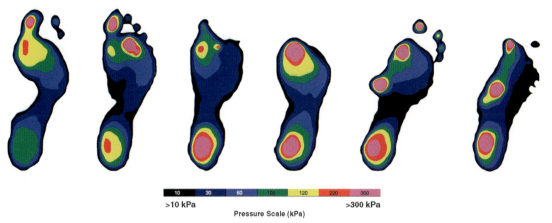

Color Plate 2.32 Peak pressure distribution profiles for six patients with varying severity of pes planovalgus.

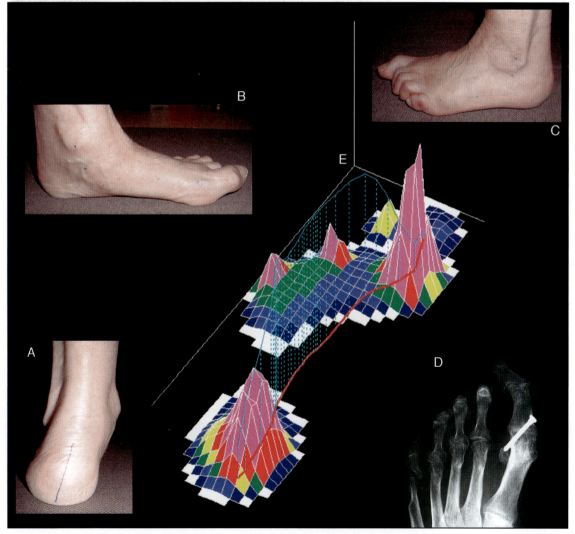

Color Plate 2.33 (A) The heel is in valgus. (B) The medial longitudinal arch height is low but not fully collapsed and the midfoot joints are stiff. (C) The lesser toes are retracted, deformed and non-weight bearing. (D) The 1st MTP is arthrodesed, the 2nd, 3rd and 4th MTP joints are severely eroded, and the 5th MTP has undergone excision of the metatarsal head and proximal phalanx. (E) Peak pressure profile with vertical ground reaction and centre-of-pressure line superimposed.

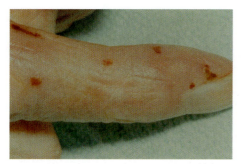

Color Plate 3.3   Small vessel digital arteries manifesting as nail fold infarcts.

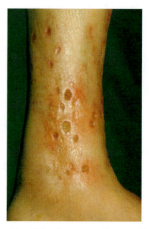

Color Plate 3.6   Vasulitic ulcers are often multiple with sharply demarcated punched out edges.

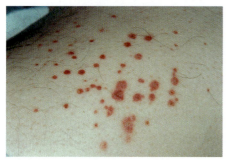

Color Plate 3.4   Inflammation of venules and small arteries usually manifests as a purpuric rash.

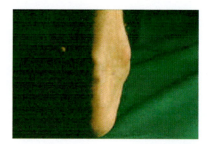

Color Plate 3.7   Rheumatoid nodules in the Achilles tendon.

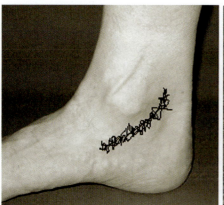
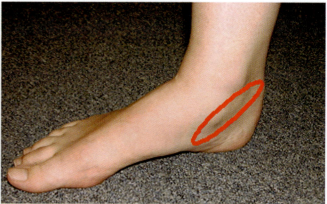

Color Plate 4.2   This patient was referred to the podiatry department with persistent medial ankle pain. She had been diagnosed with rheumatoid arthritis for 18 months and her disease activity was generally low. A copy of her completed foot map can be seen above. The photograph shows obvious swelling along the muscle tendon of tibialis posterior. The area was painful and felt warm and 'boggy' on palpation. The patient has a low medial arch profile and failure of the calcaneus to invert when standing on tiptoe. High-resolution ultrasound scanning showed tibialis posterior tenosynovitis. Provision of functional orthoses along with an ultrasound guided corticosteroid injection fully resolved the tenosynovitis.

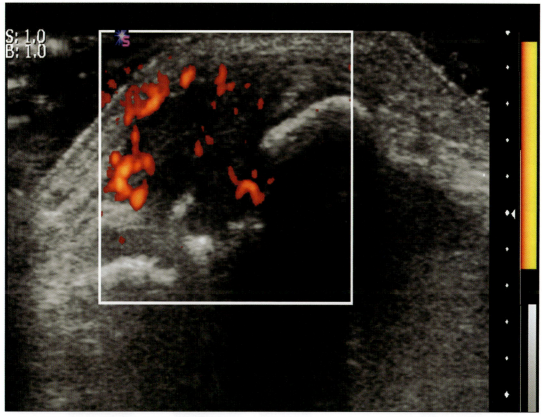

Color Plate 5.4   Sagittal power Doppler sonogram. There is disruption of the bone cortex in keeping with erosion. Hypoechoic synovitis is present adjacent to and within the erosion. This synovial tissue is vascularized as demonstrated by power Doppler.

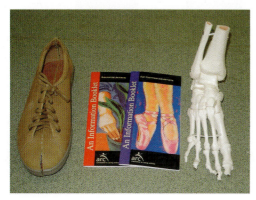

Color Plate 6.22   Patient education tools.

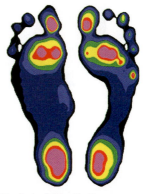

Color Plate 6.25   Early rigid orthotic management in an early case of rheumatoid arthritis. Acquired pes planovalgus in the early stages of rheumatoid arthritis. See text for details.

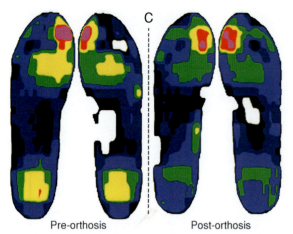

Pre-orthosis   Post-orthosis

Color Plate 6.26 Pre- and post-orthosis in-shoe pressure profiles are shown (C).

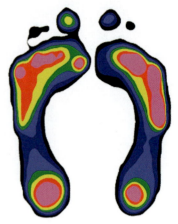

Color Plate 6.27 Management of varus heel deformity with orthoses and footwear modifications. See text for details.

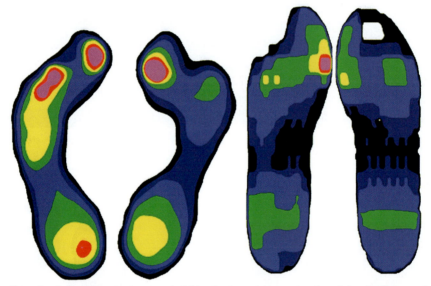

Color Plate 6.28 Example of management using a semi-rigid orthosis to accommodate foot deformity. See text for details.

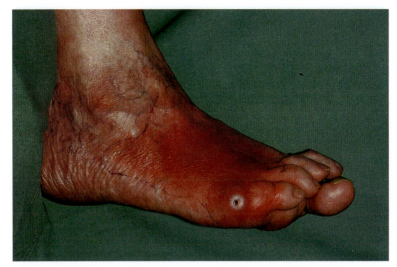

Color Plate 6.33 Rapid spreading infection in a patient currently on biological therapy. Cellulitis spread to this extent within a 24-h period.

Chapter 5

Imaging of the foot and ankle in rheumatoid arthritis

Dr S J McKie and Dr P J O'Connor

INTRODUCTION: THE IMPORTANCE OF IMAGING

Rheumatoid arthritis (RA) is a chronic progressive systemic inflammatory disease of synovial tissue. Its aetiology is poorly understood, although autoimmune and biomechanical factors are implicated. The overall incidence in the general population is in the region of 1% (Symmons et al. 2002, Lawrence et al. 1998). Females are affected approximately three times more commonly than males (Symmons et al. 2002).

Approximately 90% of patients have involvement of the foot or ankle at some point during their disease and 20% of patients present with foot problems (Resnick 2002). Symptoms of the foot usually precede the hands and are affected more severely. Therefore, not only are the feet frequently affected by RA, but also the symptoms often predate other areas.

Plain film radiography is the mainstay of imaging of the ankle and foot. In recent years the use of other imaging modalities such as ultrasound (U/S) and magnetic resonance imaging (MRI) have become more important and provide an improved abnormality detection rate due to their ability to image in multiple planes rather than the 2D representation seen with plain film (McGonagle et al. 2001). They are important in not only the diagnosis, but also the follow-up and evaluation of RA (Ostergaard and Szkudlarek 2003). Imaging also plays a pivotal role in diagnosis confirmation in patients with confusing presentations or negative serology.

Because bone and cartilage destruction is largely irreversible, a definite radiological diagnosis can drastically alter the patient's prognosis. The goal of the rheumatologist is to arrest the disease before this stage.

Clinical examination is often negative in the early stage of RA. MRI and U/S can both detect subclinical disease (Wakefield et al. 2004). Twenty per cent of patients presenting with sub-clinical disease can be shown to have synovitis at presentation, allowing earlier treatment options (Wakefield et al. 2004). Synovitis and erosive change are used to arbitrate diagnosis and treatment protocols. They are the hall-marks of disease progression and severity.

Present-day treatment with pharmacological agents such as biologics is dependent on a firm diagnosis of erosive disease or synovitis. There is a trend to treat rheumatoid disease earlier and more aggressively, often with expensive pharmacological agents, in order to improve outcome levels and reduce morbidity. Disease-modifying drugs can then be initiated early in a preventative and potentially curative manner. Imaging can help to confirm the diagnosis at the sub-clinical stage (Ostergaard et al. 1996). The most appropriate modality depends on the stage of disease and clinical question to be addressed.

Periarticular soft-tissue disease is a consequence of the joint inflammatory process; MRI and U/S are also of value in the assessment of the extrarticular pathology.

This chapter describes the common pathological changes and the techniques used to assess rheumatoid disease of the foot and ankle.

HOW TO LOOK FOR RHEUMATOID DISEASE OF THE FOOT AND ANKLE

Intraarticular disease

How to detect erosions
Bone erosions are cortical breaks that are the corner-stone of the diagnosis of inflammatory arthropathy and one of the most important prognostic indicators (Winalski 1996). Erosions are, however, only identified in 40% of new-onset RA and so cannot be relied upon to give a definitive diagnosis (Conaghan 2003).

Erosions on radiographs are characterized by corti-cal discontinuity with diagnosis reliant on a tangential orientation of the X-ray beam to the eroded cortex (Fig. 5.1). Where erosion is not projected tangentially, a clear cortical break is not demonstrated. These en-face erosions are seen as focal areas of reduced bone density (Fig. 5.2). Erosion activity can be determined by assessing the erosion margin. Inactive and active erosions are distinguished by sclerotic and non-sclerotic margins (Fig. 5.1). Plain radiography is, how-ever, an insensitive tool in the detection of erosions, which are only detected when a substantial amount of bone is destroyed. It may take months or years for the plain film to detect the osseus changes of the disease.

This lack of sensitivity results in a significant temporal delay between presentation and radiological diagno-sis, a delay that is potentially detrimental to patient morbidity. Poor peripheral bone density or overexpo-sure of the radiograph can result in the artefactual impression of cortical disruption.

MRI is, however, considered the gold standard in the detection of erosive disease (Tehranzadeh et al. 2004). MRI detects approximately three times as many erosions than the plain radiograph and at an earlier stage. The multiplanar imaging utilized in MRI is, in part, responsible for the improved erosion detection rate (McQueen 2000). It is only on rare occasions that plain film detects erosion not visualized with MRI.

It is apparent that only one in four erosions detected by MRI actually progress to erosions seen on the plain radiograph. However, if a large amount of erosion is visualized on MRI then the likelihood of later plain film erosive detection is higher (McQueen et al. 2001, Ory, 2003).

MRI produces more false positives due to the mul-tiple planes. Contrast enhancement should routinely be employed to increase diagnostic accuracy.

Bone-marrow oedema is often seen as a precursor of future erosion and can be used to predict change (McQueen et al. 2003).

Erosions appear as areas of cortical discontinuity on MRI. They are of low signal on T1 weighted in the marrow adjacent to the bony surface or under the cartilage. The contents are fluid or synovium and are bright on T2. Erosions are seen to enhance with gadolinium contrast. Longitudinal follow-up of ero-sions can, however, be difficult due to repositioning error (Fig. 5.3) (Winalski 1996).

Ultrasound is also of use in the detection of ero-sions. It has the advantage of being a multiplanar modality and is imaged in real time. It is best utilized in site-specific joints, when only one or two joints require to be imaged and as an adjunct to plain radiography (Fig. 5.4).

It can detect 6.5 times as many erosions in 7.5 times as many patients in early RA compared with 3.4 times as many erosions in 2.7 times as many patients in late RA than plain film (Wakefield et al. 2000).

In addition, it has been shown to be useful in site specific asymptomatic joints (e.g. MTP), which fre-quently reveal erosive change (Lopez-Ben et al. 2004).

How to detect synovitis
The histo-pathological hallmark of RA has been described in Chapter 1. Synovial inflammation is the primary pathological process. Synovitis predates bone damage and the amount of synovitis predicts future bone damage.

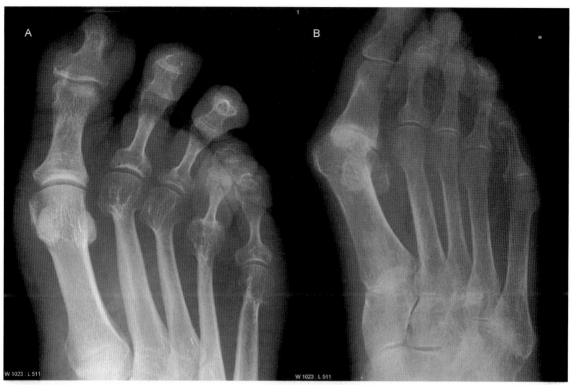

Figure 5.1   AP forefoot radiographs. This demonstrates typical rheumatoid changes in the forefoot mainly affecting the fourth and fifth MTP joints. (A) Shows a relatively inactive disease with well-defined somewhat sclerotic margins to the erosions. (B) Shows inactive disease characterized by decreased peri-articular bone density with ill-defined erosion.

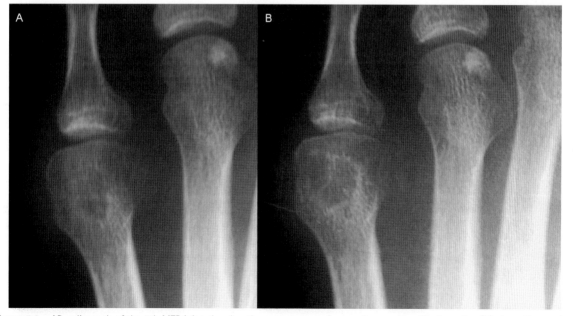

Figure 5.2   AP radiograph of the 5th MTP joint showing the appearances of an en-face erosion. The base-line (A) shows the erosion as a focal lucency within the metatarsal head that enlarges on the follow-up film 6 months later (B).

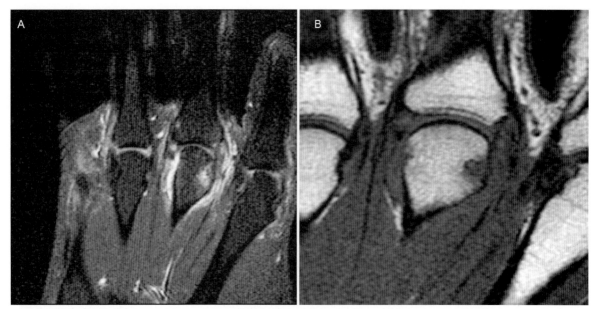

Figure 5.3   MR demonstration of early erosion. (A) T2 fat suppressed coronal scan with synovitis and effusion within the joint associated with bone-marrow oedema. (B) T1 weighted coronal MR scanning shows loss of cortical definition with the area of bone marrow oedema in keeping with an associated erosion.

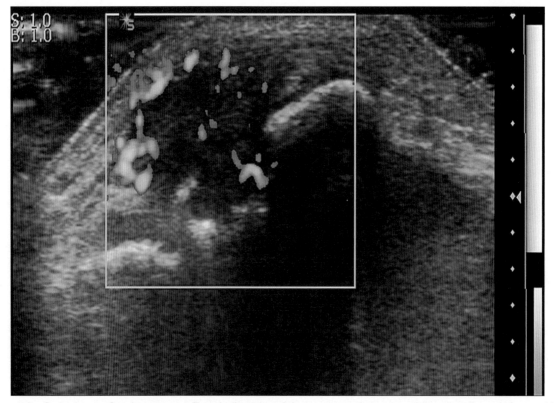

Figure 5.4   Sagittal power Doppler sonogram. There is disruption of the bone cortex in keeping with erosion. Hypoechoic synovitis is present adjacent to and within the erosion. This synovial tissue is vascularized as demonstrated by power Doppler.

Imaging of the synovium allows direct assessment of the therapeutically targeted abnormality. In addition to its ability to detect erosive change, MRI is considered the gold standard at detecting synovitis. It is able to detect the abnormally inflamed synovium before the irreparable cartilage destruction. It is significantly more sensitive than clinical examination and will show synovial pathology before a plain film (Goupille et al. 2001).

Normal synovium is difficult to differentiate from fluid. It does, however, have a very slightly lower signal on T2 and differentiation is possible on a heavily weighted T2 study. Synovium is of intermediate signal on T1.

Synovium enhances after intravenous injection of gadolinium. The degree of enhancement is proportional to its blood supply, the extracellular fliud volume and capillary permeability (Fig. 5.5). Optimal synovial enhancement occurs within 5 min. After this window, the effusion within a joint will start to enhance, which may overestimate the volume of synovium present. Synovial fluid enhancement occurs later than the synovium, which then plateaus and persists for about 1 h (Ostergaard and Klarlund 2001). Data from the joint, therefore, requires to be collected relatively early in order to be able to differentiate synovial tissue from synovial fluid. MRI can help characterize the nature of the synovitis with fibrous pannous enhancing more slowly on T1 weighted contrast enhanced dynamic sequences than acutely inflamed synovium.

The degree of enhancement of the synovium is a secondary indicator of synovial inflammation. Dynamic MRI allows evaluation of the degree and rate of synovial enhancement to be assessed. Early enhancement and high rate of enhancement of the synovium correlates well with inflammatory markers and with the histological asssessment of synovitis. (Ostergaard et al. 1998).

Quantitative measurements can also be used to measure the volume of synovium within the capsule (Ostergaard et al. 1999). The volume can be measured by manual outline or computer processing (Ostergaard 1997). Both techniques are of use in the early detection, predictor of disease severity and follow-up to assess joint response and remission. The quantification of the synovitis correlates well with the clinical signs of inflammation, the histopathology assessed by biopsy and the rate of progression of the disease (Ostergaard et al. 1997, Ostergaard et al. 1999).

These qualitative and quantitative measures of synovial disease are, however, at present experimental techniques that are not yet utilized in routine clinical practice.

MRI scoring is a method of semi-quantifying disease severity on the basis of erosive disease, synovitis

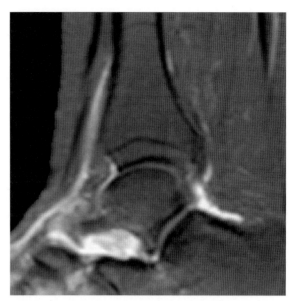

Figure 5.5 Sagittal T1 weighted fat suppressed post iv gadolinium image showing synovitis in the subtalar joint.

and bone oedema. Outcome determined by OMERACT is the recommended scoring system for synovitis and bone damage (Ostergaard et al. 2003). The scores correlate well with the clinical state and have become the gold standard in monitoring disease activity. These scoring systems have been developed for the hand, but are easily transferable to the assessment of metatarsophalangeal joint disease.

Ultrasound can also detect synovitis. Synovium is not seen at ultrasound unless it is abnormal. Synovial tissue, however, usually appears hypoechoic and is defined by OMERACT as 'hypoechogenic thickened intra-articular tissue that is non-displaceable and poorly compressible which may exhibit Doppler signal.'

It can be differentiated from joint effusion by pressure that will disperse an effusion, but distort synovium (Fig. 5.6) (O'Connor 2002). Differentiating synovitis from fluid may, however, be difficult, although colour or power Doppler can be used to visualize the increased vascularity in hyperaemic synovitis (Rubin 1999).

The volume of synovium within a joint can also be assessed with ultrasound. It is limited, however, by technical factors and reproducibility. Doppler U/S, however, appears to provide a potential method of semi-quantitative assessment of synovial tissue, though the data are preliminary and sometimes conflicting (Szkudlarek et al. 2003, Szkudlarek et al. 2001, Newman et al. 1996).

U/S allows direct assessment of the synovium and can visualize erosions. It images in real time with high

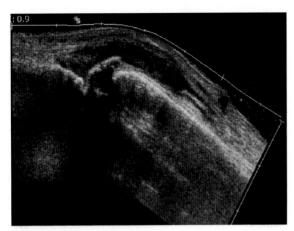

Figure 5.6   Sagittal grey scale sonogram demonstrating dorsal erosion associated with synovitis.

resolution and has advantages over MRI in cost savings, multisite assessment and patient compliance, which make a compelling argument for the use of U/S in the assessment of RA (O'Connor 2002). U/S scoring systems are currently being evaluated by the OMERACT group.

How to detect a joint effusion

U/S and MRI can both detect joint effusions with high sensitivity. U/S, however, is deemed the gold standard in the accessible joint. Joint effusions are anechoic with distal acoustic enhancement. Joint motion is particularly important in the demonstration of small joint effusions. Active or passive joint movement whilst scanning causes redistribution of any fluid present and can push fluid into ultrasonically visible areas (O'Connor 2002).

Simple fluid is anechoic with no internal echoes. The fluid is compressible and can be moved with probe pressure and demonstrates distal acoustic enhancement with no demonstrable vascularity.

The presence of effusion is a sensitive predictor of joint disease, but is unfortunately completely non-specific (O'Connor 2002). The main therapeutic impact is in the exclusion of intra-articular fluid, making artic-ular disease much less likely. This is especially impor-tant in the setting of infection where the absence of joint effusion effectively excludes septic arthritis. Ultrasound has a role in this setting allowing guided aspiration or wash-out of the joint to be performed, helping differen-tiate synovitis, complex fluid and infection.

Extraarticular disease

How to detect tendon and ligament pathology

Tendon pathology and tenosynovitis are commonly due to the direct effects of synovial inflammation. Eroded bone may also fray tendons by a process of

attrition and periarticular inflammation, thus weaken-ing ligaments and tendons. Tendon rupture is a serious consequence of tenosynovitis and may further exacerbate an already unstable joint

U/S is an excellent tool in the assessment of the tendons particularly around the ankle (Martinoli et al. 2002, Rawool and Nazarian 2000). Full- and partial-thickness tears are readily diagnosed. Tendons should be examined routinely in both the transverse and longitudinal planes.

Tendons have an organized fibrillar appearance. Tendinopathy manifests itself as loss of the normal organized tendon structure with increased tendon thickness. Increasing amounts of glycoprotein matrix produce an increase in the water content of the tendon, fibroblast and tenocyte proliferation and neovascular-ization. The tendon becomes more hypoechoic due to the increased water content and heterogenous, tissue (O'Connor 2002). Neovascularity during the reparative process in tendinopathy can also be demonstrated with power or colour Doppler; excess pressure may, how-ever, obliterate subtle blood flow. Neovascularization is related to an unfavourable outcome.

Tenosynovitis may be evident with fluid or syn-ovial thickening within the synovial sheath. Artefacts are, however, common in musculoskeletal ultrasound. Anisotropy and beam edge artefacts are important causes of potential error. Linear array ultrasound probes are, however, particularly prone to anisotropy. Anisotropy results from tissues that contain multiple parallel linear sound interfaces such as tendons or muscles that cause preferential reflection of the beam in one direction. If the probe is not perpendicular to the fibre axis, then it results in a dramatic reduction in echogenicity of the tissue. Angulation of the probe or beam steering can overcome the artefact (Connolly et al. 2001). Scrupulous technique must be adopted to ensure the ligament or tendon is imaged parallel to the face of the ultrasound transducer (O'Connor 2002).

Beam edge artefact results in a characteristic appearance at the edge of particularly large tendons, such as the Achilles, with loss of signal and distal acoustic shadowing that can mimic or obscure fluid or inflammation in the paratenon.

Both anisotropy and beam edge artefact may mimic disease to the unwary ultrasonologist and represents a pitfall in the ultrasound assessment of tendons and ligaments.

Ligaments are also vulnerable to anisotropy. Dynamic stressing of ligaments, such as the lateral col-lateral ligament of the ankle, can be used to assess its integrity and joint stability with U/S.

MRI is also used in the assessment of ligaments and tendons in the foot and ankle. It is, however, a static examination and stressing of the structure is not possible. It provides exquisite images of the anatomy of both tendons and ligaments, and is highly sensitive at exploring the full spectrum of tendon pathologies.

Tendons are homogenously of low signal on all MRI sequences. T1, T2* and STIR sequences are often used in several planes to optimize imaging. Tendinopathy results in intermediate signal, thickening and sheath fluid often with surrounding oedema (Tuite, 2002). Contrast is not routinely administered to diagnose tendinopathy or ligamentous rupture. Focal enhancement of tendon sheaths is a marker of tenosynovitis.

In summary, MRI is better at staging large area anatomy (e.g. tendon retraction) and inflammatory change. U/S best demonstrates architectural disruption and movement-related pathology. These modalities must be considered complementary and should be used in combination for the assessment of tendon pathology.

How to detect cysts, ganglia, bursa and peri-articular masses

Fluid collections around the foot and ankle can be detected with both U/S and MRI, and differentiated from solid masses. As with joint effusions, simple encysted fluid is anechoic with acoustic enhancement deep to the fluid. Fluid structures are high signal on MRI T2 and STIR sequences and low signal on T1.

Large effusions lead to distension and decompression into synovial cysts. Ganglion cysts are often seen adjacent to joints and are particularly common around the ankle. They are mucin filled and frequently septated (O'Connor 2002). On U/S and MRI they appear as well-defined cystic lesions and may communicate with the joint or adjacent tendon sheath.

Bursae are pouches of fluid that facilitate movement between adjacent structures by reducing friction. Two types of bursae are recognized, those with a synovial lining and adventitial bursa that have no synovial lining. An adventitial bursa is acquired as the result of friction between two structures leading to the collection of fluid within the intervening soft tissue. Synovial inflammation may cause bursitis in those lined with synovium. The bursa becomes distended, the thickened synovium may be evident on both U/S and MRI, and mimics the characteristics of joint synovitis (O'Connor 2002). Inter-metatrasal bursitis can be one of the first features of RA mimicking forefoot joint disease. Rheumatoid nodules have also been described within synovial bursae (Fig. 5.7).

Necrotic cellular debris may sometimes develop within the bursa forming multiple intraarticular fibrinous deposits, known as rice body bursitis. The nodules can be visualized within the bursa on U/S

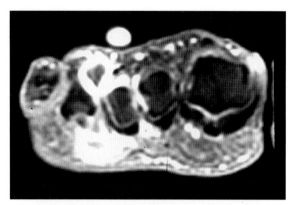

Figure 5.7   Transverse forefoot T1 weighted fat suppressed post iv gadolinium enhanced image. There is intermetatarsal bursitis with pathological proven rheumatoid nodule formation within this bursa. This was the presenting feature of this patient's rheumatoid arthritis.

and appear as low signal on both T1 and T2 weighted MRI (Spence et al. 1998).

The imaging characteristics of bursal or cystic fluid may differ if infected or haemorrhagic. Abscess collections may appear as cystic masses with the fluid containing debris. The abscess cavity will appear avascular with Doppler imaging and low signal without enhancement on T1 weighted MRI imaging.

However, the wall of the abscess, which may be thick and irregular, may appear hypervascular owing to increased perfusion about the collection. This will enhance avidly with gadolinium. U/S is particularly useful in guiding aspiration and drainage of cystic collections, especially when infection is suspected.

Rheumatoid nodules occur in periarticular extensor surfaces prone to mechanical irritation. They appear as non-cystic masses within the subcutaneous tissues, especially over the heel. Their appearance on MRI is variable, but is usually a low signal on T1 and T2 with solid or ring enhancement post contrast (Fig. 5.8) (Scutellari and Orzincolo 1998, Starok et al. 1998, el-Noueam et al. 1997). The nodules may also undergo cystic degeneration.

How to image the complications of rheumatoid arthritis.

MRI is often the optimal examination when the focus of the pathology cannot be firmly defined. Inflammation is inseparable from oedema and this appears as high signal on T2 and STIR examination. This often localizes the site of pathology when the symptoms and signs are non-specific (Narvaez et al. 2002).

Infection should be suspected in a disproportionately inflamed joint. A large joint effusion, bone destruction, marrow oedema and periarticular oedema are signs of

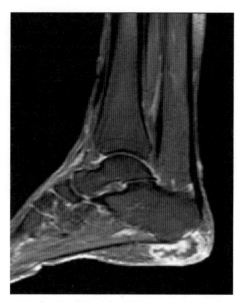

Figure 5.8 Sagittal T1 weighted fat suppressed post iv gadolinium enhanced image. There is an enhancing rheumatoid nodule in the fat pad of the heel. The nodule has a somewhat irregular non-enhancing centre in keeping with central necrotic change.

septic arthritis, but differentiation from active RA can be difficult. In these cicumstances U/S-guided aspiration or biopsy may be of use (O'Connor 2002). The degree of marrow enhancement and amount of marrow oedema are the best indicators of extent of infection. Differentiation may, however, be difficult from non-infected joints and clinical correlation is necessary (Jelinek et al. 1996). Often U/S-guided aspiration for microbiogical examination of the effusion is required.

Insufficiency fractures occur due to osteoporosis and altered ankle and foot mechanics (Narvaez et al. 2002). These may be visualized on plain film, but are notoriously difficult to see. On MRI, the marrow at the site of fracture if usually oedematous and the fracture reveals itself as a band like low signal on T1.

Avascular necrosis is a complication of the vascular compromise and steroid administration in rheumatoid patients (van Vugt et al. 1996). MRI changes predate the plain film. MRI shows a subchondral low signal line on T1 with a surrounding ring or double halo on T2. Bone infarcts may also occur and appear as serpiginous medullary areas of low signal on T1.

GENERAL FEATURES OF THE RHEUMATOID JOINT OF THE FOOT AND ANKLE

All the joints and the surrounding soft tissues of the foot and ankle may be affected by RA (Weishaupt et al. 1999, Resnick 2002, Vidigal et al. 1975).

On the plain radiograph, periarticular soft-tissue swelling is often one of the first signs of disease and predates the bony changes. The swelling is usually fusiform and symmetrical. It is due to joint effusion, synovial hypertrophy, oedema and tenosynovitis.

Thickening of the synovium, joint effusion and oedema of the cartilage may cause an initial and transient increase in joint space seen on the plain film before progressive cartilaginous destruction leads to joint space loss.

Juxta-articular osteoporosis is characteristic of RA, but not specific. With chronicity and steroid administration generalized osteoporosis may occur, but is frequently not visualized unless profound.

Synovial inflammation predates any bony change (Conaghan et al. 2003). As synovial proliferation turns to pannus, punched out para-articular, central or peripheral erosions develop. Subchondral sclerosis is minimal around the erosions. Erosions actually take years to develop and are indicative of irreparability.

Joint space narrowing indicates irreversible cartilage destruction. Osteophytes are lacking in the rheumatoid joint, unless there is secondary osteoarthritis.

With chronic inflammation, structural deformities occur owing to capsular contraction and ligamentous laxity. Tendon pathology and tenosynovitis is commonly due to direct destruction and may lead to rupture further exacerbating joint instability. This causes abnormal mechanics and secondary degenerative changes.

Ancillary features such as neuropathy, vasculitis, stress fractures, bursitis, infection, oedema, and rheumatoid nodules may also occur in the foot and ankle. Excess synovial fluid within the joint may decompress into synovial cysts.

DISEASE OF SPECIFIC JOINTS

Disease of the forefoot

Metatarsal joint disease
The foot is more frequently affected than the ankle. Forefoot pain is the presenting feature in 10–20% (Resnick, 2002).

The lateral metatarsophalangeal joints are affected earliest in the disease with the 5th metatarsophalangeal joint most commonly affected. The metatarsal head abnormalities generally antedate the phalanges. Erosions tend to occur on the medial aspect of the metatarsophalangeal joints with the exception of the 5th; this is more commonly eroded on its lateral side. The 1st metatarsal phalangeal joint is the least commonly affected in RA (Resnick 2002).

Erosions tend to be para-articular at the cartilage–synovial interface in the bare area, named due to a lack of cartilaginous cover (Maini 1979). There may also be localized porosis, extreme thinning or a translucent zone within the cortex, which is the precursor of erosion.

Migration of pannus below the articular surface results in subchondral erosion and articular collapse resulting in surface irregularities.

The sesamoids of the 1st MTP joint may be displaced by synovial mass and also become eroded and inflamed (Resnick et al. 1977).

Chronic synovial inflammation disrupts and weakens the ligamentous structural integrity of both the ankle, but particularly, the foot. This together with bone destruction and tendinous attrition results in joint malalignment. Disruption of the transverse ligaments between adjacent metatarsals results in widening and splaying of the forefoot. The phalanges become laterally deviated and subluxed, and may eventually dislocate dorsally in a valgus position (Fig. 5.9) (Kerschbaumer et al. 1996).

The plantar capsule and plate becomes destroyed by synovial disease and the metatarsal heads herniate downwards particularly those of the 2nd and 3rd metatarsal heads. The fat pad covering the metatarsal heads becomes atrophic and fails to cushion the soft tissues from bone resulting in painful callosities.

Hallux valgus is common and worsens with the duration of the disease (Haas et al. 1999). The extensor hallucis longus tendon becomes displaced into the first web space and the altered forces during contraction acts as an adductor increasing the valgus deformity.

Stress fractures most commonly affect the second metatarsal neck and shaft, due to weakening of the bone with chronic steroid administration (Elkayam et al. 2000). Plain film may fail to show the fracture for several weeks. MRI is the investigation of choice in the equivocal cases. Oedema is visualized in the bone marrow on STIR sequences and a low signal line on both T1 and STIR at the fracture site.

Interphalangeal joints
The interphalangeal joint of the 1st toe is the most commonly affected. The other proximal interphalangeal joints are commonly affected with joint space loss and erosion. The distal interphalangeal joints are usually spared (Halla et al. 1986).

Subluxation of both the metatarsophalangeal joints and interphalangeal joints results in an imbalance of the intrinsic and extrinsic muscles of the toes, this in combination with contraction of the extensor muscles results in mallet, hammer and claw toes. Hyperextension often occurs at the interphalangeal joints. Painful callosities may also occur on the dorsal aspect of cock up toes due to pressure.

Disease of the midfoot and hindfoot

Talonavicular, calcaneocuboid and subtalar joints
Midfoot involvement in RA is common. Synovitis is, however, a less conspicuous feature than in the forefoot. Joint space narrowing is prominent with sclerosis and secondary osteophytosis more common (Resnick 2002).

In the midfoot, RA has a predilection for the talocalcaneonavicular joint. Plain films often fail, however, to demonstrate the degree of early cartilage loss or erosive disease. MRI is of use to visualize the synovitis and erosive change in the midtarsal joints. Erosions are infrequently visualized and are generally small. Complete bony ankylosis of the talocalcaneonavicular joint may occur with chronicity.

The calcaneonavicular, intercuneiform, cuneocuboid and cuboideonavicular tend to be less severely, but similarly affected, as the joints are communicative. Weakness of the musculature and ligaments results in pes planus and pes planovalgus as the arch of the foot becomes unsupported.

The tendon of tibialis posterior may become weakened by the intensity and duration of activity placed upon it in an attempt to support the longitudinal arch. This is the most common tendon affected by RA (Coakley et al. 1994). A full-thickness tear results in acquired unilateral flatfoot, valgus hindfoot, forefoot abduction and talonavicular subluxation.

Synovial proliferation may involve the subtalar joint producing a subtalar mass in the posterior recess. Subtalar disease tends to occur prior to the ankle disease. Progressive deformity occurs due to slow destruction on the surrounding supporting tissues.

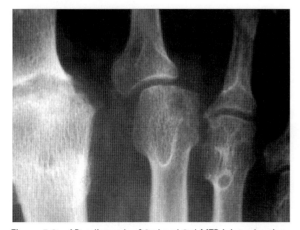

Figure 5.9   AP radiograph of 2nd and 3rd MTP joints showing erosion of the metatarsal heads with early medial subluxation of the 2nd MTP joint.

Sinus tarsi syndrome may also result from inflammed synovial tissue in the subtalar and talo-calcaneonavicular joints. This gives rise to local pain and reflects true subtalar joint involvement.

Synovial cysts or synovitis within bursa may extrude from the subtalar region causing large posterior masses, which can be visualized with both U/S and MRI.

Ankle

The tibiotalar joint is less frequently involved than the subtalar and midtarsal joints (Abdo & Iorio 1994). Osseous changes occur infrequently and late (Resnick 2002).

Valgus deformity, pronation and eversion of the hindfoot result from exaggerated forces on the inflamed subtalar joint. Subluxation, osteoporosis and stress fractures occur late in disease.

Disease of the surrounding soft tissues

Achilles tendinopathy

The surrounding soft-tissue structures of the heel are frequently diseased in RA. Heel pain is often due to Achilles tendinopathy and frequently chronic. Thickening and fusiform swelling of the tendon is frequently present (Jarvinen et al. 2001). Tendon thickening can be related to tendinopathy, paratendonitis or focal rheumatoid nodules. U/S is the most effective way of differentiating these entities in the rheumatoid patient. Tendon degeneration tends to occur in the middle third of the Achilles tendon. The swelling converts the normal ellipsoid cross-sectional area of the tendon into a circular configuration in the transverse plane. The tendon becomes heterogenous and darker in echotexture due to increased fluid content within the tendon (Fig. 5.10).

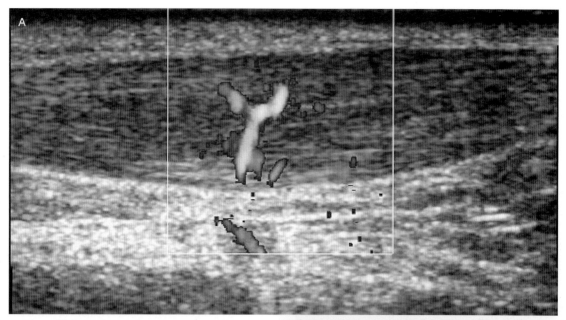

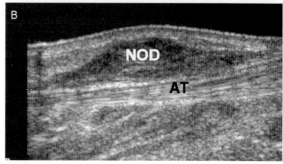

Figure 5.10   (A) Sagittal power Doppler sonogram of the Achilles tendon. There is diffuse tendonopathic change present with thickening and hypoechogenicity of the tendon associated with neovascularity. (B) Sagittal grey scale Doppler sonogram of the Achilles tendon. Rheumatoid nodule in the paratendon simulating tendonopathy.

Weakness of the Achilles occurs 2–6 cm proximal to the insertion, at the enthesis and at the muscle/tendon interface. Rupture most frequently occurs in the most hypovascular region 2–6 cm from the insertion. Suspected clinical tears of the Achilles can be readily diagnosed with U/S and MRI (Stiskal et al. 1997).

Steroid injection of the tendon under U/S guidance is of questionable value and may predispose the tendon to rupture. New therapies using dry needling, autologous blood injection and lithotripsy in the treatment of tendonopathy are under clinical assessment.

Achillles bursitis

Retrocalcaneal and subcutaneous bursitis is more common than Achilles tendinosis (Stiskal et al. 1997).

A small amount of fluid may be visualized in the retrocalcaneal bursa in Kager's triangle deep to the distal third of the Achilles. Synovial hypertophy and effusion may lead to expansion of the joint capsule and expansion of the retrocalcaneal bursa, which extends out of Kager's triangle in a teardrop fashion (Fig. 5.11). This produces a painful mass on the posterosuperior aspect of the heel, which causes impingement on the peroneal tendons. Occasionally, the superficial calcaneal bursa becomes distended.

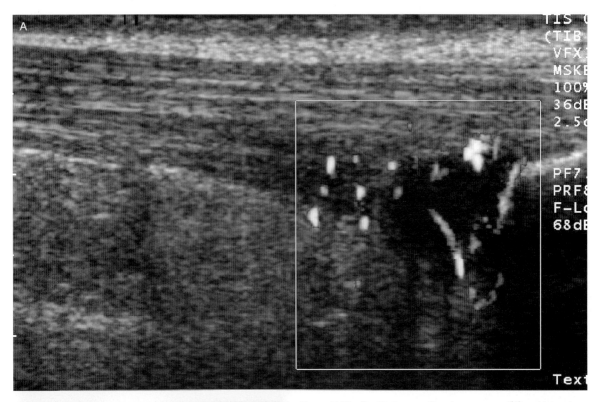

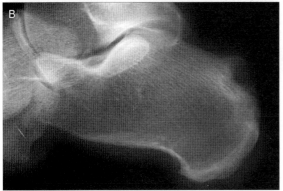

Figure 5.11 Sagittal power Doppler sonogram (A) and lateral calcaneal radiography (B) demonstrating retrocalcaneal bursitis. The ultrasound shows hypoechoic thickening of the retrocalcaneal bursa associated with hyperaemia. The radiograph shows the plain film changes of retrocalcaneal bursitis with erosion of the posterior corner of the calcaneus.

Impingement can be assessed with MRI. A synovial mass or bursa may be visualized on the lateral or posterior aspect of the ankle with fluid identified in the peroneal tendon sheaths.

Peroneal tendons

Lateral pain is the hallmark of peroneal tendon pathology with eventual loss of eversion and cavovalgus deformity. Problems arising within the peroneus longus include tenosynovitis, tendinopathy and tendinous disruption. Longitudinal tears of the tendon are commonly seen in peroneus brevis.

Longitudinal tears and ruptures of the peroneal tendons can be readily identified on MRI and U/S (Rasmussen 2000, Diaz et al. 1998, Tuite 2002). Imaging features include a chevron-shaped tendon, increased signal on T1 and T2, flattened peroneal groove, abnormalities of the lateral ligament complex, and fibular spurring.

The peroneal tendons are most vulnerable from adjacent synovial inflammation in three specific tunnels, the calcaneotrochlear process, in the region of the inferior peroneal retinaculum and the cuboid notch where the tendon sharply changes direction passing the plantar surface of the foot.

Subluxation of the peroneal tendons may occur following an acute traumatic episode or chronically after disruption of the inferior peroneal retinaculum. Dynamic U/S can visualize the tendon flicking over the fibular into its aberrant position (Neustadter et al. 2004).

Plain radiography fails to directly visualize the tendons. Tenosynovitis may be identified on U/S and MRI with fluid identified within the tendon sheath (Bare & Haddad 2001). Fluid may be visualized in the normal sheath, but if the tendon is completely surrounded, this denotes pathology.

Plantar fascia

Plantar fasciitis is a common cause of subcalcaneal heal pain, which may be related to the biomechanical alterations of the foot and is seen particularly in pes planus and pes cavus.

It is, however, a misnomer and is, in fact, a tendonitis of the common tendinous aponeurosis of the superficial intrinsic muscles of the foot. On U/S examination, there is thickening of the plantar 'ascia' to greater than 4 mm (normally 3 mm) measured in the sagittal plane at the point of it crossing the inferior calcaneal border. The contralateral side is often also thickened, but asymptomatic; however, a discrepancy of greater than 1 mm is abnormal. The echogenicity of the 'fascia' also decreases and becomes heterogenous like other tendinopathies. Occasionally, fluid is seen deep or superficial to the fascia (Gibbon & Long 1999). U/S-guided steroid injection is useful in treatment.

MRI can also be used to delineate the pathology with oedema and intermediate signal change identified of the fascia (Theodorou et al. 2001).

SUMMARY

Imaging allows the demonstration of the hallmarks of rheumatoid disease, notably erosions and synovitis. It also allows the complications of the disease on the foot and ankle to be assessed and, potentially, treated, even before clinically evident.

The role of the radiologist is integral to the diagnosis, management and prognosis of the patient with rheumatoid arthritis. Plain film radiography was previously the sole technique available. With the advent of MRI and U/S the role of the imager has taken on a new relevance. Diagnosis can now be confirmed earlier and treatment protocols initiated to try to control the disease prior to the irreparable damage to bone, cartilage and joint, with the antecedent morbidity.

MRI and U/S should be routinely employed by the rheumatologist in order to optimally treat the foot and ankle in rheumatoid arthritis.

References

Abdo RV and Iorio LJ Rheumatoid arthritis of the foot and ankle. The Journal of the American Academy of Orthopedic Surgeons 1994; 2: 326–332.

Bare AA and Haddad SL Tenosynovitis of the posterior tibial tendon. Foot and Ankle Clinics 2001; 6: 37–66.

Coakley FV, Samanta AK and Finlay DB Ultrasonography of the tibialis posterior tendon in rheumatoid arthritis. British Journal of Rheumatology 1994; 33: 273–277.

Conaghan PG, O'Connor P, McGonagle D et al. Elucidation of the relationship between synovitis and bone damage: a randomized magnetic resonance imaging study of individual joints in patients with early rheumatoid arthritis. Arthritis and Rheumatism 2003; 48: 64–71.

Connolly DJ, Berman L and McNally EG The use of beam angulation to overcome anisotropy when viewing human tendon with high frequency linear array ultrasound. British Journal of Radiology 2001; 74: 183–185.

Diaz GC, van Holsbeeck M and Jacobson JA Longitudinal split of the peroneus longus and peroneus brevis tendons with disruption of the superior peroneal retinaculum. Journal of Ultrasound Medicine 1998; 17: 525–529.

Elkayam O, Paran D, Flusser G, Wigler I, Yaron M and Caspi D Insufficiency fractures in rheumatic patients: misdiagnosis and underlying characteristics. Clinical and Experimental Rheumatology 2000; 18: 369–374.

el-Noueam KI, Giuliano V, Schweitzer M E and O'Hara BJ Rheumatoid nodules: MR/pathological correlation. Journal of Computer Assisted Tomography 1997; 21: 769–796.

Gibbon WW and Long G Ultrasound of the plantar aponeurosis (fascia). Skeletal Radiology 1999; 28: 21–26.

Goupille P, Roulot B, Akoka S et al. Magnetic resonance imaging: a valuable method for the detection of synovial inflammation in rheumatoid arthritis. Journal of Rheumatology 2001; 28: 35–40.

Haas C, Kladny B, Lott S, Weseloh G and Swoboda B Progression of foot deformities in rheumatoid arthritis – a radiologic follow-up study over 5 years. Zeitschrift fur Rheumatologie 1999; 58: 351–357.

Halla JT, Fallahi S and Hardin JG Small joint involvement: a systematic roentgenographic study in rheumatoid arthritis. Annals of the Rheumatic Diseases 1986; 45, 327–330.

Jarvinen TA, Kannus P, Paavola M, Jarvinen TL, Jozsa L and Jarvinen M Achilles tendon injuries. Current Opinion in Rheumatology 2001; 13: 150–155.

Jelinek J, Pearl AB, Kominsky SJ and Schultz PM Magnetic resonance imaging of the foot. Rheumatologic disorders mimicking osteomyelitis. Journal of the American Podiatric Medicine Association 1996; 86: 228–231.

Kerschbaumer F, von Salomon D and Lehr F The rheumatic forefoot. Orthopade 1996; 25: 354–361.

Lawrence RC, Helmick CG, Arnett FC et al. Estimates of the prevalence of arthritis and selected musculoskeletal disorders in the United States. Arthritis and Rheumatism 1998; 41: 778–799.

Lopez-Ben R, Bernreuter WK, Moreland LW and Alarcon GS Ultrasound detection of bone erosions in rheumatoid arthritis: a comparison to routine radiographs of the hands and feet. Skeletal Radiology 2004; 33: 80–84.

Maini RN Immunopathological mechanisms in rheumatoid arthritis at the dual interface of the synovial membrane: the joint cavity and the pannus. Rheumatology Rehabilitation 1979; 20–29.

Martinoli C, Bianchi S, Dahmane M, Pugliese F, Bianchi-Zamorani MP and Valle M Ultrasound of tendons and nerves. European Radiology 2002; 12: 44–55.

McGonagle D, Conaghan PG, Wakefield R and Emery P Imaging the joints in early rheumatoid arthritis. Best Practice and Research. Clinical Rheumatology 2001; 15: 91–104.

McQueen FM Magnetic resonance imaging in early inflammatory arthritis: what is its role? Rheumatology (Oxford) 2000; 39: 700–706.

McQueen FM, Benton N, Crabbe J, Robinson E, Yeoman S, McLean L and Stewart N What is the fate of erosions in early rheumatoid arthritis? Tracking individual lesions using x rays and magnetic resonance imaging over the first two years of disease. Annals of the Rheumatic Diseases 2001; 60: 859–868.

McQueen FM, Benton N, Perry D et al. Bone edema scored on magnetic resonance imaging scans of the dominant carpus at presentation predicts radiographic joint damage of the hands and feet six years later in patients with rheumatoid arthritis. Arthritis and Rheumatism 2003; 48: 1814–1827.

Narvaez JA, Narvaez J, Roca Y and Aguilera C MR imaging assessment of clinical problems in rheumatoid arthritis. European Radiology 2002; 12: 1819–1828.

Neustadter J, Raikin SM and Nazarian LN Dynamic sonographic evaluation of peroneal tendon subluxation. AJR American Journal of Roentgenology 2004; 183: 985–988.

Newman JS, Laing TJ, McCarthy CJ and Adler RS Power Doppler sonography of synovitis: assessment of therapeutic response – preliminary observations. Radiology 1996; 198: 582–584.

O'Connor PJ, Grainger A J Ultrasound imaging of joint disease. British Journal of Radiology, Imaging 2002; 14: 1–14.

Ory PA Radiography in the assessment of musculoskeletal conditions. Best Practice and Research. Clinical Rheumatology 2003; 17: 495–512.

Ostergaard M and Klarlund M Importance of timing of post-contrast MRI in rheumatoid arthritis: what happens during the first 60 minutes after IV gadolinium-DTPA? Annals of the Rheumatic Diseases 2001; 60: 1050–1054.

Ostergaard M and Szkudlarek M Imaging in rheumatoid arthritis – why MRI and ultrasonography can no longer be ignored. Scandinavian Journal of Rheumatology 2003; 32: 63–73.

Ostergaard M Different approaches to synovial membrane volume determination by magnetic resonance imaging: manual versus automated segmentation. British Journal of Rheumatology 1997; 36: 1166–1177.

Ostergaard M, Gideon P, Stoltenberg MB, Henriksen O and Lorenzen I Volumes of synovial membrane and joint effusion determined by MR imaging. Markers of severity and/or activity in rheumatoid arthritis? Ugeskrift for Laeger 1997; 159: 3956–3961.

Ostergaard M, Hansen M, Stoltenberg M, Gideon P, Klarlund M, Jensen KE and Lorenzen I Magnetic resonance imaging-determined synovial membrane volume as a marker of disease activity and a predictor of progressive joint destruction in the wrists of patients with rheumatoid arthritis. Arthritis and Rheumatism 1999; 42: 918–929.

Ostergaard M, Peterfy C, Conaghan P et al. Rheumatoid Arthritis Magnetic Resonance Imaging Studies. Core set of MRI acquisitions, joint pathology definitions, and the OMERACT RA-MRI scoring system. Journal of Rheumatology 2003; 30: 1385–1386.

Ostergaard M, Stoltenberg M, Henriksen O and Lorenzen I Quantitative assessment of synovial inflammation by dynamic gadolinium-enhanced magnetic resonance imaging. A study of the effect of intra-articular methylprednisolone on the rate of early synovial enhancement. British Journal of Rheumatology 1996; 35: 50–59.

Ostergaard M, Stoltenberg M, Lovgreen-Nielsen P, Volck B, Sonne–Holm S and Lorenzen I Quantification of synovitis by MRI: correlation between dynamic and static gadolinium-enhanced magnetic resonance imaging and microscopic and macroscopic signs of synovial inflammation. Magnetic Resonance Imaging 1998; 16: 743–754.

Rasmussen OS Sonography of tendons. Scandinavian Journal of Medicine and Science in Sports 2000; 10: 360–364.

Rawool NM and Nazarian LN Ultrasound of the ankle and foot. Seminars in Ultrasound, CT and MR 2000; 21: 275–84.

Resnick D Diagnosis of Bone and Joint Disorders, 4th edn WB. Saunders, 2002, vol 5, chap. 21.

Resnick D, Niwayama G and Feingold ML The sesamoid bones of the hands and feet: participators in arthritis. Radiology 1977; 123: 57–62.

Rubin JM Musculoskeletal power Doppler. European Radiology 1999; 9(Suppl 3): S403–406.

Scutellari PN and Orzincolo C Rheumatoid arthritis: sequences. European Journal of Radiology 1998; 27(Suppl 1): S31–38.

Spence LD, Adams J, Gibbons D, Mason MD and Eustace S Rice body formation in bicipito-radial bursitis: ultrasound, CT, and MRI findings. Skeletal Radiology 1998; 27: 30–32.

Starok M, Eilenberg SS and Resnick D Rheumatoid nodules: MRI characteristics. Clinical Imaging 1998; 22: 216–219.

Stiskal M, Szolar DH, Stenzel I, Steiner E, Mesaric P, Czembirek H and Preidler KW Magnetic resonance imaging of Achilles tendon in patients with rheumatoid arthritis. Investigative Radiology 1997; 32: 602–608.

Symmons D, Turner G, Webb R et al. The prevalence of rheumatoid arthritis in the United Kingdom: new estimates for a new century. Rheumatology (Oxford) 2002; 41: 793–800.

Szkudlarek M, Court-Payen M, Strandberg C, Klarlund M, Klausen T and Ostergaard M Contrast-enhanced power Doppler ultrasonography of the metacarpophalangeal joints in rheumatoid arthritis. European Radiology 2003; 13: 163–168.

Szkudlarek M, Court-Payen M, Strandberg C, Klarlund M, Klausen T and Ostergaard M Power Doppler ultrasonography for assessment of synovitis in the metacarpophalangeal joints of patients with rheumatoid arthritis: a comparison with dynamic magnetic resonance imaging. Arthritis and Rheumatism 2001; 44: 2018–2023.

Tehranzadeh J, Ashikyan O and Dascalos J Advanced imaging of early rheumatoid arthritis. Radiologic Clinics of North America 2004; 42: 89–107.

Theodorou DJ, Theodorou SJ, Farooki S, Kakitsubata Y and Resnick D Disorders of the plantar aponeurosis: a spectrum of MR imaging findings. AJR American Journal of Roentgenology 2001; 176: 97–104.

Tuite MJ MR imaging of the tendons of the foot and ankle. Seminars in Musculoskeletal Radiology 2002; 6: 119–131.

van Vugt RM, Sijbrandij ES and Bijlsma JW Magnetic resonance imaging of the femoral head to detect avascular necrosis in active rheumatoid arthritis treated with methylprednisolone pulse therapy. Scandinavian Journal of Rheumatology 1996; 25: 74–76.

Vidigal E, Jacoby RK, Dixon AS, Ratliff AH and Kirkup J The foot in chronic rheumatoid arthritis. Annals of the Rheumatic Diseases 1975; 34: 292–297.

Wakefield RJ, Gibbon WW, Conaghan PG et al. The value of sonography in the detection of bone erosions in patients with rheumatoid arthritis: a comparison with conventional radiography. Arthritis and Rheumatism 2000; 43: 2762–2770.

Wakefield RJ, Green MJ, Marzo-Ortega H et al. Should oligoarthritis be reclassified? Ultrasound reveals a high prevalence of subclinical disease. Annals of the Rheumatic Diseases 2004; 63: 382–385.

Weishaupt D, Schweitzer ME, Alam F, Karasick D and Wapner K MR imaging of inflammatory joint diseases of the foot and ankle. Skeletal Radiology 1999; 28: 663–669.

Winalski CS, Palmer WE, Rosenthal DI and Weissman BN Magnetic resonance imaging of rheumatoid arthritis. Radiologic Clinics of North America 1996; 34: 243–258.

Chapter **6**

Treatment of rheumatoid arthritis

SYSTEMIC DRUG MANAGEMENT

Historical aspects

The medical management of rheumatoid arthritis (RA) and other inflammatory arthritides is changing from year to year. From a 'sleepy' sub-specialty of medicine, with origins in rehabilitation and physical medicine, rheumatology has become a 'high tech' specialty with escalating costs and, for the first time, a genuine hope of cure. Traditional approaches to RA are now completely outdated and the therapeutic scene is changing fast. Without a doubt, the origin of these changes was the more complete understanding of the mechanisms of disease, outlined in Chapter 1, together with the technology to 'target' key molecules in the inflammatory cascade. But equally striking, and possibly more dramatic, advances may come from an understanding of the genetic mechanisms behind the onset of rheumatoid arthritis. Already in early RA we are able to observe the profile of activated genes out of several thousand using new microchip technology (Olsen et al. 2004). Gene arrays such as this may be useful to indicate different prognostic groups and, ultimately, it may become possible to 'turn off' these genes at an early stage and so prevent the chronic inflammatory cascade that we know as RA.

However, at the present time these developments are on the horizon and not yet in clinical practice. It will be of some illustrative use to review the historical approach to early-onset inflammatory disease and to contrast this with current practice. In the 1970s a person with early-onset inflammatory arthritis would have visited their general practitioner and would probably have been given an anti-inflammatory drug (NSAID) such as indomethacin, phenyl butazone or ibuprofen. No other treatment would have been given and no referral to hospital would have been made at that stage. In fact, referral to secondary care occurred late in comparison to the present time; this reflected the lack of rheumatologists as much as the lack of effective treatment. Once referral had been made the options were limited: treatment with NSAIDs and a few second-line drugs, most notably gold injections and corticosteroids. Patients with established inflammatory disease would have been referred to a regional rheumatology centre: in Yorkshire this was situated in the old spa town of Harrogate adjacent to the beautiful Valley Gardens. A typical stay in the Royal Bath Hospital, Harrogate was several weeks long and involved long periods of bed rest. In addition to the mainstream therapy, patients also received a mixture of the traditional spa treatments including drinking sulphurous water, hot and cold baths, Vichy douches and bathing in mud. In fact, the latter treatment continued to be used right up until the hospital was closed in the early 1990s. Sadly, with the advent of tighter purchasing and budgetary control, and accountability reverting to individual Health Authorities, such regional centres became obsolete. The absence of a well-established evidence base didn't help.

By the mid 1980s things had started to change. The traditional second-line drugs had been supplemented by a number of others, notably sulphasalazine and methotrexate. Many new NSAIDs appeared each claiming to be better than the next. Patients were referred earlier and evidence was emerging that joint and bone damage could be retarded with appropriate treatment. Less emphasis was placed on the physical treatments: evidence in favour of these interventions was still awaited. People were less likely to be admitted to hospital and more likely to receive day-case treatments.

Revised criteria for RA (see Chapter 1), new outcome criteria (fostered by the OMERACT initiative (Bellamy 1999)), early arthritis clinics and new information on the pathophysiology of rheumatoid synovitis marked a change in the approach to inflammatory arthritis. Evidence started emerging on the benefits of early aggressive treatment so that instead of the traditional pyramidal approach to treatment (where treatment is 'stepped up' according to the patient's response) treatment is often given with multiple DMARDs initially and then 'stepped down' as the patient responds (see Fig. 6.1). The latter approach is akin to that used in haematological malignancies where remission is induced by multiple chemotherapy regimes and then maintained by single agents, if necessary, or the patient remains drug free. The advent of biological drugs has taken this a step further in that this targeted therapy can induce a rapid remission at an early stage totally reversing the inflammatory process and retarding the progress of erosions (Olsen and Stein 2004). The problems now revolve around cost, side-effects and the relapse that occurs if the drug is stopped.

However, without doubt, the major step forward has been with early referral to specialist clinics. Recent support for this approach in the UK has come from the Arthritis and Musculoskeletal Alliance (ARMA). ARMA has developed national UK standards of care for RA requiring that all patients with suspected inflammatory arthritis are seen by a rheumatology specialist within 12 weeks of first presentation, and preferably within 6 weeks (Arthritis and Musculoskeletal Alliance 2004). The standards also outline the standard of care that is expected, including access and referral to podiatry. Such endeavours may help to redress some of the imbalances that currently exist in the availability of podiatry care in the UK (see Chapter 8).

Analgesics

The prime symptom of RA is pain and analgesics are the first drug people take when symptoms develop. If symptoms persist then analgesics will continue to be taken. Many analgesics are now non-proprietary and can be bought 'over the counter', paracetamol being the prime example. If this is insufficient, escalating strengths of analgesics may be required, and often these are opiate based: codeine (in co-codamol), dihydrocodeine, tramadol and nefopam. Side-effects are common and include nausea, vomiting, drowsiness and constipation. To overcome these problems transdermal analgesic preparations are now available and have been shown to be useful in RA: these include fentanyl and buprenorphine patches. It is worth noting, however, that in early RA if a patient has to take large amounts of analgesia it represents a failure of treatment. In late disease, where pain may be caused by joint damage, analgesics may be required to help control the symptoms of secondary osteoarthritis.

Non-steroidal anti-inflammatory drugs

Sir John Vane (1927–2004) was awarded a Nobel Prize for showing that aspirin works by blocking prostaglandin synthesis and for discovering prostacyclin and its biological significance (Vane 1971). His discoveries led directly to the development of the newer NSAIDs. The newer NSAIDs (diclofenac, piroxicam, flurbiprofen, sulindac) were found to have an efficacy equivalent to the older ones but with less side-effects. Nevertheless, some patients still preferred to take the traditional NSAIDs and some, such as

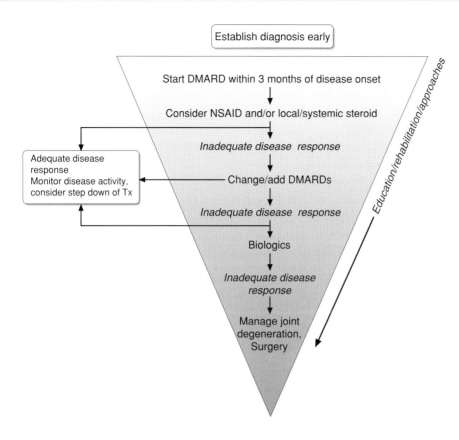

phenylbutazone, were reserved solely for use by rheumatologists in ankylosing spondylitis. NSAIDs act as both analgesics and anti-inflammatory drugs and are, without doubt, very effective drugs for the control of symptoms in inflammatory and non-inflammatory arthritis. However, side-effects have limited their use. The most important of these is gastro-intestinal ulceration (not only upper GI ulceration, but also in the small and large bowel). NSAIDs were identified as the major risk factor for admission of elderly people with bleeding or perforated ulcers in a major study in 1988 (Faulkner et al. 1988).

The considerable morbidity and mortality from gastro-intestinal-related side-effects was the prime reason for the development of the COX-2 specific NSAIDs (coxibs). To understand the reason for this, some elementary knowledge of cyclo-oxygenase (COX) biochemistry is required. COX-1 and COX-2 are both enzymes that catalyse the conversion of precursors to prostaglandins (Fig. 6.2). COX-2 occurs largely at sites of inflammation and is termed 'inducible'. COX-1 is termed 'constitutive' as it can be found in tissues in the

Non-steroidal anti-inflammatory drugs (NSAIDs)

- NSAIDs are effective against the symptoms of inflammatory arthritis and have been used as first line treatment for over 40 years
- NSAIDs act by blocking the action of cyclo-oxygenase thus preventing the synthesis of prostaglandins
- Side effects include upper gastrointestinal ulceration, fluid retention, hypertension, deterioration in renal function and many others
- COX-2 specific NSAIDs were developed to avoid the upper GI side-effects of these drugs. However, their use has been limited by their adverse cardiovascular risk profile (which is to a certain extent also true for non-COX-2 specific NSAIDs)
- Although effective short term symptom control is possible with these drugs they are now being used with more caution

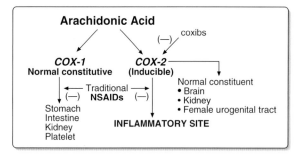

Figure 6.2 The biochemical pathways involved in inflammation.

absence of inflammation and, therefore, has a physiological role independent of inflammation. Constitutively, COX-1 is found mainly in the stomach (where prostaglandins have a protective effect), kidney (where PGs help maintain blood flow), and platelets (where PGs have a role in adherence) (Hawkey 1999). Interestingly, COX-2 is also found constitutively in certain tissues: the kidney the female urogenital tract, where it is involved in ovulation, and the vascular system, where COX-2 sustains prostacyclin production. Traditional NSAIDs disrupt the action of COX-1 and COX-2 and, therefore, cause stomach and intestinal ulceration, a rise in serum creatinine and have a platelet anti-coagulant effect (a beneficial side effect). Selective COX-2 drugs largely avoid the risks of upper gastro-intestinal ulceration (although this benefit has been exaggerated), but still carry the risk of the other side-effects including renal impairment, and problems with ovulation. Unfortunately, the delicate balance of prostacyclin and thromboxane in the blood vessel wall is disrupted by COX-2 drugs (Maxwell and Webb 2005) and, as a result, their action may, in addition to being anti-inflammatory, be pro-thrombotic. Results from the first large study of rofecoxib hinted at this and subsequent longer term studies have confirmed the excess risk of cardiovascular side-effects resulting in the withdrawal of rofecoxib from the market in 2004. Although this may be a 'class' effect, where all drugs in this class share this property, it appears that rofecoxib was particularly disadvantaged in this way (Juni et al. 2004). A further coxib (valdecoxib) has recently been withdrawn and the other members of this class of drugs (celecoxib, etoricoxib, lumaricoxib) remain under close scrutiny (Fitzgerald 2004). Prescribers are, therefore, advised to be cautious and to avoid these drugs in anyone with a high risk, or history of, cardiovascular or cerebrovascular disease.

It is also worth noting that both COX-1 and COX-2 NSAIDs share adverse events on the kidney, ovary, lower GI tract and liver and must be used with caution in 'at-risk' groups. Although the guidelines drawn

up by the National Institute for Clinical Excellence (NICE) for use of COX-2 specific drugs identify groups at risk for upper gastro-intestinal ulceration, these same groups of people are often vulnerable to the other side effects shared by both groups of drugs, particularly renal impairment and consequent fluid retention. There may also be a group of people with other risk factors for vascular disease (such as hypertension, hyperlipidaemia and diabetes).

NICE guidelines for the use of COX-2 selective (NSAIDs)

- People over 65 years old
- History of dyspepsia/peptic ulcer
- Co-therapy with steroids
- Smokers
- Asthma
- Cardiovascular disease, e.g. CCF, hypertension
- Heavy alcohol

Traditional disease modifying drugs

Serendipity and misconceptions resulted in the discovery of many of the traditional DMARDs. Gold salts were originally thought useful as a treatment for tuberculosis and tried in RA as it was thought to be a similar disease. Anti-malarials were found to be effective in affected patients living or travelling in endemic areas. Sulphasalazine was also originally used as a treatment for RA in the mistaken belief that it had an infective aetiology. The logic behind the use of methotrexate was more rational in that it was known to have important effects on dividing cells and macrophages via its action on purine synthesis.

Gold salts

Gold salts have been used for a long time to treat RA. The main preparation is a water-soluble salt called sodium aurothiomalate (Myocrisin). About one-third of people suffer from side-effects (rash is the commonest, less commonly neutropenia and proteinuria), one-third receive no benefit and one-third experience a good level of benefit. Patients in the latter category often stay on the drug for many years. Gold salts were the subject of one of the first randomized controlled trials in rheumatology, funded by the forerunner of *arc*, the Empire Rheumatism Council (Research Committee of the Empire Rheumatism Council 1961). They are rarely used now in the UK, except in those people already established on them and still obtaining benefit from them. An oral preparation of gold was introduced in the late 1980s (auranofin), but is probably less effective than the injectable form and has not found general acceptance.

Anti-malarial drugs

Chloroquine phosphate (originally) and hydroxychloroquine (now) are still used widely in rheumatic diseases, both as a treatment for RA and for connective tissue diseases. Anti-malarial drugs have several in vitro actions on the immune system and, theoretically at least, should be very effective against autoimmune disorders. In practice, their contribution to controlling disease activity is relatively small, but they are still used as 'cornerstone' therapy in drug combinations (see below). These drugs are relatively safe but may cause photosensitivity, nausea and, with increasing doses over the long term, irreversible retinopathy. For the latter reason doses are kept below 5 mg/kg/day and patients are advised to monitor their central and peripheral vision, and to have regular eye checks. Retinopathy is probably more likely with chloroquine phosphate and so hydroxychloroquine is the drug of choice when anti-malarials are indicated.

D-penicillamine

In a similar way to gold salts the patients who are able to tolerate this drug, and get good benefit from it, will often remain on it for many years (Day et al. 1974). However, like gold salts and anti-malarials, there is little evidence from randomized-controlled trials of retardation of disease progression. Its use is, therefore, limited in current UK practice. Common side-effects are nausea, helped by dose reduction, and rash. Less common, but more important side-effects are thrombocytopenia and proteinuria.

Sulphasalazine

Although this drug is still used widely in the UK the availability of more effective therapies mean that patients are quickly moved off the drug if improvement is sub-optimal or slow. Sulphasalazine is an interesting drug. It is chemically a combination of aspirin like moiety (5 amino salicylic acid) and a sulphonamide antibiotic (sulphpyridine). It is used successfully for inflammatory bowel disease and is particularly useful for seronegative spondyloarthritis, possibly because there is a high prevalence of 'hidden' bowel inflammation in the latter disorders (Mielants and Veys 1990). Studies have shown that the active part of the drug is different for inflammatory bowel disease and inflammatory arthritis; that is aspirin-like moiety for bowel disease (now marketed separately for this condition) and sulphonamide moiety for arthritis, although the combination molecule is much

more effective in arthritis (Neumann et al. 1986). The commonest side-effects are nausea and rash, but the most important side-effect is agranulocytosis, which can occur idiosyncratically but usually within the first 3 months of therapy.

Methotrexate

Originally used in the 1950s as an anti-cancer drug, low-dose weekly therapy was later used to treat RA and has now become the standard DMARD to which others are compared. Methotrexate is well tolerated, can be taken orally or parenterally, has a good safety record and is effective in controlling disease activity and preventing progression of erosions (Weinblatt et al. 1992). As the drug can cause bone marrow suppression, regular blood checks are necessary, varying in frequency from weekly to bimonthly depending on the situation. Nausea and diarrhoea may limit its tolerability, but liver and pulmonary side-effects are the most problematic. Elevated liver enzymes are an indication to reduce the dose and this can be exacerbated by other hepatotoxic agents, notably alcohol. There is an association between long-term methotrexate use and cirrhosis; the need for liver biopsy in patients taking cumulative doses of this drug exceeding 2 g is controversial. An acute pulmonary inflammation (pneumonitis) can occur early in treatment and pulmonary fibrosis may be linked to long-term use, thus obligating the physician to make regular checks on the lungs.

Newer treatments

Leflunomide

Introduced in the late 1990s as an inhibitor of pyrimidine synthesis, leflunomide was thought to be the ideal drug companion to methotrexate (Olsen and Stein 2004). In fact, the combination, although effective, was initially reported to cause severe toxic reactions in the liver. Since then, more judicious selection of patients and smaller doses has resulted in the drug combination returning with good results (Kremer et al. 2004). Leflunomide has an exceptionally long half life of several weeks and must be 'washed out' if toxicity occurs. Hypertension, diarrhoea and raised liver enzymes are the major side-effects.

Other drugs

There has been a vogue for using cyclosporine in RA, although continued use is limited by hypertension and renal toxicity. Cyclosporine continues to be used in drug combinations (see below). Minocycline has activity against metalloproteinases and has a mild antirheumatic activity (O'Dell et al. 2001). Thalidomide, removed from the market in the late 1960s because of its teratogenic potential is still available for use on a named patient basis and is thought to work as a moderate inhibitor of TNF. Apart from the restriction of use to women of child-bearing potential it may cause a peripheral neuropathy: patients taking this drug should have pre-treatment electrophysiology and paraesthesiae developing on therapy are an early warning sign of toxicity.

Biological drugs

The new biological drugs inhibit cytokine activity high up in the inflammatory pathway and can be highly effective even in patients who have failed conventional DMARD therapy (O'Dell 2004, Olsen and Stein 2004). The most common drugs are the agents active against tumour necrosis factor α (TNFα); marketed as infliximab, etanercept, and recently adalimumab (Olsen and Stein 2004). The effect of anti-TNF therapy is often striking, with some patients showing a positive response within days or even hours. However, biologic DMARDs are expensive, costing £8000 to £10 000 for a year of treatment and so their publicly funded use is restricted to those patients with active disease who have already failed conventional DMARDs (http//www.rheumatology.org.uk). A case has been made for their use in early disease because of their superior efficacy (Emery et al. 2003, Breedveld 2004) where it is contended that the significant reduction in (work related) disability associated with biologic therapy makes these therapies cost effective when viewed in the context of savings to the country from lost work days (9.4 million days, equivalent to £833 million p.a. for RA alone (Arthritis Research Campaign 2002)) and decreased dependence on the benefits system. However, a direct comparison of etanercept and methotrexate in early RA found only marginal superiority in those patients achieving ACR-20 scores (see Chapter 8), although the percentage of patients with no increase in erosion score (72% for etanercept, 60% for methotrexate) was significantly in favour of etanercept (Bathon et al. 2000). Further, when anti-TNF drugs are assessed for cost-efficacy the cost per quality adjusted life year may not be as favourable as initially thought (Bansback et al. 2004). It is clear that this debate will continue to run for many years but, on the positive side, the cost of these drugs is likely to fall in the future.

The major side effect of anti-TNF drugs is an increased susceptibility to infection. In fact, the increased susceptibility is compounded by the masking of the usual signs of infection such as fever and pain. Both these problems result from the pivotal role of TNF

> ## Biological drugs
> - A new class of disease modifying drug targeted against key molecules involved in inflammation
> - These drugs are expensive, typically costing £8,000 – £10,000 per year
> - The major side-effect is infection
> - Latent tuberculosis may be re-activated by these drugs, particularly the anti-TNF drugs
> - Any foot infection or ulcer must be regarded as a medical emergency for people taking these drugs
> - Main classes of drugs are:
>   - Anti-TNF drugs (infliximab, etanercept, adalimumab)
>   - Anti-IL1 (anakinra)
>   - Anti-CD20 (rituximab)

in the immune response (see Chapter 1). Patients taking these drugs are vulnerable to catastrophic and rapidly progressive infection. As the drugs are new this susceptibility to infection may not always be appreciated by attending physicians and other health-care workers unfamiliar with their use. An alert card, which patients carry with them and show to all health professionals they consult, may help to avoid this problem. The importance of therapy with these drugs extends into the podiatry profession: infected lesions in the foot must always be a source of concern in patients taking biological drugs (see Clinical note opposite).

Two other scenarios must be mentioned in this context. TNF plays a major role in the containment of tuberculous lesions. Tuberculosis may remain present in the body after an infection is treated, the immune system ensuring that the bacterium is kept under control. For this reason anti-TNF drugs may cause recrudescence of dormant tuberculous lesions and rapidly progressive clinical infection. Everyone starting these drugs should be screened for previous infection with tuberculosis and they should be used with caution if infection has occurred in the past. Secondly, the drugs must be temporarily discontinued during major surgery: the period of time that the drug should be stopped prior to surgery will vary with the drug, as some have a longer half life than others. Exactly what constitutes major surgery is not clear, but this advice will probably extend to surgery on the foot.

As the name implies, tumour necrosis factor also has a role in the body's normal mechanisms for

It is essential that those involved in the care of the feet of people with inflammatory arthritis are aware of the medication being taken by their patients, and the implications of the drug therapy. Patients with inflammatory arthritis are twice as likely as the general population to develop an infection and there is a further increase in infection risk in patients taking DMARDs (Edwards et al. 2004, Olsen and Stein 2004). Patients undergoing biologic immunotherapy are particularly at risk from infection as they can be susceptible to unusually rapid progression. It is absolutely essential that the foot health clinician liaises with the rheumatologist where there is any risk of infection, e.g. from ulceration, or prior to minor surgery. Otter has made the point well that this should not erode the practitioner's autonomy, but it does allow the appropriate precautions to be taken: including antibiotic cover and, if necessary, temporary alteration of anti-rheumatic therapy (Olsen and Stein 2004, Otter 2004).

tumour surveillance and removal. At the outset, there were concerns that these drugs would increase the incidence of malignancies, particularly lymphoreticular malignancies such as lymphoma. The incidence of lymphoma is increased in RA, so this was a real source of concern in patients. The use of these drugs is realistically still in its infancy, although registers of patients taking them have been established partly to answer these questions: early results are inconclusive (Symmons and Silman 2004). Biological drugs should be used with caution in people who have already had a tumour, even if treated successfully.

Other problems with anti-TNF drugs include the potential to cause autoantibodies such as anti-nuclear factor (Krause et al. 2003). These antibodies are important since they can attenuate clinical efficacy of the drugs, cause hypersensitivity reactions and auto-immune phenomena, including lupus-like syndromes. An association with neurological problems occurring on anti-TNF drugs (such as paraesthesia, weakness, optic neuritis and frank demyelination seen in multiple sclerosis) and the development of these antibodies is not yet clear, but these drugs should be used with caution in patients with demyelinating syndromes. Co-prescription of methotrexate will help prevent the development of auto-antibodies and this combination is usually the norm for treatment with infliximab.

Other biological drugs are anti-IL1 (anakinra) and an anti-B cell therapy, rituximab. Anakinra is probably less effective than anti-TNF drugs, but provides a useful alternative to patients who have 'failed' treatment with other biological drugs. Anakinra has also been used with benefit in drug combinations (see below). Rituximab targets a cell surface marker in a sub-population of B lymphocytes and has shown good efficacy in RA (Edwards et al. 2004). Although cost is still an important issue, as with the other biological drugs, the alternative mode of action may make this drug preferable to anti-TNF drugs as the key cytokine pathways are not targeted by this therapy. Hypersensitivity reactions to the infusions may, however, occur.

Steroids

When synthetic adrenocortical hormones (corticosteroids or steroids) were introduced in the late 1940s they were hailed as wonder drugs and miracle cures. Images of severely disabled people suddenly finding themselves pain free and with boundless energy are very reminiscent of the scenes that accompanied the introduction of the new biological drugs. It soon became apparent that there was a downside to steroid therapy: weight gain, diabetes and osteoporosis. These drugs are still in widespread use with about one-third of all patients with RA in any one cohort taking these drugs long term. There has been renewed interest in the drugs as disease modifying agents in RA (Kirwan 1995) and they are still widely used to treat extra-articular disease in combination with immunosuppressive drugs. Used judiciously, many of the side-effects can be minimized: oral doses are kept below 7.5 mg daily or administration is by intermittent intra-muscular or intra-articular injection. Co-prescription with anti-resorptive agents such as bisphosphonates can attenuate the bone loss if given early, at the same time as the steroids are given if 'long term' treatment is planned. Steroids have retained a prominent place in the rheumatologist's therapeutic armamentarium and will continue to do so. As experience grows the unfortunate side-effect profile will be minimized.

Combination regimes

A number of combination regimes have been tried, some empirical and some based on a knowledge of pharmacology, such as the methotrexate/leflunomide combination. Hydroxychloroquine is often given in combination and, because of a relatively benign side-effect profile, is often retained when other drugs are changed. A strategy known as the 'inverted pyramid' or 'step-down' approach to initial therapy in RA uses an initial combination of hydroxychloroquine, methotrexate and sulfasalazine (Pincus et al. 1999) or steroids, methotrexate and sulfasalazine (Landewe et al. 2002). A number of combinations have been compared with the triple combinations achieving the best results (O'Dell et al. 2002). Other combinations include sulphasalazine/methotrexate, sulphasalazine/azathioprine, methotrexate/cyclosporine, and gold/penicillamine (Schwarzer et al. 1990).

With the introduction of biological drugs, other combinations have appeared. Methotrexate is often used in combination with a biological drug to prevent the development of auto-antibodies, but other drugs such as leflunomide have also been used in this way. Combinations of biological drugs have also been used, notably a combination of etanercept and anakinra, although the results were no better than with the individual drugs alone and more side-effects were recorded with the combination (Genovese et al. 2004).

The current optimal approach to treating a case of new onset rheumatoid arthritis

In inflammatory arthritis, the goal at first presentation is to establish and maintain disease remission, and this can often be achieved with standard (i.e. traditional, non-biologic) therapies (Bukhari et al. 2003). There is good evidence that instigation of DMARD therapy within 3 months of disease onset is highly effective in controlling RA (American College of Rheumatology Subcommittee on Rheumatoid Arthritis 2002) and so patients are normally started on a suitable DMARD immediately. The most commonly used DMARDs at present are hydroxychloroquine, methotrexate, leflunomide and sulphasalazine.

Methotrexate is usually the DMARD of first choice because of its significant therapeutic effects when used in isolation, and because of its adjunctive effects when used in combination with other drugs (notably other DMARDs) (O'Dell 2004, Verstappen et al. 2003). Doses of methotrexate should be escalated rapidly over a 6–8 week period to a maximum of 20–25 mg weekly depending on tolerance (Smollen et al. 2005). Methotrexate is the best tolerated DMARD for long term therapy, and patients often use methotrexate for many years. Used in this way, methotrexate is often referred to as an 'anchor drug' (Pincus et al. 1999).

Oral corticosteroids are no longer recommended for long-term treatment because of the systemic side-effects, but are useful in early disease as a 'bridging therapy' before the DMARDs take effect, and for short-term suppression of disease flares (O'Dell 2004).

Biological drugs are highly effective in about two-thirds of people, but their cost restricts their use to those who have failed or can't tolerate at least two of the conventional drugs. Although arguments have been evinced for their early use prior to conventional DMARDs, professional bodies such as the British Society for Rheumatology and NICE are currently advising their use as tertiary agents (see comments above).

Standard treatment regimes for new onset rheumatoid arthritis

- Instigation of treatment in rheumatoid arthritis within 3 months of diagnosis is highly effective in controlling the disease
- Methotrexate is the DMARD of first choice in most cases of rheumatoid arthritis
- Oral steroids are no longer used as maintenance therapy but may be used in early disease as 'bridging' therapy until other treatments begin to work
- Biological drugs are currently used as tertiary agents after other DMARDs have failed. Even so, benefit may only be seen in 75% of patients

Factors influencing clinical response to disease modifying drugs

A drug may be deemed ineffective or the patient may be intolerant but the end result is the same: the patient 'fails' on that particular drug. The reasons for drug failure are many and include non-compliance, drug–drug interaction, toxicity, and disease non-response. Predictors of response include long disease duration, multiple previous DMARDs and genetic factors influencing drug metabolism (Hider et al. 2005). Genetic factors can influence both non-response and side-effects. An example of the former is glutathione-S-transferase deficiency and response to penicillamine. The latter problem is exemplified by acetylation status and sulphasalazine. Ethnic variation in response to disease modifying drugs may be genetic, but is more likely a cultural problem, although the data to support this are not yet available (Helliwell and Ibrahim 2003).

Summary of medical management of rheumatoid arthritis

The clinical course of RA has been improved markedly with improvements in DMARD therapy in the 1980s and 90s, and, more recently, with the advent of biological immunotherapy. Patients treated with conventional

DMARDs will typically do moderately well with some 13% going into long-term remission, and just under one-half following a moderated disease course with episodes of remission and relapse (Young et al. 2000). Patients following this disease course will do better than those untreated or on NSAIDs only, but joint degeneration does accrue in the long term (>10 years) and disability remains a factor in established RA (Gordon et al. 2001). About one in eight patients do not respond satisfactorily to conventional DMARDs. For biological agents this figure is about one in four. Steroids continue to be used with about one in four patients taking these drugs orally at any one time. Systemic steroids are used to induce rapid remission prior to the onset of other DMARDs and they are particularly useful for intra-articular use.

INTRA-ARTICULAR THERAPY IN THE FOOT AND ANKLE

Introduction

Administering steroids by the intra-articular and intra-lesional route has many advantages. The patient is not exposed to the usual systemic side-effects of these drugs, the improvement is almost immediate and usually long lasting, and this option has a low incidence of side-effects. Injections are generally used as therapy, but may be used as a diagnostic aid using local anaesthetic and selective injection to determine which structure is the most troublesome. This is sometimes a problem in the foot, where the close proximity of joints may make accurate clinical localization of the pain difficult (Hay et al. 1999).

General principles

General principles of injections in the foot and ankle are given below:

- Although Dixon has warned of a higher incidence of infection associated with injections in the foot

and ankle the authors' experience is otherwise. However, meticulous attention should be given to skin preparation with an alcohol-based preparation (Dixon St.J and Graber 1981). The evidence base for both these viewpoints is sparse. Elsewhere in the body it appears to make no difference what skin preparation is used (Cawley and Morris 1992).

- The content of the injection can vary. Long- or short-acting corticosteroids may be used (see Table 6.1). It is generally advisable to use the shorter-acting, more soluble steroid preparations for injections in the proximity of tendons. Again the evidence base for this statement is lacking, but it is 'common sense' to avoid long-acting depot steroid preparations in such locations. An exception to this advice might be a florid 'hypertrophic' tenosynovitis, which provides a large mass of inflammatory tissue for location of the steroid preparation. The advantage of the depot 'long-acting' preparations is, of course, their longer duration of action. These preparations are microcrystalline and can not leave the joint by simple diffusion. The crystals 'leach' their steroid component over time. Some are ingested by inflammatory cells such as polymorphs, which subsequently die, releasing pro-inflammatory cell contents. This sometimes manifests as a brief 'flare' of the joint post injection (see below).

- It is sometimes, but not always, advisable to use lignocaine before the therapeutic injection. Lignocaine can be used to either:
  - perform a nerve block prior to the procedure (see below). As some of the procedures performed in the foot and ankle can be painful it would seem logical to perform anaesthetic nerve blocks. The main disadvantage with this technique is the delay between placing the local anaesthetic and the onset of anaesthesia. For example, when performing a block of the tibial nerve at the ankle it takes 15 min for full anaesthetic effect to be

Table 6.1   Preparations for intra-articular and soft-tissue injections.

Preparation	Trade name	Duration of action (based on solubility)	Dose for large joint e.g. knee or hip	Dose for medium joint e.g. wrist or ankle	Dose for small joint such as metatarsophalangeal joint	Dose for soft-tissue injections
Methyl prednisolone	Depo-Medrone	Long	80–120 mg	40–60 mg	10–20 mg	20–40 mg
Prednisolone	Deltastab	Medium	25–50 mg	25 mg	12.5 mg	25 mg
Triamcinolone acetonide	Adcortyl and Kenalog	Long	40–60 mg	20 mg	10 mg	10–20 mg
Hydrocortisone	Hydrocortistab	Short	N/A	N/A	25 mg	25–50 mg

apparent. In the only study to examine this procedure (tibial nerve blocks were used for injections of the plantar fascia) patients did not report any less pain with the nerve block (Crawford et al. 1999).

or

– perform local anaesthesia at the site of the injection. This is the method of choice for most rheumatologists. It allows anaesthesia of the skin and subcutaneous structures and it allows the operator to 'feel' for the joint cavity prior to administering the therapeutic injection. It also allows the operator to aspirate the target joint or bursa prior to injection. The only theoretical disadvantage is the higher risk of infection as syringes have to be changed on the same needle but in practice this doesn't seem to be a problem.

or

– administer local anaesthetic along with the therapeutic injection to confirm correct diagnosis and placement with immediate relief of symptoms. This has some advantages and allows the patient some immediate relief of symptoms with the promise that further relief will follow as the therapeutic injection starts to work.

- Local injection therapy of the foot and ankle is indicated for acute inflammation at specific sites, but is generally combined with attempts to correct any structural deformity using orthoses. For this reason it is generally best to delay the injection until such orthotics have been made to the satisfaction of both orthotist/podiatrist and patient. They can then be worn immediately following the injection.

- It is advisable to rest weight-bearing joints that have been injected with steroids. The optimal period of rest is 24–48 h (Chakravarty et al. 1994). The reason for rest is to ensure the steroid preparation stays in the joint, for maximum benefit.

- In the 1960s a number of publications raised the possibility that repeated injections of steroids may cause joint damage and a 'Charcot like' arthropathy (Chandler et al. 1959). In fact, the senior author of this book had the opportunity to discuss one of these cases with the authors of one of those reports. One of the cases, a lady with osteoarthritis whose husband was a general practitioner, had received weekly injections of steroid over a period of several years; clearly an unusual practice. More recent reports have demonstrated the safety of repeated injections, such that the 'rule of thumb' now is that weight-bearing joints are injected no more than four times a year (Raynauld et al. 2003). There is

evidence that the steroid injections are in fact protective against cartilage damage due to the inflammatory process per se (Williams and Brandt 1984).

- Success of inta-articular and other soft-tissue injections depends on accuracy of placement. In the foot accurate placement is sometimes difficult and some injections are, therefore, performed using a guided technique with either ultrasound (U/S) or X-ray screening. Studying a variety of injection sites Jones et al. found that the clinical response was associated with accuracy of injection placement (Jones et al. 1993). Unfortunately, neither technology nor expertise is widely available at the present time. Some centres rely on radiologists to guide the injections, but this inevitably means delay and the patient returning for a further appointment. In future, U/S-guided injection is likely to occur more frequently as more clinicians are trained in this technique and as the technology becomes cheaper and more accessible (Brown et al. 2004).

- The duration of benefit of a steroid injection varies and depends on a number of factors:
  - Accuracy of placement (and, therefore, in an unguided situation, the experience of the operator (Jones et al. 1993))
  - Physicochemical properties of steroids used (see Table 6.1)
  - The bulk of inflamed synovial tissue
  - The period of rest post-injection.

Cortico–steroid injections of the foot and ankle

- The patient is not exposed to the usual systemic side effects of these drugs
- Improvement is almost immediate and usually long lasting
- There is a low incidence of side effects.
- While useful for articular inflammation they should generally be used in conjunction with orthotic management
- People are usually advised to rest weight bearing joints for 24-48 hours after injection
- Some form of imaging (ultrasound or CT) helps accurate placement of the injection
- Local anaesthetic may be used prior to injection to ease the procedure for the patient and with the injection to confirm accuracy of placement

Adverse effects

Generally speaking, this is a treatment with a low incidence of side effects. The risks are summarized below:

- Infection. This is the major concern, but post therapeutic injection septic arthritis is very uncommon. Reported figures vary from 1 in 10 000 to 1 in 20 000 (Hollander 1985). The risk is minimized by ensuring meticulous attention to aseptic technique using an alcohol-based skin preparation. Injecting through skin lesions (such as psoriatic plaques), which are likely to be colonized by bacteria, is inadvisable. If there is any suspicion about pre-existing infection then this should be excluded before therapeutic injection is performed. If the patient has an intercurrent infection elsewhere with the possibility of septicaemia then the injection should be deferred until the remote infection is under control.

- Bleeding. It is inadvisable to inject weight-bearing joints in people with a coagulopathy either inherited (such as haemophilia) or acquired (such as people taking warfarin therapy). The risk of bleeding into the injected joint is minimized by correcting the coagulopathy or omitting the anti-coagulant for a few days prior to the procedure.

- Post-injection flare. An increase in symptoms within 24 hours of the injection is sometimes experienced. There is a belief that this results from a transient crystal synovitis induced by the steroid crystals (Hollander 1985). Helliwell was able to demonstrate an increase in stiffness of the injected joint at 24 h, which resolved gradually over the next week (Helliwell 1997).

- Post injection systemic symptoms. Depending on the dose of steroid used some people will experience flushing in the days following the steroid injection due to some systemic absorption of steroid. Women may report menstrual irregularity for the same reason.

- If the patient is diabetic it is advisable to warn them that there may be some loss of normal diabetic control in the days following the steroid injection. This is seldom a serious problem.

- Subcutaneous tissue atrophy may occur, particularly if the steroid injection is not correctly placed in the joint. This is seen usually following subcutaneous injections elsewhere, such as at the lateral epicondyle. With time the tissue atrophy will return to normal, but it may take several months and look unsightly during this time.

- Long-acting depot steroid injections should be avoided in the proximity of and within tendons as tendon rupture may follow. This is mainly of concern for the Achilles tendon and the other major tendons around the ankle: the tibialis posterior, long flexor and extensor tendons, and the peroneal group.

Other drugs for intra-articular use

Hyaluronic acid has been found to be of some benefit for osteoarthritis of the knee and hip, but there are no reports of it being used in the foot (Hochberg 2000). In some cases of inflammatory arthritis the synovitis is responsive to intra-articular steroids, but the effect is not very prolonged. In these cases it is sometimes worth considering more permanent methods of controlling synovitis, providing the joint is not too damaged. The two agents that have been used are osmic acid and radiocolloids.

Osmic acid has been used to induce a chemical synovectomy since the 1960s. It was developed as an alternative to radiosynovectomy for use in children where there were concerns about long-term safety of radiation. The preparation is rather difficult to handle as exposure to air may produce toxins and contact with the skin can produce blistering and burns. Preadministration anaesthesia of the joint must be performed and there is almost always a florid synovitis resulting from the injection, sometimes necessitating aspiration. Nevertheless, results in the knee at least are reasonable and fairly long lasting (Cruz-Esteban and Wilke 1995).

Radiation synovectomy in the UK is exclusively with a colloidal preparation of Yttrium (Y^{90}), which is a pure β emitter and has a half life of 2.7 days. If there is any doubt about the needle placement (such as in a 'dry' joint) the intra-articular injection *must* be guided to ensure correct placement of the isotope. To ensure that the isotope remains in the joint it must be immobilized and rested for 3 days after the injection. There have been no randomized-controlled trials of these agents, but anecdotal series using Yttrium and other radiocolloids have been encouraging. This form of therapy is more widely used in Europe where a greater range of isotopes is available (Cruz-Esteban and Wilke 1995).

Intra-articular injections in detail

General observations

In established RA, and particularly in the rear foot, normal joint integrity may be compromised. This results in communication between joints, such that injection into one joint may result in passage of the injected material into other joints. We have frequently seen communication between sub-talar and talo-crural joints and even between the ankle joints and the major tendon sheaths passing around the ankle. Local steroid injections are indicated for troublesome joints; especially where one joint is inflamed, but if several joints are inflamed it is important to pay attention to disease management with systemic drugs as outlined in the previous section.

Talo-crural joint (Fig. 6.3)

This joint is usually approached anteriorly with the entry point of the needle just medial to the tendon of tibialis anterior and the direction of the needle perpendicular to the skin pointing backwards and slightly laterally into the joint cavity. Use a 21-gauge 'green' or a 23-gauge 'blue' needle. There is a little resistance as the joint is penetrated. Use 40 mg of methyl prednisolone or triamcinolone and advise rest after the injection for 48 h. There are a number of potentially vulnerable structures underneath the extensor retinaculum, including the superficial and deep peroneal nerves and the dorsalis pedis artery, which are situated lateral to the injection site.

Sub-talar joint (Fig. 6.4)

The subtalar joint is a complex synovial joint with anterior and posterior 'facets' separated by a well developed ligament. The joint is generally felt to be relatively difficult to enter without some form of imaging. The traditional approach to the subtalar joint is either medially using the sustentaculum tali as a bony landmark, where the needle can be directed anterior or posteriorly to enter the respective parts of the joint, or posteriorly approaching just lateral to the

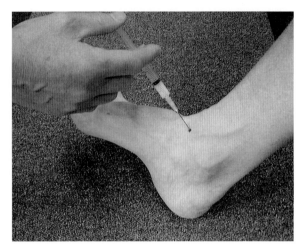

Figure 6.3 Injection of the talo-crural joint.

Achilles tendon and entering the posterior part of the joint (Dixon St.J and Graber 1981). An alternative approach laterally, via the sinus tarsi, provides a simpler approach through which aspiration and injection can be performed without imaging (Canoso 1998). The sinus tarsi is located by palpation just anterior to the lateral malleolus. If the location is tender local anaesthetic can be used. The needle (either a 21 or 23 gauge) is directed towards the sustentaculum tali, medially. The joint space is entered at a depth of 1–2 cm. The approach should encounter no bony obstruction and the injection is performed without

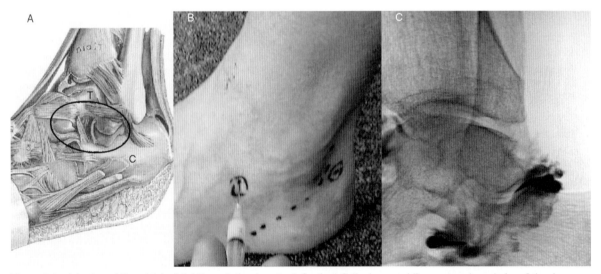

Figure 6.4 Injection of the subtalar joint through the sinus tarsi. On the left the bony and ligamentous boundaries of the sinus tarsi are shown. The central panel illustrates the approach for injection – direct the needle tip towards the sustentaculum tali medially. On the right radiological contrast has been injected via the sinus tarsi in a 65-year-old man.

resistance. Such an approach, using radio-opaque contrast, is illustrated.

Talo-navicular joint (Fig. 6.5)
This joint is a common source of symptoms in RA, but is not always easy to inject. Identify the tuberosity of the navicular and the joint line of the talo-navicular joint just posterior to this landmark. Inject perpendicular to the skin, but the joint is usually quite near the surface so use a 25-gauge 'orange' needle. This is not a very capacious joint and 20 mg methyl prednisolone or equivalent is recommended.

First metatarsophalangeal joint (Fig. 6.6)
The aim is not to place the needle tip within the joint cavity, but to place it within the joint capsule. As the injection is given for an inflamed and swollen joint usually all that is required is to slip the needle under the joint capsule using an oblique dorsal approach.

The needle tip is placed under the extensor tendon, which is contiguous with the dorsal 'hood' of capsule. The approach to the joint may be obstructed by large amounts of new bone if severe hallus abductovalgus is present and the use of imaging and guided techniques has obvious advantages in such cases. A fine 23-gauge or 25-gauge needle should be used.

Lesser metatarsophalangeal joints (Fig. 6.7)
By analogy to the technique for injecting the first metatarsophalangeal joint the aim is not to enter the joint cavity but to place the needle within the capsule using the dorsal approach, injecting beneath the extensor tendon. Use a fine needle such as a 23-gauge or 25-gauge needle. If required a nerve block of the superficial peroneal nerve prior to the injection will help reduce the discomfort during the procedure: in practice we rarely find this necessary.

Proximal inter-phalangeal joints (Fig. 6.8)
These are sometimes particularly troublesome, but more often require special attention in psoriatic arthritis where one or two proximal and distal interphalangeal joints may be a problem. A fine 25-gauge 'orange' needle is required. The approach is similar to the metatarsophalangeal joints: the joint is approached dorsally from either side and the needle slipped under the extensor tendon to rest within the joint capsule. When the injection is made a bulge is felt on the opposite side of the joint. If the needle is placed dorsal to the extensor tendon the bulge appears at the tip of the needle and the needle should be repositioned. The joint, like those of the metatarsophalangeal joints, will only accept a small volume of fluid (0.5 ml maximum).

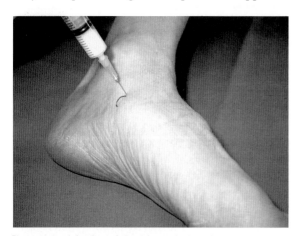

Figure 6.5 Injection of the talo-navicular joint.

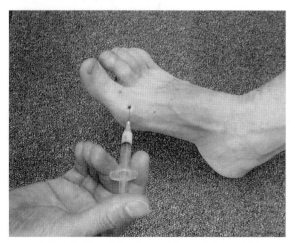

Figure 6.6 Injection of the first metatarsophalangeal joint.

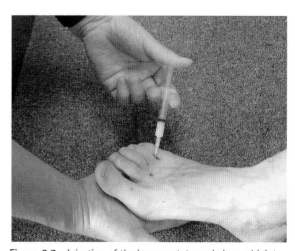

Figure 6.7 Injection of the lesser metatarsophalangeal joint.

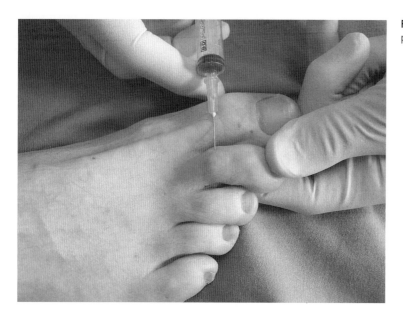

Figure 6.8   Injection of the proximal inter-phalangeal joints of the foot.

Injection of bursae

Retrocalcaneal bursa (Fig. 6.9)

The retrocalcaneal bursa, situated between the Achilles tendon and the posterior-superior aspect of the calcaneum can become inflamed in RA and may, occasionally, require injection with steroids. More often this injection is required in seronegative spondyloarthritis such as psoriatic arthritis. The bursa is approached at an angle to one side of the Achilles tendon close to its insertion into the calcaneum. There are no neurovascu-

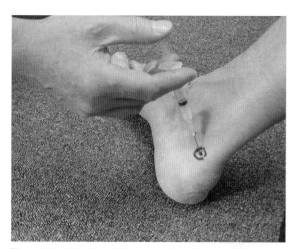

Figure 6.9   Injection of the retro-calcaneal bursa. Although this injection can readily be performed 'blind' the proximity to the Achilles tendon makes an ultrasound-guided injection the recommended procedure.

lar tissues to be concerned about, although exact placement may be difficult because of the variable depth of the bursa. This injection is readily and probably best performed with U/S guidance. Once the (23-gauge) needle is correctly positioned the injection is 'easy': use 20 mg of methyl prednisolone or equivalent.

Adventitious bursae (see DVD)

Adventitious bursae may develop to protect underlying tissues when deformity results in prominence of a bony structure. The full clinical picture involves an area of high pressure, an overlying callus and beneath this, but lying over the bony prominence, an adventitious bursa. These sometimes become inflamed and they benefit from aspiration and injection with steroids (Dixon St.J and Graber 1981). These bursae may also become infected and, therefore, caution should be exercised in injecting these structures. If there is any doubt try and aspirate before performing a therapeutic injection.

Injection of soft tissues and tendon sheaths

Plantar fascia (Fig. 6.10 and DVD)

Patients with rheumatoid arthritis may experience painful lesions at the medial tubercle of the calcaneum where the longitudinal plantar fascia is attached. This is more commonly seen in the seronegative spondyloarthropathies, but has been shown to occur with a similar frequency in RA (Falsetti et al. 2003). The traditional approach to this injection has been directly on

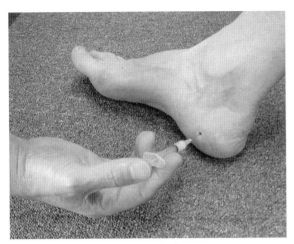

Figure 6.10 Injection of plantar fascia.

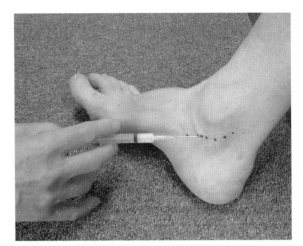

Figure 6.11 Injection of tibialis posterior tendon.

to the painful spot through the heel pad, but this approach is painful, may result in excessive bleeding and may also promote rupture of the plantar fascia. The alternative technique is to inject the attachment from the medial aspect of the ankle aiming to target the needle tip at the medial calcaneal tubercle. This technique is slightly harder as some degree of 'triangulation' is necessary. Either procedure may be made more comfortable by performing a tibial nerve block at the ankle, but the results of this are disappointing and incur a delay of 15 min when performing the injection, as noted above. An alternative to local steroid injection has been proposed: extracorporeal shock-wave therapy, but a recent trial of this technique found it to be ineffective for this condition (Haake et al. 2003).

Tibialis posterior tendon (Fig. 6.11 and DVD)
The tibialis posterior tendon is frequently involved by florid tenosynovitis as it passes around the medial condyle of the ankle. Instability at the rearfoot with eversion of the calcaneum on weight bearing will exacerbate this. If the tenosynovitis is to be treated by local steroid injection it is imperative to address the sub-talar instability at the same time. The injection is made with a 23-gauge needle along the axis of the tendon, using a distal approach. If the needle is correctly sited the injected material can be seen and felt to pass up the tendon sheath. If the needle appears to be correctly sited, but injection is difficult, it is possible the needle tip is within the substance of the tendon and the needle should be withdrawn slightly.

Peroneal tendons (Fig. 6.12)
A similar technique is used to the injection of tibialis posterior, but it is not uncommon to visualize the peroneus longus and brevis tendons as they pass around

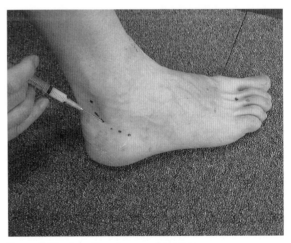

Figure 6.12 Injection of peroneal tendons.

the lateral malleolus. In such circumstances, the injection can be made using a proximal approach. With either of the approaches it should be possible to see and feel the injected material as it passes along the tendon sheath.

'Morton's interdigital neuroma' (Fig. 6.13)
As already discussed, the use of the term 'Morton's neuroma' is a misnomer in RA, as the condition is reproduced by inflammatory tissue in the inter-digital space. In some cases a rheumatoid nodule occurs at the site. For either of these conditions an injection of a long-acting steroid is efficacious. The injection is made from the dorsal approach directly through to the inter-digital space using a 23-gauge needle. If necessary a nerve block of the deep peroneal nerve can be made prior to the injection.

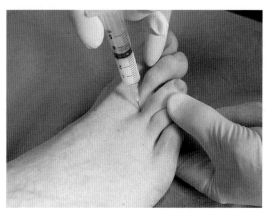

Figure 6.13 Injection of 'Morton's interdigital neuroma'. As with the retro-calcaneal bursa it is recommended that ultrasound guidance is used for this procedure, unless circumstances dictate that the injection be performed 'blind'.

Tarsal tunnel (Fig. 6.14)

The tarsal tunnel lies on the medial side of the ankle and is bounded by the calcaneus, the flexor retinaculum (ligamentum lacinatum) and the tendinous arch of abductor hallucis. Also found passing through the 'tunnel' are the posterior tibial artery and the tendons of tibialis posterior and flexor hallucis longus. Tenosynovitis in the sheaths of the latter is the most likely cause of the tarsal tunnel syndrome in RA. As discussed in Chapter 3, this condition is not infrequent on neurophysiological testing, yet it is seldom diagnosed in the clinic situation. The injection is made from either proximal or distal aspects of the site using a 23-gauge needle, attempting to avoid the neurovascular structures; placement of the needle 'blind' at the inferior aspect of the ligament is the best way to do this, but if in doubt use a U/S-guided technique. If the condition persists despite injection, and the problem is

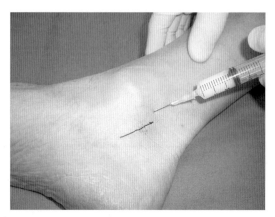

Figure 6.14 Injection of tarsal tunnel. The palpable course of the posterior tibial artery is indicated.

confirmed by electrophysiology, surgery may be contemplated.

Rheumatoid nodules

From time to time a patient will present with a painful rheumatoid nodule over a bony prominence or within soft tissue, the commonest sites being the Achilles tendon and the heel pad. In the latter case it may be helpful to inject a small dose of steroid directly in to the nodule. Nodules on the Achilles are best avoided with steroids to avoid the risk of tendon rupture.

Nerve blocks for the foot and ankle

There are several indications for nerve blockade in the foot in RA:

1. Temporary relief of pain from synovitis or tendonitis. It has been noted that interrupting the pain chronic pain cycle even temporarily has some longer-term benefits for some patients (Arner et al. 1990).
2. As a diagnostic aid helping to identify painful structures or to estimate joint degeneration (Hay et al. 1999, Mitchell et al. 1995)
3. Prior to more invasive procedures or painful injections such as local corticosteroid infiltration.

The most widely used local anaesthetic agents are lignocaine, mepivicaine and bupivicaine. They are used *without* adrenaline in end structures such as the foot to avoid compromising the arterial supply.

Lignocaine is used at concentrations typically of 1 or 2% and may be used alone or mixed with other agents such as corticosteroid. The onset of analgesia is fairly rapid, usually within 1–2 min in a joint or soft tissue, but relatively longer (20–30 min) for a nerve such as the tibial or peroneal. Lignocaine provides relatively short-duration analgesia, typically of 2–3 h. Mepivicaine, usually administered at a concentration of 1.5 or 3% can have a slightly more rapid onset and has a similar duration of effect. For a longer-lasting blockade Bupivicaine (typically 0.25 or 0.50%) will provide analgesia for up to 10 h, although its onset of action is slow at 20–40 min, and its toxicity is greater than Lignocaine or Mepivicaine.

Local analgesia is most often administered subcutaneously to desensitize the skin local to the site of a more painful procedure. Local anaesthetic may also be introduced directly into a painful structure such as a joint or soft tissue lesion. Intravenous regional analgesia provides widespread analgesia, but is medically more complex and is not a technique suited to routine use in rheumatology outpatient clinics.

A skilful operator can, however, use local anaesthetic to blockade individual nerves at the level of the
ankle and so provide analgesia with a single injection
to the moderately large areas of the foot associated
with each dermatome.

There are as many as seven ankle nerve blocks that
may be used, but most indications in rheumatology
require only analgesia of the plantar foot (tibial nerve)
or the dorsum of the forefoot (common peroneal
nerve). All can be performed with the patient in a
supine position, although the operator might find
access better for the two posterior approaches if the
patient is put in a prone position.

Tibial nerve blockade

The tibial nerve is a branch of the sciatic nerve. Its sensory dermatome includes the plantar surface of the
foot (via the medial and lateral plantar nerves), and
the lateral side of the foot (via the sural nerve)
(Fig. 6.15). A single injection blockading the tibial
nerve at ankle level gives satisfactory analgesia of the
whole of the plantar surface of the foot, making this
technique potentially suitable for painful plantar procedures such as for plantar fasciitis or ulcer debride-

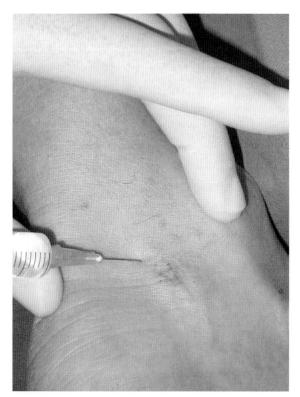

Figure 6.15 Local anaesthetic block of the tibial nerve at
the ankle.

ment. The tibial nerve passes from the popliteal fossa,
deep to the calf musculature and passes posteriorly
around the medial malleolus retained by the flexor
retinaculum.

It is blocked at the level of the malleolus using a posterior or medial approach. If the patient is supine the
foot should be abducted to expose the postero-medial
aspect of the ankle. It may be possible to palpate or roll
the nerve to identify its location precisely, although this
is not common. The nerve lies medial to the rest of the
neurovascular structures and so the approach should
stay close to the medial side of the tendo-Achilles. The
needle is introduced mid-way between the tip of malleolus and the medial border of the tendo-Achilles and
advanced toward the posterior aspect of the tibia. The
patient should be advised to warn the operator if
paraesthesia is felt, as this indicates that the needle tip
has touched the nerve itself. If this occurs then the
needle tip should be withdrawn a few millimetres
prior to completing the injection. If the needle tip
advances without encountering the nerve, then it will
come to rest on the posterior aspect of the tibia.

At this point the needle should again be withdrawn
a few millimetres prior to completing the injection.

Once the desired spot is reached aspiration *must*
be performed to ensure that the needle tip is not
lying within any of the vascular structures closely
associated with the tibial nerve in this region. If there
is no aspirate, the injection is completed by infiltrat-
ing 2–5 ml of solution around the nerve, the amount
depending on concentration used. The diameter of
the tibial nerve slows the rate of onset of analgesia
and satisfactory analgesia may take 20–30 min at this
site.

Common/superficial peroneal nerve blockade

The common peroneal nerve also derives from the
sciatic nerve dividing into a superficial and deep
branch at mid-tibia. The superficial branch passes
anterior to the lateral malleolus to supply the majority of the dorsum of the foot, while the deep branch
passes through the tibio-fibular interosseous membrane along the dorsum of the foot to supply the
1st/2nd toe interspace. If the area of required anaesthesia includes the 1st/2nd toe interspace, then blockade is best achieved proximal to branching at the level
of the fibular styloid process. If analgesia of the
1st/2nd toe interspace is not required, the common
peroneal nerve can be blocked at the fibular styloid or
the superficial branch alone can be blocked at the
lateral malleolus.

The block at the fibular styloid is straightforward
(Fig. 6.16). The nerve is usually directly palpable
1–2 cm distal to the styloid process of the fibular and

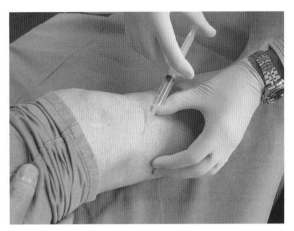

Figure 6.16 Local anaesthetic block of the common peroneal nerve at the head of the fibular.

the nerve may be rolled under the fingertips. It is blocked with a straightforward subcutaneous injection close to the nerve. Onset of action is typically in the 15–20-min range.

Blockade of the superficial branch is undertaken on the anterolateral aspect of the lateral malleolus. The nerve can often be palpated directly or may even be seen and if so a direct subcutaneous deposition is made close to the nerve. If the nerve cannot be located precisely then an alternative technique is used. The course of the nerve can be quite variable in this region, so a common technique is to pass the needle tip subcutaneously across the likely course of the nerve for 2–3 cm (Fig. 6.17). The local analgesic is deposited as the needle is slowly withdrawn leaving a 2–3 cm sausage of local anaesthetic subcutaneously. Blocking the nerve directly at the ankle can give rapid onset of action.

Saphenous and sural nerves

These are not commonly used, but may allow for a more direct medial or lateral approach in some cases, or may be required to provide analgesia when tibial or peroneal nerve blockade has provided incomplete regional coverage.

The saphenous nerve arises from the femoral nerve and passes anteriorly down the leg in association with the saphenous vein. It passes anterior to the medial malleolus and innervates the dorso-medial border of the foot (Fig. 6.18). It is blocked by an anterior approach over the medial malleolus, with the needle tip inserted immediately medial to the tendon of tibialis anterior, and between this tendon and the saphenous vein. The saphenous nerve is quite superficial at this point and so the needle does not need to be advanced far. Aspiration must again be performed prior to depositing the LA, and deposition of no more than 2–3 ml will usually achieve satisfactory analgesia.

The sural nerve is a branch of the sciatic nerve but may branch at mid calf and be part missed by the standard tibial nerve blockade. The sural nerve passes down the posterior aspect of the calf and around the lateral malleolus to innervate a relatively small region on the lateral side of the fore foot (Fig. 6.19).

The sural nerve rarely needs individual blockade, but is easily targeted using a posterior approach mirroring that used for the tibial nerve.

Using a postero-lateral approach, the needle is inserted midway between the lateral aspect of the tendo-Achilles and the tip of the lateral malleolus, and is directed toward the posterior aspect of the tibia. The sural nerve is relatively superficial and the needle tip does not need to penetrate as far as the tibial surface, the site is aspirated and 1–2 ml of local anaesthetic deposited. Analgesia is again rapid at this site.

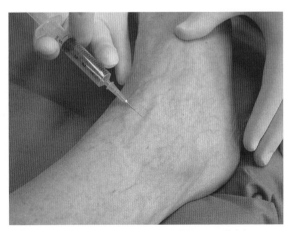

Figure 6.17 Local anaesthetic block of the superficial peroneal nerve at the ankle.

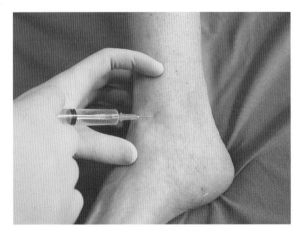

Figure 6.18 Local anaesthetic block of the saphenous nerve at the ankle.

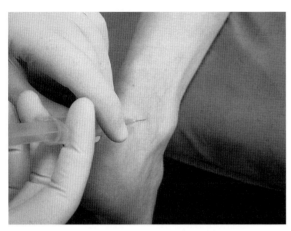

Figure 6.19   Local anaesthetic block of the sural nerve.

CONSERVATIVE PODIATRY MANAGEMENT

Introduction

The WHO ICF has been championed as the basis for multi-professional patient assessment, goal setting, intervention management, and evaluation (Stucki and Ewert 2005). Multidisciplinary rehabilitation of RA foot problems fits this model well and in Figure 6.20 the

medical and therapy delivered components, as well as current outcome tools used to evaluate the effectiveness of these interventions, are linked to each domain. In the model, delivery of conservative care is not prescribed by therapy professions, as this is less clear throughout European rheumatology centres, but this section will focus on the podiatrist in this role. For convenience, surgical intervention (Chapter 7) has been arbitrarily separated from the model, but it must be considered as an important part of the care continuum.

As we know physician management of the disease and local treatment of inflammatory lesions forms the major component of rheumatoid arthritis treatment. Although the focus may be on rehabilitating foot problems, global disease activity, medication and response to medication must be considered in the care pathway. Why is that? Well, consider the newly diagnosed patient referred with forefoot symptoms related to MTP disease. Is there heightened activity in these joints when other sites are quiescent or is the disease more active generally? What disease modifying anti-rheumatic drug regime does the patient have, when was it started and how effective is it? Armed with this information the podiatrist may be able to tell if the disease is more localized suggesting mechanical factors, or

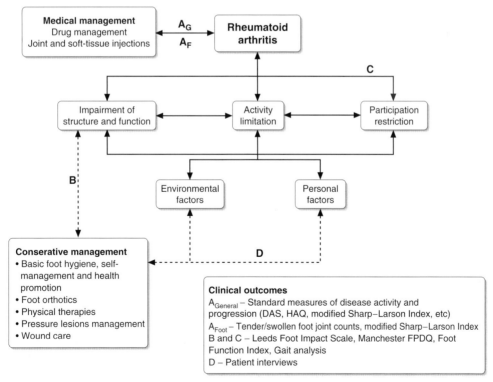

Figure 6.20   ICF framework for disability with interaction shown between framework components and medical and conservative management of the foot in rheumatoid arthritis (adapted from Stucki and Ewert 2005).

whether the foot involvement may simply be part of a general disease flare where therapy has just been initiated. Either way, there is no strong supporting evidence to support the optimal timing for any of the interventions in the armoury of the therapist. Off-loading inflamed MTP joints is a reasonable approach in both scenarios and this can be undertaken using footwear modifications and orthoses. Attenuating mechanical stresses would be beneficial in joints that are acutely inflamed or in those where disease remains locally persistent.

In the ICF framework, typical podiatry interventions such as footwear and orthoses, callus debridement and wound care take place at the level of impairment of structure and function. As yet we have little information on how these may affect underlying disease mechanisms, or drive changes at higher-level domains for activity limitation and participation restriction. Evidence of reasonable quality is emerging to drive an evidence-based approach to conservative footcare in RA, yet podiatry, like other therapy groups, will continue to struggle to provide evidence in sufficient quantity to fully understand the effectiveness of interventions in important sub-cohorts. Nevertheless, progress is being made. For example, custom foot orthoses were shown to have no benefit over placebo on foot pain and disability in RA (Conrad et al. 1996). Alone, these findings were not widely generalizable, since the cohort comprised older male patients with long-standing disease, yet who had no severe foot impairments or comorbid conditions affecting gait. Contrast this, then, with data from Leeds, where a randomized controlled trial showed a significant clinical improvement when the orthoses were used in patients with early disease (Woodburn et al. 2002). Furthermore, new insights are continually emerging into the relationship between mechanical foot function and physical interventions in clinical studies of foot orthoses and footwear (Fransen and Edmonds 1997, Hodge et al. 1999, Shrader and Siegel 2003, Woodburn et al. 2003). In the following pages footwear and orthoses will be discussed in detail.

In the clinical setting, the ICF framework is also appealing as it includes environmental and personal factors and these significantly influence the physical interventions undertaken by podiatrists and others. Furthermore, if treatment of the impairment is undertaken without addressing all the framework components, in a multidisciplinary approach, then treatment may ultimately be less successful.

Aspects of coping, well-being, motivation, etc., are factors identified at the personal level in the ICF framework and these have a significant effect on foot care. Yet we do not formally assess this nor call on the services of others, for example clinical psychology, to assist. Other factors, such as appearance and fashion-consciousness are also potential barriers to effective treatment. For example, consider the well-educated patient, knowledgeable about their disease and empowered in self-care who refuses to change their footwear because of the prevailing fashion. She tells her podiatrist, 'I'm giving in to it – its forcing me to make changes, but one change I wont make is to wear horrible shoes.' This is a common clinical problem and best solved by working on footwear education and support since the evidence suggests that inappropriate shoes will be seen only on clinic days or consigned to the patient's wardrobe (Williams and Meacher 2001). The problems with footwear for patients will be discussed further later in the chapter.

The implementation of the ICF framework in clinical practice may be aided by the use of model sheets (Steiner et al. 2002). This has been adapted for podiatry in Figure 6.21 to illustrate how to structure foot problems from the patient and podiatrist point of view and to set goals for the rehabilitation programme. This is a 67-year-old female patient with 15 years' disease duration, managed on methotrexate, sulphasalazine and a non-steroidal anti-inflammatory drug. Her disease activity is low and she has just been referred to the Foot Health Department at her hospital outpatient unit. Using the model, the patient's main problem with her right foot can be identified and listed (upper section) along with the podiatrist's findings and observations (lower section). Along with environmental and personal factors, relationships between these factors can be explored and links made (indicated with lines) so that the most important problems become the goals of the initial treatment. Briefly, in the case presented, callus debridement, custom orthosis and extra-depth shoes are all indicated to accommodate and functionally stabilize the foot to treat the forefoot deformity, callosities, pes planovalgus and tibialis posterior tenosynovitis. The goal here is to decrease pain and improve function. Muscle strengthening is required for the calf muscle weakness and collaboration is sought with the rehabilitation team for the right knee problem. The goal here is to improve function. Information on the benefits and risks of foot surgery must be provided to help alleviate those fears. Since the plantar callosities may be at risk of ulceration when the patient has peripheral vascular disease, self-assessment strategies are taught so the patient or relative can regularly inspect the feet. The goal here is patient education and empowerment.

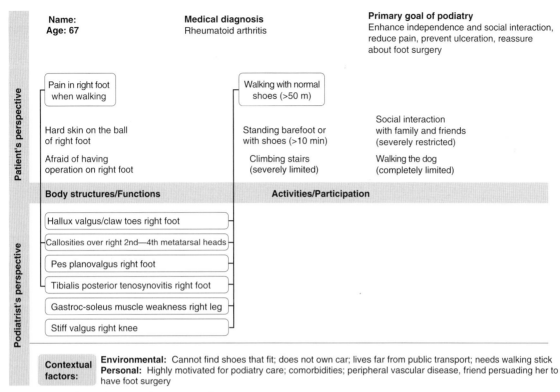

Figure 6.21   An ICF model sheet adapted for podiatry.

Patient education and self-management

Over the last few years, new policies to modernize the NHS have consistently emphasized the importance of the patient in the design and delivery of health services (see Chapter 9). Fundamental changes are taking place not only to provide patients with health education, but to empower patients and recognize that patients and professionals each have their own area of knowledge and expertise and need to work together. One of the key messages of the chronic disease management and self-care National Service Framework (NSF) (DOH 2002) is to ensure that patients with chronic disease fully understand and are empowered to manage their condition. All of the NSFs emphasize the importance of self-care in managing long-term disease and the promotion of independence. Evidence supports the idea that self-management of chronic conditions leads to improved psychological well-being, reduction in pain and lower levels of depression. In addition, training in self-management programmes at early stages of a condition may help prevent the onset of compounded conditions and further disability.

Patient education has been described as any set of planned educational activities designed to improve patients' health behaviours, and, through this, their health status and, ultimately, long-term outcome (Hill 1997). Patient education and self-management have been advocated in chronic diseases, including RA for their information provision and therapeutic potential. Patient education should be portrayed not only as a 'nice extra', but should be accepted as an important part of the management of patients with a chronic rheumatic disease (Lorig 1995). Lorig and colleagues at the Stanford University School of Medicine have frequently identified the benefits of a Chronic Disease Self-management Plan which include improved health behaviours and health status, fewer hospitalizations and days of hospitalization as well as reduced health-care costs.

A Cochrane Systematic review of patient education for adults with RA, carried out by Riemsma et al. (2004), assessed the effectiveness of patient education interventions on health status in RA. Patient education was shown to have small short-term effects on disability, painful joint counts, patient global assessment, psychological status and depression. However, the review highlighted that in practice many patient education programmes have not been disease specific and there has been the assumption that all effects are generic. Patient education and self-management programmes are always delivered in addition to usual medical care, which is often of a very high standard in research centres where these trials are carried out. Furthermore, it is believed that patient characteristics play a role in the beneficial effects of education. Patients in trials are invited to take part, whereas patients in routine clinical practice are more likely to be willing volunteers for education programmes. Delivering education to patients requires behavioural change on the part of the patient; however, there are barriers to behavioural change that may arise. The level of education of patients with RA has been shown to contribute to the use of walking aids such as orthopaedic footwear (Van der Esch et al. 2003). This may be explained by the fact that education is an indicator of socio-economic status and, therefore, these patients could afford to purchase such aids or that higher-educated patients are more assertive in acquiring aids to help themselves.

A lack of self-care of the feet by patients with RA can have severe implications. Health promotion and education are required at all stages of the disease process and can be delivered in a variety of forms. It is not only important that patients are provided with health promotion and education but those providers are knowledgeable and confident in delivering the advice. Even if patients have appropriate knowledge and the motivation to apply that knowledge, benefits may not occur unless their health providers also take appropriate actions (Spraul 2000). With finite funding for provision of footcare services, many patients with RA are classified by current podiatry referral guide-lines as not having 'at-risk' feet and, therefore, do not qualify for practitioner led podiatry care. However, because of other joint impairments they are unable to reach their feet or use appropriate equipment to pro-vide their own care. The FOOTSTEP self-management programme (discussed in further detail later in this chapter) was developed by podiatrists in order to pro-vide a programme of self-care for patients that do not require practitioner-led care (Waxman et al. 2003). Practitioners are typically not aware of the benefits of developing patient partner networks and alternative ways of providing self-care, which will enable the patient to remain independent. Thus, the thrust of current educational efforts should be given to the education of health-care providers.

Unfortunately there is little evidence in favour of podiatric education programmes for rheumatology patients. Sari-Kouzel et al. (2001) reported the inci-dence of foot problems in systemic sclerosis and sug-gested that patient education and increased awareness

about foot problems in primary care may reduce the frequency of surgical amputations in such patients by reducing the incidence of ulcers. However, putting knowledge into practice is the 'Holy Grail' of educa-tion: one of the most commonly reported outcomes for all patient educational interventions is that of improved knowledge, yet it is now widely accepted that knowledge alone bears a very poor relationship to positive behaviour change (Stuart and Wiles 2000).

Diabetic Patient Education Programmes have been widely tested and their value is recognized within the podiatry profession. Diabetic foot-care education and primary preventive measures provided individually by a podiatrist have been shown to result in significant improvements in knowledge and foot self-care scores and in a decrease in the prevalence of some minor foot problems (Ronnemaa et al. 1997). Different disease processes lead to different disease outcomes, there-fore, the strategies for providing patient education may vary extensively between patient groups. The neuropathic diabetic patient (where numbness of feet leads to trauma that may go unnoticed by the patient) will have different perceptions of foot problems in comparison to the patient with RA who experiences significant foot impairments as a result of their disease process. Hence, the current diabetic patient education programmes may not address the issues appropriate for patients with RA and, therefore, should be adapted accordingly. As with other chronic diseases, there is a gradual decline in physical functioning, but with relapses and remissions such that the requirements for foot care provision are likely to change. Ability to self care and risk status will be dependent on changes in disease activity, changes to drug treatment regimes and development of complications such as vasculitis or peripheral vascular disease.

It is frequently perceived that health professionals specializing in their field of work are the most appro-priate people to provide patients with the advice and education that will help them to successfully manage their condition. However, the traditional model of patients as the passive recipients of care is beginning to change, especially for those with chronic diseases, who often can be more informed about their condition than the practitioners caring for them. The data pro-duced by Branch et al. (1999) showed that arthritis patient educators can provide a meaningful and useful addition to traditional rheumatology care by posi-tively affecting the patient's satisfaction with clinic services. The Expert Patients Programme, available at http//www.ohn.gov.uk is led by volunteer course tutors who are themselves patients that have previ-ously undertaken the Expert Patients Programme. The programme covers a variety of self-management skills helping patients to seek possible solutions and achieve goals. These programmes are not specific to RA patients or to foot health, but are available to anyone with chronic or long-term health conditions, who wishes to learn skills for managing and improving their general health.

The method by which education can be delivered can vary from written information in the format of booklets/leaflets left in patient waiting areas to formalized educational sessions aimed at a group or individual level. The value of providing leaflets in patient waiting areas should not be underestimated. One study showed that knowledge of systemic lupus erythematosis can be significantly improved with a comprehensive guide-book (Konttinen et al. 1991). Furthermore, it has been shown that patients instructed by a health professional show no greater knowledge over patients who were just simply provided with the booklet alone (Maggs et al. 1996). The Arthritis Research Campaign (*arc*) provides a number of leaflets, mindmaps and fold-out guides for patients with RA on all aspects of the disease including information on drug therapies, alternative therapy and exercise, and, specifically, has a foot-related leaflet entitled 'Feet, footwear and arthritis'. This leaflet is an ideal education tool that can be given to patients at diagnosis prior to receiving foot care or given in conjunction with foot care advice or management therapies. The leaflets can be obtained directly from *arc* or can be downloaded from the *arc* website (http//www.arc.org.uk). The leaflets are updated on a regular basis and are written in a language that is easy for patients to understand, they are also available in different languages.

Leaflets such as these, provided by *arc*, which detail strategies for self-management, have been shown to be the commonest source of self-management information for patients with RA (Hammond 1998).

In the Leeds rheumatology foot clinic, a variety of patient education tools are incorporated into everyday routine clinical practice (Fig. 6.22). Examples of different types of footwear are available to demonstrate to patients the benefits of extra room in the toe box area for accommodating foot deformity, the differences in the cushioning properties of outsoles with different styles of shoe, and the advantages of Velcro fastenings when they are unable to tie shoe laces. Anatomical foot models help patients to understand how the foot functions and helps to explain why they are experiencing foot problems. Currently, there are no courses specifically run for the basic self-management of foot problems in patient with RA. The FOOT-STEP self-management programme (SMP) was the

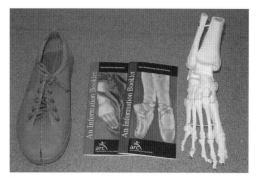

Figure 6.22   Patient education tools.

first comprehensive self-management, education and training programme to be developed and tested in the area of routine podiatry care (Waxman et al. 2003). The FOOTSTEP SMP has provided evidence that management of routine foot care at the primary level can be reoriented towards a system of patient-directed decision-making concerning treatment timing and options without compromising care. The FOOTSTEP SMP was designed for people aged 60+ years seeking self-initiated or primary referred podiatric consultation, and it has been suggested that the FOOTSTEP SMP could be extended to other target groups such as those with arthropathies. We routinely assess patients who find it difficult or are unable to provide their own foot care. Frequently we find that these patients do not fit the criteria for treatment set out by podiatry departments, for example they are too young, they are not diabetic and they do not have any potentially harmful lesions on their feet. But patients with RA frequently experience difficulty using everyday scissors or nail clippers to cut their own toenails because of hand deformity or loss of grip strength. An SMP could potentially provide a solution for these struggling patients and provide a more patient-led approach to care, empowering patients and their partners and reducing the potential for urgent appointments because of problems caused by inappropriate self-management or neglect.

There are many potential barriers to patients providing self-care of their feet, specifically related to RA. Hand deformity, stiffness, pain and muscle weakness can physically disable the patient. Thomson and Masson (1992) assessed the ability of elderly patients to co-operate with foot care advice. Using small self-adhesive red spots, foot lesions were simulated and patients advised and prompted to detect and inspect these 'lesions'. The outcome revealed that only 14% of all the elderly patients could detect the simulated plantar lesions and

EDUCATION

- The importance of self-care and patient empowerment should not be underestimated and can be delivered in a variety of formats. Health promotion and patient education should be provided at all stages of the disease process and should be patient group specific.
- Assessments should be undertaken to establish the patient's ability to provide basic foot care. When the patient is unable to do this the development of patient partner networks provides an alternative to costly practitioner led foot care and enables the patient to remain independent.
- Patient educators can provide a meaningful addition to traditional rheumatology care by positively affecting the patient's satisfaction with clinic services.
- A variety of patient education tools should be available to be incorporated into everyday routine clinical practice.

were able to respond to them. It is likely that patients with RA, particularly those with joint stiffness and hand deformity, may find it even more difficult to identify potential problematic lesions on the plantar aspect of their feet. In many instances, it is helpful to provide patients with some practical advice of how to overcome potential barriers. Such advice may include using a mirror to inspect the plantar surface of the foot, suggestions on the correct sitting position for cutting nails, stockists of equipment for providing foot care and training family members to provide basic foot care will allow the patient to self manage. In the early stages of disease patients will benefit from written and verbal foot care information, providing details of basic skin and nail care, the development of and training for patient partners to facilitate basic foot care when patients find it difficult to provide self care, the importance of daily foot inspections and what action to take if they develop a problem supplemented with rapid podiatry support when necessary. In some instances, practitioner-led podiatry care is indicated due to the high-risk status of the patient related to medication, the presence of co-morbidities including vascular disease, diabetes and previous ulceration, even in these instances appropriate self-management for basic foot hygiene and inspection should be encouraged.

Foot orthoses

The provision of foot orthoses is an area of specialist expertise for the podiatrist, although by no means is it exclusive since customized foot orthotics are provided by orthotic/appliance departments, physiotherapists, occupational therapists and others. Pain can be a significant factor in promoting self management. In a quest for comfort many patients will seek out non-prescribed devices, which are now widely available in 'High Street' chemists, sports shops, advertised in newspapers/magazines and through the internet. In some cases, patients will go to ingenious lengths to fabricate their own devices (Fig. 6.23). At Leeds the approach to orthotic provision is to use customized devices appropriate to the stage of disease, with increased focus on early disease in an attempt to stabilize the foot and prevent deformity or to protect the at risk foot in established disease. This section will be centred on indicators for treatment (impairments of structure and function), constraints for treatment (patient and environmental factors) and indicators for treatment response.

ORTHOSES

Disease staged management is advocated with foot orthoses provision.

In early disease the aim of orthoses is to preserve and maintain function and to prevent and lessen deformity.

In early disease clinical experience has shown that those patients most likely to benefit from orthoses are those with:

- pre-existing foot deformity
- tenosynovitis, particularly of tibialis posterior
- poor rearfoot alignment
- low medial arch profile
- residual foot impairments even when disease activity has been suppressed.

In more established foot disease the aim of orthoses management will be to:

- reduce pain
- maintain function
- accommodate existing deformity
- prevent further deformity
- maintain tissue viability in conjunction with accommodative footwear.

There are many types of orthotic devices available ranging from simple, flat, cushioning insoles, to rigid customized orthoses. In our experience, the flat cushioning insoles are the types of devices patients will seek

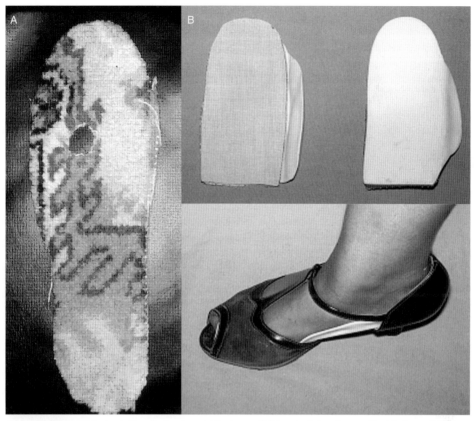

Figure 6.23   Some patient initiated solutions to insoles and footwear. (A) Insoles taken from patients' shoes at first assessment appointment. The patient presented with fatty padding under the MTP joints and a subluxed MTP joint with an overlying pressure-induced lesion. These insoles show the level of the patient's perception of their needs; the carpet material provides much needed cushioning under the ball of the foot with a cut out to attempt to deflect pressure away from a painful callosity. (B) This patient had noticed that her arches had fallen and she was developing arch and ankle pain, she recognized that she needed support within the arch area, particularly when she went out ballroom dancing with her husband. This rigid plastic orthotic was made to support the medial longitudinal arch and also had a cushioning top cover. It was constructed from a cut down piece of plastic guttering pipe, heat-moulded to fit the foot using a gas cooker ring and adapted to discretely fit into her dancing shoes. This case highlights the high level of sophistication and ingenious lengths some patients will go to in order to obtain comfort.

out for themselves as they perceive that they need extra cushioning under the foot for comfort. Rigid customized devices are usually prescribed in early disease aiming to optimize foot function and to resist the deforming forces resulting from repeated episodes of inflammation. In established disease where fixed deformity predominates, orthotic devices are individually contoured to provide support and to fully accommodate deformity and are referred to as total contact inlays.

The rationale for the use of foot orthoses in patients with RA with foot impairments generally centres on the following concepts.

- Joint stabilization (control)
- Anatomical positioning (correction)
- Pain reduction
- Prevention of deformity (joint protection)

- Improvement of function
- Improved range of movement
- Rest anatomical structures (joints and soft tissues)
- Reduce inflammation.

Few orthotic interventions have been subjected to rigourous evaluation under clinical trial conditions. Table 6.2 provides a summary of the studies to date. Previous work in this area has been directed towards specific foot deformities, mainly in established disease. Selective inclusion of specific patient groups and different methodological approaches hampers the clinical translation of current research. In the absence of general design principles for foot orthoses in patients with RA and a limited number of studies on efficacy, general recommendations for orthotic treatment can not be made. As a general rule the orthotic design and

Table 6.2 Summary of literature for orthoses efficacy.

Graded on evidence based on Shekelle et al. (1999)

Author	Evidence level	N	Disease duration (years)	Outcome measures	Effect
Locke (1984)	III	25	–	Pain	+
				Gait	+
Hunt (1987)	III	1	20	Pain	+
				Gait	+
Budiman-Mak (1995)	Ib	102	10	HAV progression	–
Conrad (1996)	Ib	102	Males 'Long'	Pain disability	–
Shrader (1997)	IV	1	Female Long standing		
Hodge (1999)	IIb	12	22	Pain	+
				Gait	+
MacSween (1999)	IIb	8	11	Comfort	+
				Gait	+
Chalmers (2000)	IIb	28	15	Pain	+
Li (2000)	III	12	–	Pressure	+
Woodburn (2002, 2003)	Ib	101	3	Pain, disability	+
				3D AJC motion	+
				Pressure	+
Kavlak (2003)	IIb	18	–	Pain	+
				Gait	+
				Energy expenditure	+
Shrader (2003)	IV	1	Female 10	Pain	+
				Pressure	+
Jackson (2004)	IIb	10	–	Pressure	+
Mejjad (2004)	Ib	16			

materials chosen must match the intended function. In the early stage of rheumatoid arthritis, pain and stiffness are the predominant foot impairments, whereas in established disease impairments include pain, stiffness, deformity and muscle weakness. To date, there are no prospective studies specifically investigating the natural progression of foot impairments in rheumatoid arthritis. Furthermore, the extent to which foot impairments can be predicted and prognosis determined from disease-related factors, biomechanical factors and environmental/societal factors is yet to be established.

Early disease

Rearfoot deformity in RA occurs at different rates with perhaps 25% of all cases vulnerable to moderate-to-severe valgus heel deformity within the first 5 years. Often in this early stage of disease, the valgus heel deformity is still mobile and can be corrected to a vertical position. Therefore, during this period there is an opportunity to intervene before irreversible changes to structure and function occur. Figure 6.24 shows a hypothetical model for states of foot deformity progression adapted from standard models of outcomes proposed by Woodburn (2000). The course of deformity (Y1) is

plotted against time (X) from disease onset alongside treatment strategy (Y2). Patients who develop severe deformity within 5 years from disease onset (Pathway C) have only a short time period in which to initiate preventative management. Others may develop progressive deformity (Pathway B) following repeated inflammatory attacks (hence the 'saw tooth' appearance). Finally, a smaller group (Pathway A) resist cumulative damage and deformity until the later stages of disease and then rapid development of deformity occurs following some acute incident (perhaps rupture of tibialis posterior tendon).

In early disease the aim of orthotic management would be aimed at preserving or maintaining function and to prevent or lessen deformity. With the advent of early arthritis clinics and targeted aggressive treatment of synovitis, in the future it is hoped that less patients will go on to develop severe foot deformity. Recent data for RA suggest that 50% of patients have active synovitis involving their feet and this includes patients with early disease. Regression models show that clinical factors predict approximately 50% of the variance for the presence of swollen and tender foot joints (Farrow et al. 2004). A large proportion of

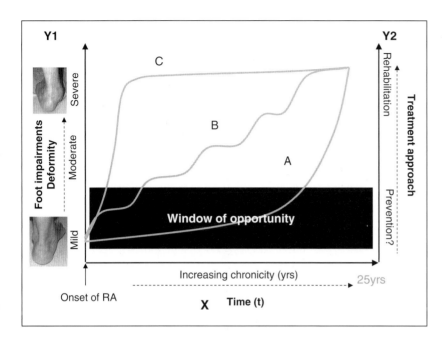

Figure 6.24 Hypothetical model for states of foot-deformity progression.

patients referred to podiatry are patients who despite having low disease activity have persistent foot impairments. This group forms 90% of the current podiatry caseload at Leeds, and many patients benefit from mechanically based therapies such as orthoses and footwear. This suggests that biomechanical factors may be important and measures to prevent or delay the progression of the typical valgus deformity must combine management of both the joint and soft tissue synovitis and any underlying mechanical dysfunction (Woodburn et al. 2002).

To date, there has only been one randomized clinical trial specifically investigating the effect of functional rigid orthoses for the management of painful correctable valgus heel deformity in early stages of disease (Woodburn et al. 2002). Woodburn and colleagues prospectively followed 98 patients over a period of 30 months. The patients were randomized to receive customized rigid carbon graphite orthoses, with in-built correction according to the degree of deformity (n=50) or to the control group (n=48). Measures of foot pain and disability using the Foot Function Index along with measures of disease activity, tolerance, and adverse reactions were taken at 3, 6, 12, 18, 24 and 30 months. The orthotic intervention group demonstrated a reduction in foot pain, disability and functional limitation compared to the control group. The use of orthoses resulted in an immediate clinical improvement with the effect peaking at 12 months.

Following the findings of the above study, the approach at Leeds is to use rigid customized orthoses with correction according to the level of deformity in patients with mobile valgus heel deformity in early disease. The median disease duration in the above study was 3 years, but, ideally, orthotics should be used to stabilize the rearfoot complex at the earliest phases of this disease. There are early changes in axes of rotation of the talus and calcaneus and inflammation weakens the periarticular structures and soft tissue retaining systems, which make the rearfoot complex less stable and less able to resist the forces across the joint. As many patients report foot involvement in early disease it is logical to assume most would benefit from treatment at the earliest opportunity.

The natural course of foot disease in early arthritis is largely unknown and predictors for those most likely to develop persistent foot impairments are not known. It is not feasible to provide every patient with foot orthoses, nor is it advocated in the absence of evidence. Findings from clinical experience have primarily led to the development of clinical red flags to guide practitioners as to which patients may need or are likely to benefit from orthotic intervention. The red flags include those patients with pre-existing foot deformity, tenosynovitis particularly of tibialis posterior, poor rearfoot alignment, low medial arch profile and those patients who have residual foot impairments even when disease activity has been suppressed.

Established disease

In more established foot disease the aim of orthotic management will be to reduce pain, maintain function, accommodate existing deformity, prevention of further deformity and maintain tissue viability. Patients, particularly with advanced forefoot deformity, typically complain of the feeling of walking on pebbles or marbles. These patients often have toes that are non-weight bearing with associated anterior displacement of the fibro-fatty pad, erosions and subluxation at the MTP joints, and pressure-induced plantar lesions. As discussed previously in Chapter 2, these patients often develop an antalgic gait pattern, typically decreased gait velocity, increased periods of double limb support and decreased contact loading in the forefoot region. The use of specialist footwear and orthoses has been shown to be effective at reducing levels of foot pain, decreasing associated functional limitation and reducing plantar pressures in patients with established forefoot disease (Fransen and Edmonds 1997, Hodge et al. 1999, Chalmers et al. 2000). The main aim of orthotic devices in these patients is to support the medial arch profile, transfer and reduce pressure from the metatarsal heads, increase shock absorption and reduce shear forces. In these cases attempts to fully correct rear-foot alignment may not be possible or may not be tolerated by the patient and less rigid devices are indicated.

A very small percentage of patients develop a varus heel deformity. These patients commonly report that they had aggressive disease in the foot during the early stages of the disease. They often recall that they had pain in the forefoot especially on the medial side and in an attempt to avoid pain they walked on the outside of the foot (in an inverted position) to avoid loading the painful MTP joints. Over time, the sub-talar joint becomes stiff and fixed in this inverted position. Clinically, these patients will usually present with lateral instability, often reporting frequent inversion sprains and pain around the lateral malleolus. The arch profile is usually high and the lesser toes retracted, resulting in anterior displacement of the fibro-fatty pad and prominent metatarsal heads. As the patient has a high arch and retracted toes the total weight-bearing contact area of the foot is greatly reduced and plantar pressures are usually elevated under the MTP joints. As these patients often present with fixed deformity, rigid control is generally not tolerated; these patients usually respond well to a semi-rigid orthotic device to redistribute pressures from the metatarsal heads into the midfoot and cushioning materials under the MTP joints. Owing to the inverted position of the calcaneus and resultant lateral instability external modification to footwear is usually required.

Deciding on orthotic management, from assessment to fitting   The science behind orthotics is still in its infancy. There is little good evidence to guide the practitioner on which materials to use, how to combine them, how thick they should be, or the specific orthosis for any particular foot type. Practitioners will often refer to using functional or accommodative devices. However, this terminology can be confusing as any type of orthosis will have some functional effect on the foot.

Functional devices generally are those devices that are used in the presence of a deformity that is not fixed and is still correctable, for example the presence of a mobile valgus heel deformity. The aim of the device is to control abnormal motion, optimize foot function and, hopefully, prevent or slow down the progression of development of foot deformity.

Accommodative devices are used in the presence of fixed deformity (a deformity that can not be fully corrected), thus the aim of the device is to accommodate the existing deformity and maximize existing functional potential. In reality, most orthotic devices will incorporate both functional and accommodation principles.

Orthoses can also be described on the basis of the materials used, for example, soft/flexible, semi-rigid/semi-flexible or rigid and also by the density of material, low medium or high density. The degree of rigidity or hardness of the orthosis is dependent on the intended function; generally, the more rigid the material, the more control it will provide. In some instances the intended function is to provide cushioning and shock absorption, in these cases a soft/flexible material would be required.

The overall patient assessment is detailed in Chapter 4. Key aspects from the assessment will be those related to the structural aspects of the foot (presence of deformity, structural alignment, presence of pressure induced lesions, shoe wear patterns) functional aspects of the foot (range, direction and quality of joint motion, muscle strength) and the likely consequences during gait and activities of daily living. Strategies for managing foot impairments in patients with RA are similar to the general principles in rehabilitation which are to control pain, prevent or slow down the progression of deformity, maximize functional potential and to promote general well being (Gerber 1994). The timing and rationale for referral to a foot health specialist, ideally, should be made prior to significant decline in function, or before the development of fixed deformity and muscle atrophy. In reality, referral is usually made when patients present with significant foot deformity, pain and associated disability.

As a general rule, where possible, attempts should be made to fully correct joint mal-alignments using rigid materials. In some instances deformity may not be fully correctable or rigid materials may not be tolerated by the patient. If there is a limited range of joint motion it may be desirable to try and assist or increase motion, for example at the 1st MTP joint. If there is a limited range of motion that is causing pain, the orthosis may be aimed at controlling the movement and reducing pain. Semi-rigid devices can be used in these instances to offer some degree of control, but to also offer a degree of shock absorption and pressure redistribution.

An orthosis may be required to achieve different goals at different points in the gait cycle. An example of this would be some shock absorption at initial contact, functional control of abnormal frontal plane motion at the sub-talar joint from loading response through to mid-stance, and increased shock absorption and pressure redistribution at forefoot loading and terminal stance. This can be achieved by combining materials with different mechanical properties within the same orthosis.

The mechanical properties of materials can be determined by performing tests under controlled conditions. Clinicians who want to use materials in footwear or orthoses need to know how materials react when subjected to compression and shear forces. Materials selected must be suitable for the intended purpose. When functional control is needed the material must be sufficiently rigid and lightweight, such as carbon graphite. When the aim is to provide substitution for depletion of soft tissue under prominent, painful and eroded MTP joints then materials should provide shock absorption and cushioning properties. Materials such as polyurethane, poron and the visco-elastic polymers resist shear-compression forces better than the polyethylene foams.

As discussed, in reality different types of materials may be combined in an orthosis in order to achieve different functions at different regions of the foot or at different phases in the gait cycle. There are concerns related to decreased shock absorption associated with rigid devices. To overcome this, they are used in conjunction with a soft top cover with forefoot extension, in addition to footwear that offers good shock absorbing characteristics. Plastazote is useful as a top covering for orthoses when patients have vasospastic disorders, as it has good thermal properties. However, due to its limited lifespan it must be replaced frequently. Leather top covers are often utilized because they can be easily cleaned and this is particularly important for patients with active ulceration when there is the possibility of exudate leaking from dressings and coming into contact with the orthosis.

When the intended function of the orthosis is to provide cushioning and pressure reduction the aim would be to achieve optimum pressure relief, for minimum thickness of material (the amount of room in the shoe is limited especially in the presence of lesser toe deformity). To date, there has not been any study that has systematically investigated the effects of insole thickness on pressure relieving properties in a large group of patients. It is likely that peak pressures will be decreased further as insole thickness increases. However, a point will be reached where there will be not much extra benefit in terms of pressure reduction for an extra increase in thickness of insole material. Usually, constraints associated with footwear are the key factor that determines the depth of cushioning material used in orthoses.

Consideration should also be given to how the properties of the material may alter over time with repeated use. With rigid orthoses it is very unlikely these will fatigue: in the RCT by Woodburn and colleagues patients were followed for 30 months and in that period none of the insoles had to be replaced due to excessive wear. It is more likely that changes in foot posture may require alterations to be made to the shell. With cushioning materials long-term use can cause degradation of the material. The mechanical properties of materials commonly used in foot orthoses have been studied, where materials have been subjected to both sustained and cyclic loading. The thickness of materials has been recorded before and after loading as an indicator of performance. Generally, materials similar to poron demonstrate little reduction in thickness, whereas plastazote shows around a 50% reduction in thickness. Brodsky and colleagues studied five commonly used materials, subjected to 10 000 cycles (Brodsky et al. 1998). The loss of thickness ranged from 0 in polyurethane (PPT) to 55% in plastazote. Pratt et al. assessed different materials for their shock absorbing properties; they found that Plastazote was poor at absorbing shock, whereas Poron and Viscolas were best at absorbing shock (Pratt et al. 1986). Generally, one can assume materials will experience losses in performance with repeated use. One study has suggested that generally the greatest losses in performance occur within the first 10 000 cycles (equivalent to approximately 2 weeks of usual wear) (Foto and Birke 1998).

Material testing can provide the clinician with an idea of how material will perform. However, it can not allow prediction of efficacy as this is dependent on many other factors, such as foot structure, function and compliance. In-shoe plantar pressure measurement systems allow measurements to be recorded at the foot/orthosis interface. It allows practitioners to evaluate orthoses objectively and has led to an increased understanding about the influence that orthoses have on foot function.

How to best capture the foot geometry: templates and casting Some practitioners use simple insoles and prefabricated devices. Generally, these devices can be fabricated at the time of the consultation and, therefore, have the advantage over casted devices as they can be issued immediately. For simple insoles depending on the type of device it is often possible to use the wear patterns on the insoles from the patient's current footwear. Many shoes now have insoles that are completely removable and high pressure points can be easily detected from increased wear at the site, and these can be easily transferred onto a template for a simple insole. Where this is not possible patients can be given thin plastazote insoles to fit into their existing shoes and asked to wear them until the wear patterns become evident, as plastazote bottoms out relatively quickly.

Pre-fabricated moulded devices can be useful, but are not often used in Leeds. Clinical experience has shown that they do not provide enough rigid support in the medial longitudinal arch. Pre-fabricated devices that can be heat moulded to conform closely to the arch may overcome this problem. Where possible, the aim is to use evidence based practice and the limited evidence in this area suggests that patients benefit from casted rigid customized devices in early disease and clinical experience supports this finding.

There are multiple methods currently available for taking a negative impression of the foot: non-weight-bearing plaster casting, partial-weight-bearing plaster casting or foam impressions (Oasis box), full-weight-bearing foam impressions and non-weight-bearing and weight-bearing laser scanning. Some of these different techniques have been compared in terms of reliability on healthy adults, but it is likely that differences would be more obvious in the presence of foot deformity. Disagreement exists as to the most appropriate technique for casting the foot and which position in which to place the foot. Most podiatrists will aim to position the foot in the subtalar neutral position. Whilst there is general recognition that there are issues related to measurement reliability and concerns regarding its usefulness in predicting foot function during gait, it is still widely used.

The casting technique will be fully dependent on the intended nature of the orthosis. When the primary intention is to provide rigid functional control then it is easier to correctly align the foot in a non-weight-bearing position than under weight-bearing conditions. In some instances, it may be necessary to capture the foot shape under weight-bearing conditions, especially when the aim of the orthosis is to deflect pressure from soft tissues, including bursae and nodules, as it is likely

these will distort when loaded. The foot does change shape considerably between non-weight-bearing and weight-bearing conditions, highlighted by the study by Tsung and colleagues. They examined the changes of foot shape under a full-body-weight-bearing condition in normal healthy subjects. They concluded that the foot length and foot width under full-body weight will increase by 3.4% (8.0 mm) and 6.0% (5.7 mm), respectively, compared with the non-weight-bearing condition (Tsung et al. 2003).

Other considerations for casting technique will include cost and time. Foam impression casting has the advantage of being quick, cheap and relatively easy to perform. Plaster casting is time-consuming, messy and difficult.

Although there is no direct head to head comparison of plaster cast versus foam impression in terms of cost and efficacy, the approach at Leeds is to use non-weight-bearing plaster casting when the aim of the orthoses is to achieve functional control, and partial or full weight-bearing casting techniques in a subtalar joint neutral position when the aim to is to provide some functional control, but also to accommodate a specific deformity or if there appears to be large changes in foot shape from non-weight-bearing to weight-bearing conditions.

Issues related to the validity of the subtalar joint neutral position and its role in foot function needs to be re-evaluated. Work in the area of gait analysis and the development of multi-segmental foot models used to analyse gait in patients with RA will undoubtedly increase our understanding of foot function in RA and ultimately the way we manage patients with foot impairments.

Treatment response Patient response to orthoses varies considerably; there is little information about prognostic indicators for treatment response. Although we have no data, our experience indicates that involving the patient with the decision-making process results in better compliance and satisfaction. In early disease, where the aim of the orthosis is to control excessive frontal plane motion and provide rigid support in the medial longitudinal arch, full consultation with the patient regarding device choice and an explanation as to why this device is necessary is of paramount importance. Often patients will perceive that they have a need for cushioning under the metatarsal head areas, and when faced with a rigid device can not understand how the device can work. The use of anatomical models and plantar pressure profiles with and without orthoses are helpful to enhance the explanation as to why a rigid orthosis should work.

Poor compliance with orthoses can be the result of several factors:

- Problems with fit of the orthoses to the foot
- Problems with fit of orthoses in footwear
- Unrealistic patient expectations of a large and immediate treatment response.

The RCT by Woodburn and colleagues showed that there was a self-reported increase in foot pain from initiation of the orthotic in 20% of the patients, and 30% of patients reported pain elsewhere in the legs Woodburn et al. (2002). Other adverse reactions in this trial included blister formation and development of thickened or callused skin in the heel region.

During the fitting appointment, care should be taken to ensure the orthosis contours well to the foot and fits into the shoes the patient intends to wear on a regular basis. Time should be taken to outline an appropriate programme of wear with a gradual build up to minimize the chances of developing adverse reactions such as blister formation. Most importantly, the patient should be given a realistic expectation as to response to treatment and the likelihood of an increase in foot pain in the initial phase of wear as the foot adapts to a new corrected functioning position.

Early rigid orthotic management in an early case is highlighted in Figure 6.25. This patient in her early thirties had a diagnosis of RA of less than 6 months. She recalls that her feet were slightly flat, but not troublesome prior to the onset of her disease. During the initial months she was greatly troubled by pain and stiffness in the medial ankle region and noticed that her instep was collapsing inwards, especially on the left side. Her disease was aggressively treated with a combination of anti-rheumatic drugs including prednisolone, methotrexate and etanercept. In the intervening time she progressed to develop bilateral flexible pes planovalgus markedly worse on the left than right side. On weight bearing, the medial longitudinal arch profile was low on both sides with evidence of complete collapse on the left side (Fig. 6.25A and B), confirmed by pressure analysis indicating weight bearing on the medial cuneiform and navicular region (Fig. 6.25C). Both heels were in valgus, left worse than right, and the ankle, subtalar and talonavicular joints were swollen and tender (Fig. 6.25 D). The gastrocnemius-solues complex was weak on both sides (grade 3-left, grade 4-right on the MRC scale) as was tibialis posterior on the left side (grade 4). The tendon was patent, but swollen and tender along its course from the medial malleolus to the insertion at the navicular. In both feet she was tender at MTP joints 1-4. Her Leeds foot Impact Scale score of 34 indicated significant foot impairment and associated participation restriction and activity limitation. Despite excellent response to medication, her DAS score was 3.14; interestingly, a number of localized and persistent sites of inflammation remained in the feet. This suggests biomechanical causes consistent with dysfunction associated with the pes planovalgus.

The treatment approach in this patient was as follows:

1. *Orthosis*: plaster cast impressions were taken of both feet, non-weight bearing and referenced in a 'corrected' position. To explain, the valgus orientation of the rearfoot relative to the leg was corrected by inverting the heel until it was aligned straight with the leg. Simultaneously, the forefoot was everted

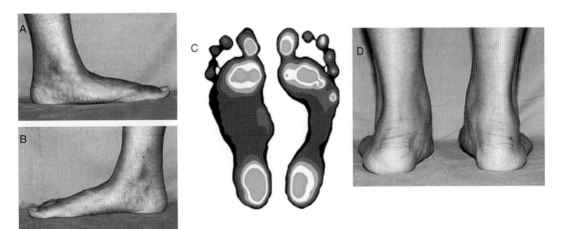

Figure 6.25 Early rigid orthotic management in an early case of rheumatoid arthritis. Acquired pes planovalgus in the early stages of rheumatoid arthritis. See text for details.

until a plane formed by the metatarsal heads was parallel with the ground. The foot was maintained in this position until the plaster cast set. From these casts, rigid carbon-graphite orthoses were constructed to stabilize the foot joint and optimize function. The key functional components of the device were: (A) deep heel to support the heel and assist motion control, (B) angled heel seat (or post) to control rearfoot motion, (C) contoured medial longitudinal arch to support the talonavicular joint and (D) cushioning material extended from behind the metatarsal heads to the toes. Given the severity of the deformity, the orthoses were designed to offer partial correction, built up sequentially over two further devices to be supplied at 4 and 8 months.

2. *Physical therapy*: referral was made to physiotherapy for muscle-strengthening exercises for the weak gastrocnemius-solues muscle complex combined with training to improve proprioception at the ankle and tarsal joints.

3. *Pain management*: tenosynovitis of the left tibialis posterior was confirmed by ultrasonography and a guided corticosteroid injection was given. Both the pathological status of the tendon and response to orthotic management will be reviewed at 4 months with further recommendation for local lesion treatment as necessary.

The intial fit and comfort of the prescribed orthosis was satisfactory and the patient noted a definite improvement in foot posture when walking, especially in the medial longitudinal arch (Fig. 6.26). Partial correction of the foot function was noted from the in-shoe plantar pressure assessment. This showed increased loading in the medial longitudinal arch and decreased focal areas of pressure in the rearfoot and forefoot. As the treatment progresses and further correction is built into the orthoses it would be expected that greater off-loading of the medial forefoot and the interphalangeal region of the hallux will occur.

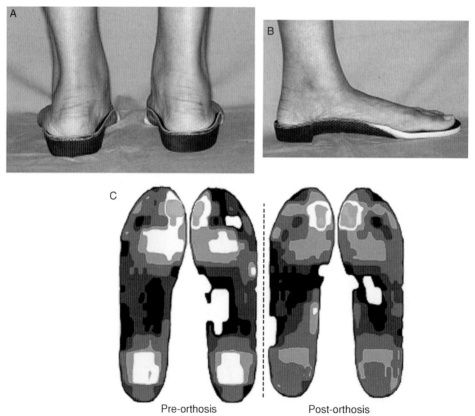

Pre-orthosis   Post-orthosis

Figure 6.26 Same patient as in Figure 6.25, after orthotics management. Custom orthoses manufactured in rigid carbon-graphite material with forefoot cushioning extension (A and B). Partial correction of the planovalgus is observed on weight bearing (B). Pre- and post-orthosis in-shoe pressure profiles are shown (C).

Orthotic management in a patient with a varus heel deformity is presented in Figure 6.27. This patient in her early forties had disease duration of 14 years. Her disease activity was high for a number of years as changes were made to her medication. She recalls that her feet were particularly painful at disease onset and even when her general disease activity was lowered as a result of medical management she had persistent foot pain. In an attempt to avoid loading the metatarsal heads she walked on the outside border of her foot. The patient has had aggressive disease and as a consequence has a history of a long-term oral corticosteroid use. The patient was referred to the foot health department due to a history of recurrent foot ulceration on the lateral MTP joints of both feet.

On weight bearing the patient had a high medial longitudinal arch profile and an inverted heel position (varus heel alignment) (Fig. 6.27A and B). There was retraction of the lesser toes and minimal soft tissue under the MTP joints. The patient reported pain under the MTP joints and lateral ankle pain and lateral instability. There was severely restricted range of motion at the subtalar joint and the calcaneus was fixed in an inverted position. Plantar pressure analysis revealed high pressure areas at the sites of recurrent ulceration (greater than 1275 kPa), a high arch profile and minimal toe loading (Fig. 6.27C).

The treatment approach in this patient was as follows:

1. *Orthosis*: partial-weight-bearing foam cast impressions were taken of both feet. From these casts, three-quarter length semi-rigid orthoses were constructed to redistribute pressure away from the metatarsal heads into the midfoot (arch area). The semi-rigid shells were covered and a forefoot extension of cushioning material provided to act as an external substitution for the lack of soft tissue under the MTP joints. The patient had previously

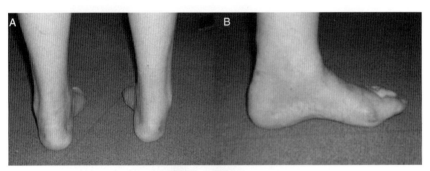
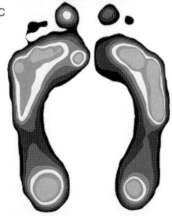
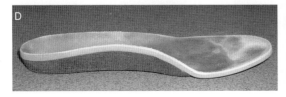
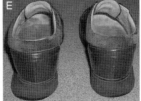

Figure 6.27 Management of varus heel deformity with orthoses and footwear modifications. See text for details.

reported problems related to the foot slipping on a leather cover, although this would be a preferred cover for ease of cleaning with the history of ulceration, a chamois leather top cover was used in this instance (Fig. 6.27D).

2. *Footwear*: Referral was made to appliance department for footwear. Extra depth shoes were provided and a lateral heel flare was used to counteract the lateral instability associated with the varus heel position. A forefoot rocker was incorporated into the outsole to further reduce the plantar pressures from the metatarsal heads (Fig. 6.27E).

An example of a clinical case where an orthotic was used to accommodate a specific foot deformity is described in Figure 6.28.

This patient had RA for 15 years. Her general disease activity was low and she was currently not taking any DMARD therapy, only analgesics when required. Her main foot problem was related to painful 4th MTP joint with overlying adventitious bursa formation on the left foot (Fig. 6.28A). She attended for regular callus debridement of the lesion. On clinical examination, the patient had limited range of motion at the subtalar and ankle joint. On weight bearing the first ray was plantarflexed and the hallux and lesser toes were retracted with minimal soft tissue present under the metatarsal heads (Fig. 6.28B). Plantar pressure analysis revealed high localized pressure over the site of the bursa and under the 1st MTP joint, absence of toe loading and a high arch profile (Fig. 6.28C). The primary aim of orthotic management in this case was to reduce

Figure 6.28 Example of management using a semi-rigid orthosis to accommodate foot deformity. See text for details.

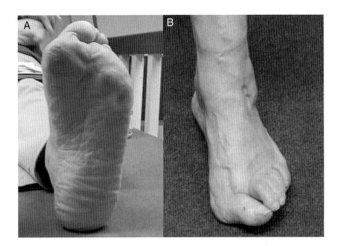

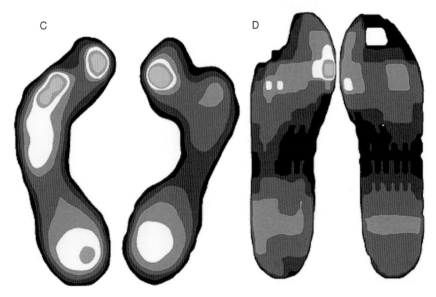

pain under the 4th metatarsal by reducing the high pressure. A secondary aim was to improve function at the 1st MTP joint. The strategy was to deflect pressure away from the bursa site and reduce pressure by increasing the weight-bearing contact area of the foot.

The treatment approach in this patient was as follows:

1. *Orthosis*: plaster cast impressions were taken of both feet. A pen was used to mark around the bursa prior to casting, so the location could be identified and additional plaster added to the positive cast to make a sink in the orthoses. A medium-density ethylene vinyl acetate (EVA) shell was fabricated with a low density EVA forefoot extension with a full-depth sink over the bursa site to deflect pressure away from the site. A polyurethane cushioning material (Poron) was used as a top cover.

The orthosis contoured well to the shape of the foot and the location of the sink appeared to be in the correct location. In-shoe plantar pressure analysis was undertaken to evaluate the effectiveness of the orthosis at reducing pressure from the bursa site (Fig. 6.28D). The in-shoe pressure profile showed the orthosis were successfully increasing the weight-bearing contact area of the foot, reducing pressure over the bursa site

Future of foot orthoses   Recent developments in the area of finite element modelling of the foot-shoe and foot-orthosis interface has emerged as a promising approach to further understand the effect that foot structure and function has on outcome measures such as plantar pressure distribution. Furthermore, this approach has the potential to investigate the effects that footwear, materials and orthoses have on overall foot function and in the future may allow the generation of general design principles for footwear and orthoses on a per case basis.

Future orthotic production may look to the mass customization process where individualized orthoses can be quickly designed and manufactured in an almost fully automated way. One technique currently being developed in our own unit seeks to capture foot geometry, which is often complex when deformities are present, using 3D laser surface scanning (Fig. 6.29). This approach negates the use of plaster and other moulding techniques and provides surface data in a digital format for transfer to the design and manufacture suite. The geometry and functional characteristics of the orthosis are generated by computer-aided designs according to the foot impairments present. This will allow, for example, stiffness to be varied throughout the orthosis to impart specific joint motion control or stress redistribution and this can be simu

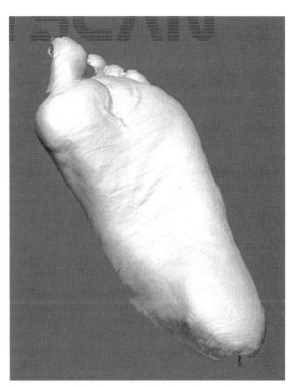

Figure 6.29   3D surface scan of the foot in a patient with rheumatoid arthritis.

lated in a biomechanical model. Manufacture is also computer controlled and we are investigating the use of selective laser sintering, where the orthoses are constructed in plastics built from powder, which is laser-heated to bond in layers (Fig. 6.30). This approach will benefit the patient in many ways and we anticipate devices, which have better fit and function and, importantly, can be supplied within a 24-hour period.

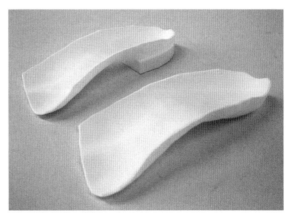

Figure 6.30   Prototype orthotics devices manufactured via selective laser sintering.

Footwear

Footwear is often considered the most problematic factor in managing foot pain and deformity both by the patient and the practitioner. Footwear can be instrumental in causing foot pain and can also be a potential barrier/constraint for management of foot impairments. It has been shown that a large proportion of the general population wear ill-fitting footwear and subsequently report increased foot pain (Burns et al. 2002). Chantelau and Gede assessed the width of feet in 568 patients and found over two-thirds of feet were considerably broader than normal footwear available on the high street (Chantelau and Gede 2002). Although there are no studies specifically addressing this issue in RA, in light of the fact many patients with RA have forefoot deformity, one can assume the proportion of patients with ill-fitting footwear or inappropriate footwear is high. Lack of appropriate commercial footwear is an important determinant of impaired mobility in RA. Indeed, it is not uncommon for many patients to have to adapt footwear to accommodate their foot deformity or wear sandals all year round. Patients will inevitably go to great lengths in order to obtain footwear that is comfortable (Fig. 6.31).

Within the WHO ICF framework footwear falls into the environment section; the requirements for footwear will be dependent on the level of foot impairments, but can be greatly influenced by environmental factors and personal factors. Footwear is linked intrinsically with fashion and body image. People relate to footwear not just on a descriptive level, but also in ways that involve making social judgments about aspects of the likely wearer; for example knee-length boots have been shown to be linked with an overtly sexual image (Wilson 2004). For these reasons instigating changes in footwear can be problematic, more so

in female patients and in some cases patients are not willing to make changes to shoes. There is no doubt that in these instances the practitioner will be unable to manage these patients effectively. A decision has to be made as to whether a compromise can be made or whether the patient should be given an open referral to come back once they are prepared to make changes in footwear. Many practitioners will start at footwear and discuss changing footwear before they have assessed the patient and may send the patient away to buy new shoes before assessing the patient and discussing treatment options. Inevitably, this approach often leads to many patients failing to come back to be assessed. An approach that seems to work better is to assess the patient and to discuss the outcome with the patient, informing them of the various treatment options and how the patient is likely to benefit. Discussing how their current footwear would negate any treatment response or prevent treatment allows the patient to make an informed decision as to whether they would like to proceed on the understanding that changing the type of footwear is an integral part of the treatment strategy.

In early disease many patients report foot pain at the MTP joints and changes in foot shape. It is not uncommon for patients to recall that they had to increase their shoe size to accommodate a wider forefoot. Some patients will visit specialist footwear manufacturers who can be very helpful in offering advice and providing wider-fitting shoes. Many patients will instigate changes in footwear in an attempt to find comfort; for example changing from a high-heeled court shoe to a flat lace up with a cushioning sole. At this stage in the disease most patients will be able to purchase appropriate footwear on the high street, but will probably benefit from some basic footwear advice.

Williams and colleagues reported that doctors who referred their patients for orthopaedic footwear felt they lacked the time and knowledge to give advice about retail footwear, suggesting that some patients could purchase their own footwear if they were given appropriate advice (Williams and Meacher 2001). Many patients associate quality with price and think 'good shoes' have to be expensive. The use of anatomical models, examples of footwear in clinic leaflets and a good local knowledge of shops and current stock lines can be useful when explaining the types of footwear characteristics they need to look for and to direct them to suppliers. The British Footwear Association (http://www.britfoot.com/) provides detailed information about the companies that make up the British footwear industry and consumer information about hard-to-find footwear suitable for all foot shapes and sizes and is a useful for patients.

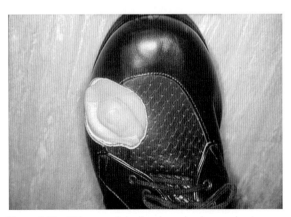

Figure 6.31   This was originally a bespoke shoe made at considerable cost to the NHS.

As foot deformity increases, patients find it increasingly difficult to buy footwear that can accommodate their foot shape and they may need to have prescribed footwear. Reasons for prescribed footwear from the patient's perspective predominantly include foot pain and associated disability. Frequently, they can no longer buy footwear on the high street to accommodate their foot shape and/or they have recurrent footwear related pressure-induced lesions, particularly on the dorsal toe region. Obtaining comfortable footwear may help patients avoid the need for surgery. In addition, practitioner factors include improvement in foot function, maintenance of tissue viability and to facilitate other treatments such as orthoses.

So what constitutes the end of high street footwear and need to go to appliance/orthotics departments for prescribed/bespoke footwear? The answer is unknown. The referral criteria for sending patients for prescribed footwear are not strong and for this reason there appears to be discordance between individual need and provision of footwear. How patients become in receipt of prescribed footwear and if they benefit from them are largely unknown. It appears that the ability to have prescribed footwear and the ability to benefit from prescribed footwear may be quite different.

Many patients with advanced forefoot disease are issued with surgical/orthopaedic accommodative footwear by an orthotist (Williams and Meacher 2001). Specially designed shoe-wear has previously been shown to increase the patient's functional capacity and reduce forefoot callosities (Barrett Jr 1976). However, surgical footwear alone does not appear to significantly reduce forefoot pain in patients with RA (Chalmers et al. 2000, Kerry et al. 1994). Unfortunately, patient dissatisfaction with prescribed footwear is a frequent occurrence and often results in poor compliance.

In an attempt to reduce dissatisfaction and poor compliance with footwear, multidisciplinary clinics have been developed involving both podiatrists and orthotists. Williams and colleagues compared outcomes of a multidisciplinary footwear clinic (MDFC) with a traditional surgical appliance clinic (SAC) (Williams and Meacher 2001). The study found that referrers to both clinics indicated that they lacked the time and knowledge to give advice about retail footwear. Discussion with patients about footwear before the prescription took place and advice regarding what to do if problems occurred were identified as key factors in ensuring effective use of footwear. The study demonstrated an association between the patient's attitude, their perception of improvement in their feet and overall satisfaction. These factors seemed to have an impact on the usage of the prescription footwear with 13 (48.1%) of the SAC group using footwear other than those prescribed, compared with 2 (7.2%) in the MDFC group. This study highlights the need for health professionals to include patients in the decision-making process for interventions.

FOOTWEAR

- Footwear can be a major contributing factor to foot impairments and can be a potential barrier to treatment.
- Footwear is linked intrinsically with fashion and body image. Therefore instigating changes in footwear can be problematic, more so in female patients
- Patient dissatisfaction with prescribed footwear is a frequent occurrence and often results in poor compliance.
- The development of multidisciplinary footwear clinics and the involvement of patients in the decision-making process helps improve compliance.

On the basis of limited information in this area, and studies reporting poor compliance and dissatisfaction with prescribed footwear, having decided that the patient needs prescribed footwear there are a number of issues discussed with the patient prior to referral:

- We attempt to inform the patient fully of the potential benefits of footwear: including comfort, optimum fit and improvements to foot function.
- However, more importantly, we discuss the potential constraints, which include limited number of colours and style, how many pairs they will be given and seasonal problems (it is difficult to achieve support and accommodate an orthosis in a sandal).
- Patients are shown a catalogue that illustrates the various shoe styles and colours and, where possible, allowed to inspect a pair.
- Liaison with other patients who have already received footwear may also be beneficial.
- The patient is given the opportunity to voice any concerns. At this point patients are asked if they feel they would wear prescribed footwear and are only referred if they are willing to try. Clinical experience has shown that the patient is referred with a more realistic expectation of footwear and this leads to better compliance once footwear is issued.

It is a fundamental requirement that there is a good working relationship between the podiatrist and other members of the MDT. Helliwell (2003) highlighted the need for a medical consultant, podiatrist and orthotist to be involved in the setting-up and practice of a multidisciplinary foot clinic in rheumatology to ensure effective management of foot pathologies. When service restrictions mean that it is not possible for orthotist and podiatrist to have joint clinics (a common occurrence in management of the diabetic foot) then it is important that each professional understands the role of the other, and that a good working relationship is formed to ensure that the patient is receiving the optimum benefits of orthopaedic footwear in conjunction with other therapeutic interventions.

There are a number of different therapeutic footwear approaches used, depending on the nature and level of foot impairment. Several modifications are particularly useful in the management of the foot:

- Deeper and wider toe box to accommodate forefoot deformity
- Modifications to the outer sole to direct high pressures away from the MTP joints
- Medial reinforcement of the upper to provide additional support
- Velcro fastenings for patients with hand deformity who find it difficult to fasten laces.

Muscle strengthening and improvement of proprioception

Muscle weakness, restricted range of motion of joints and reduced physical function are common signs in patients with RA. The benefits of exercise therapy in RA patients are as follows:

- Increasing aerobic capacity
- Increasing muscle strength
- Decreasing pain and
- Improving function.

However, the literature to support this mostly comes from studies of the knee (Chamberlain et al. 1982) and does not specifically apply to the foot. Lately, studies of general aerobic exercise and its benefits are emerging (Lemmey et al. 2001).

Historically, patients with RA were recommended to avoid weight-bearing exercise and concentrate on isometric non-weight-bearing exercises and range of motion exercise in order to avoid aggravating joint inflammation and accelerating joint damage. However, the American College of Rheumatology now recommends regular participation in dynamic exercise programmes in their treatment guidelines for the management of RA (American College of Rheumatology 2002). Long-term, high-intensity, weight-bearing exer-

cise programmes, compared with usual care physical therapy, have been shown to be effective in increasing the physical capacity and functional ability of patients with RA without causing additional damage to the large weight-bearing joints (de Jong et al. 2003, de Jong et al. 2004a). A further advantage is that such programmes help to prevent bone loss.

The effects of exercise on the smaller joints such as the hands and feet have not been formally examined until recently. Five studies (displayed in Table 6.3) have reported the effects of long-term intensive exercises on the radiological damage of the joints of the feet. Nordemar et al. (1981) reported a decreased rate of radiological damage in the joints of the feet of RA patients in the exercise group compared with the control group. However, three other studies did not show any significant difference in the rate of damage of the joints of the feet between the exercise and control group (Hakkinen et al. 2001, Hansen et al. 1993, Strenstrom et al. 1991).

de Jong et al. (2004b) investigated the effect of long-term, high-intensity, weight-bearing exercises on radiological damage of the joints of the feet and hands in patients with RA. The study concluded that long-term, intensive, weight-bearing exercises when compared to usual care physical therapy does not increase the rate of radiological damage of the feet, but appears to have a protective effect for these joints.

However, despite the existing evidence regarding the effectiveness and safety of high-intensity exercise programmes, patients, rheumatologists and physiotherapists have more positive expectations of conventional exercise programmes than of high-intensity exercise programmes and, therefore, the need for continuous education of all involved is also required (Munneke et al. 2004).

Rall et al. (1996) examined the feasibility of high-intensity, progressive-resistance training in patients with RA compared with healthy young and old patients. Subjects with RA had no change in the number of painful or swollen joints, but had significant reductions in self-reported pain score and fatigue score, improved 50-foot walking times, and improved balance and gait scores. They concluded that high-intensity strength training is feasible and safe in selected patients with well-controlled RA and leads to significant improvements in strength, pain and fatigue without exacerbating disease activity or joint pain (Rall et al. 1996). It is important that we encourage patients with RA to remain active as well as ensuring that patients are carrying out the most appropriate exercises to improve their activity.

Muscle weakness is frequently seen in patients with RA (see Chapter 3) and is considered to be partly due to muscle atrophy resulting from disuse, because pain and

Table 6.3 Summary of exercise studies.

Author	Year	Trial design	No of rheumatoid arthritis subjects	Interventions tested	Outcome – radiological damage/progression at MTP joints
De Jong et al.	2004	Randomized controlled	281	Physical therapy vs. high-intensity w/b exercises	Not increased by high-intensity w/b exercise
Hakkinen et al.	2001	Randomized prospective	70	Strength training vs. range of motion exercises without resistance	No significant between group difference
Hansen et al.	1993	Randomized prospective	75	Self training vs. training with physio vs. group training vs. group training and pool vs. no training	No significant between group difference
Strenstrom et al.	1991	Randomized	60	Intensive dynamic training in water vs. control group	No significant between group difference
Nordemar et al.	1981	Controlled	46	Physical training physio led vs. control group	Significantly less in physical training group

w/b=weightbearing

disability curtail the patient's activity. Leg-muscle strength is an important and independent determinator of walking ability. The strength of the quadriceps muscles have been correlated with floor walking and stair climbing time (Madsen and Egsmose 2001, Mengshoel et al. 2004). Therefore, it is important that the strength of the quadriceps muscles is examined and appropriate action taken.

In patients with RA proprioceptive deficits, as well as loss of muscle strength and functional ability have been shown (Bearne et al. 2002). Quadriceps sensorimotor deficits are associated with lower-limb disability and have been shown to improve with a rehabilitation programme that incorporates both physical activity and strength training without exacerbating pain and disease activity. Furthermore, it has been suggested that improvements in proprioceptive acuity may reduce harmful impact forces during gait, resulting in better timing of placement of the foot.

Gait training and re-education for patients with RA is not routinely carried out in rheumatology clinics and we have been unable to provide any evidence to support its use in patients with RA. However, gait training has been shown to be beneficial in the rehabilitation of patients who have had strokes, patients with Parkinson's disease, amputee patients using artificial limbs and reducing falls in the elderly population. Gait training using the rhythmic auditory stimulation (RAS) method consists of audiotapes with metronome-pulse patterns embedded into the on/off beat structure of rhythmically accentuated instrumental music and has been shown to increase gait velocity, stride length and step cadence in some cases.

Skin and wound care

Debridement of forefoot plantar corns and callosities in RA is a standard regular treatment undertaken by podiatrists. Prominent, subluxed and dislocated metatarsal heads are subject to excessive shear and compressive stresses during gait, stimulating the stratum corneum to produce painful callosities beneath the metatarsal heads (Klenerman 1995, Minns and Craxford 1984, Woodburn and Helliwell 1996). In patients who have normal heel alignment, it has been shown that forefoot peak pressures are equal to that of healthy adults. However, in patients with a valgus heel deformity, forefoot peak pressures are more medially directed and are accompanied by a higher prevalence of callosities (Woodburn and Helliwell 1996). The prevalence of painful and asymptomatic forefoot plantar hyperkeratosis in RA is unknown.

The rationale and therapeutic benefit of sharp scalpel debridement of plantar callosities is well established in diabetes. Furthermore, callus has been identified as a positive predictor of subsequent ulceration and debridement of plantar callosities has been shown to reduce peak pressures, prevent ulceration and facilitate wound healing (Murray et al. 1996, Young et al. 1992). In RA, hyperkeratosis is associated with significant discomfort (Woodburn et al. 2000), which in turn suggests that it causes functional changes in gait in order to compensate for the pain (Collis and Jayson 1972, Minns and Craxford 1984). Furthermore, it is suggested that changes in foot structure contribute towards reduced tissue viability, skin ulceration and delayed healing (Williams 2000). Unlike diabetes the precise relationship between callus, pain and pressure has not been established.

Anecdotal clinical evidence suggests that the debridement of forefoot plantar callosities signifi-

CALLUS

- A randomized controlled trial conducted by this group showed that sharp scalpel debridement offered no greater benefit than a sham procedure
- MTP joints with an overlying callus were more eroded than those without callus, suggesting a relationship may exist between local stresses, joint damage, callus formation and painful symptoms.
- It is recommended that callus debridement should be carried out in conjunction with other treatment modalities.

cantly reduces pain and appears to facilitate healing of plantar ulceration. A preliminary investigation (Woodburn et al. 2000) showed a large but short-lived reduction in pain following debridement (the treatment effect was lost within 7 days). In addition peak plantar pressures were increased in the majority of patients following treatment. To further explore the relationship between callus reduction, pain and function a randomized controlled trial has been recently conducted at Leeds (Davys et al. 2005). This trial involved using a sham treatment (where callus reduction was simulated but no hyperkeratotic tissue was removed) as a comparator to the normal treatment procedure. Patients were blinded to the treatment allocation. The outcome of the study contrasted the previous findings and expectations of clinicians and

patients. Sharp scalpel debridement of painful forefoot plantar callosities reduced pain and focal pressures and increased walking, as expected. However, these changes were no greater for the treatment group than for the sham procedure.

The above study revealed that MTP joints with an overlying callus were more eroded than those without callus, suggesting a relationship may exist between local stresses, joint damage, callus formation and painful symptoms. This finding is further supported by the work by Tuna and associates who reported an association between joint erosions and plantar pressure distribution (Tuna et al. 2004). In this study, patients with high joint erosion scores had higher static forefoot peak pressures. It is likely that in these cases forefoot pain may not be solely attributed to plantar callosities and further research is necessary to determine the relationship between pathology and symptoms and so to determine effective strategies for treatment.

Further, the above RCT does not support the current recommendations that podiatrists should carry out sharp scalpel debridement. However, these negative findings must be interpreted with caution. Pain associated with the lesions was only evaluated immediately post treatment and the consequences of not removing callus over a longer period of time were not assessed. It is possible that if left untreated the plantar lesions would increase in size causing more pain and potentially resulting in ulceration. Further investigation is needed before current clinical guidelines can be refuted. Clinicians should continue to debride painful forefoot plantar callosities in RA at an interval suitable for optimum pain relief and prevention of ulceration. However, regular debridement, whilst offering short-term benefits, does not address the underlying bony deformities that give rise to pressure lesions, and surgical intervention (discussed in Chapter 7) may be more clinically and cost effective.

Management of the high-risk foot in patients with rheumatoid arthritis

The pathogenesis of foot ulceration in patients with RA is poorly researched and risk factors for ulceration are as yet undetermined. Increased tissue stress at sites of prominent foot deformity is important, but this factor alone does not explain the whole picture. For example, Masson and colleagues compared plantar pressure distribution and neurological status between groups of patients with long-standing RA and diabetes. They found that the patients with RA had higher plantar pressures than the diabetic group, but none had a previous history of ulceration, compared to 32% of the diabetic group (Masson et al. 1998).

Although sub-clinical neuropathy is reported in RA (see Chapter 3), rarely does it translate to loss of protective sensation. The Masson study suggested that loss of protective sensation was the key factor in explaining why the diabetic patients ulcerate and the patients with RA do not. Significant limitations of the study were: no information was provided on systemic treatments for the cases with RA, and those with peripheral vascular disease were excluded. Observations in our own unit suggest these two factors have a significant role in the development of foot ulcers, in addition to long-term steroid treatment and poor skin nutrition associated with reduced circulation in the foot. More recently, the introduction of biologic therapy presents new challenges with spontaneous episodes of ulceration occurring at sites of fairly trivial trauma in the foot, highlighting the potentially significant role of immuno-suppression.

HIGH RISK MANAGEMENT

- Factors which predict patients who ulcerate have not yet been established but observations in our unit suggest poor vascular status, long-term steroid treatment, biologic therapy and history of ulceration.
- Subtle changes need to be monitored as the classic signs of infection may be masked by immunosuppression related to medication.
- Infection can rapidly progress in patients who are taking biologic agents. Therefore biologic therapy is usually suspended temporarily if a patient develops an ulcer.
- A multidisciplinary approach for high risk patients is advocated to facilitate rapid and effective assessment, treatment planning, intervention and follow-up.

Estimating the prevalence of foot ulceration in RA and identifying factors that are both predictive and prognostic are currently under investigation in our unit. However, the problem is common enough to merit the recent implementation of a weekly ulcer clinic. It should also be recognized that the morbidity associated with foot ulceration is less than that for diabetes. Nevertheless, it is often a chronic and painful complication of the disease. From clinical audit data at Leeds, we found 80 new cases of foot ulceration per year, representing 10% of the podiatry workload. Seventy per cent of these patients had RA and, although past treatment was difficult to account for, many reported a past history of ulceration either at the same foot site or an other. As for the diabetic foot, past history of ulceration is the strongest predictive factor for current or future ulceration. Prevention following healing is paramount in all patients.

What work is undertaken in the ulcer clinic and what are the principles and goals of treatment? Firstly, the clinic is podiatry-led by a specialist practitioner. The clinic is located in a rheumatology outpatient department and runs on the day of a general clinic to allow rapid access to other members of the medical team. This serves four main purposes:

1. The sharing of important medical information necessary to facilitate diagnosis and treatment.
2. To allow rapid prescription of antibiotics as necessary (podiatrists in the UK are currently unable to prescribe antibiotics).
3. To allow rapid medical attention to new cases of ulceration for those patients on biologic therapy.
4. To gain access to diagnostic and imaging modalities, including radiology and pressure studies.

The clinic is multidisciplinary with same-day access to orthopaedics and orthotics services. Although not formally tested, it is reasonable to assume that this approach, like that for the diabetic foot, should improve outcome. Equally important is our impression that continuity of care by the same podiatrist is vital in chronic wound and ulcer care. The principles and goals for treating ulceration are simple:

- Find the cause of the ulcer and treat accordingly
- Heal the ulcer itself
- Prevent infection in active ulcers
- Manage the painful ulcer
- Monitor progression and determine outcome (healed – yes/no, time to heal in weeks, etc.)
- Prevent further episodes of ulceration.

The distribution of ulcers by site has not been determined, but most occur at sites of high focal pressure, be that a joint deformity such as a prominent metatarsal head or a tight shoe pressing on the interphalangeal joint of a claw toe. To remove the focal pressure may require a change of footwear or a custom orthosis that redistributes pressure away from the site or changes the loading on the ulcerated site. In some cases foot surgery is indicated to correct severe deformity. There is often a reluctance to recommend this, but it should always be considered when ulceration is chronic, reoccurring and associated with complications of such as past episodes of cellulitis.

Of course, podiatrists themselves may be the cause of ulceration, as illustrated in Figure 6.32. In Figure 6.32A, a callus is left untreated and ulcerates under the plaque of callus itself whereas in Figure 6.32B, zealous debridement has left the remaining skin denuded and vulnerable (Woodburn et al. 2000). Ulceration often underlies plantar callus or callus forming over a prominent dorsal interphalangeal joint and it requires the skill of the podiatrist to identify this, often during the process of debridement. In most cases some callus must be debrided as it is often the source of severe pain in those patients reporting symptoms of walking on glass, pebbles or stones. This treatment is repeated as often as monthly and patients seldom fail to attend, such is the source of irritation and discomfort. Patients, driven to frustration, may undertake this treatment themselves using such instruments as scissors, razor blades or callus files. Therefore, this is an important area of patient education, especially in those patients with comorbidities, such as peripheral vascular disease. Recently, doubts have been raised as to the effectiveness of callus debridement and further work is required to clarify this (Davys et al. 2005). Others argue that these patients would probably benefit from forefoot arthroplasty, but many of these procedures themselves are associated with new callus formation as a recognized post-surgical complication. In ulcerated lesions, our impression that callus must be debrided to open and expose the ulcer, to reduce focal pressures and to help promote healing.

During the acute stages of a foot ulcer, traditional methods of off-loading high pressure sites can be used and these include DH Pressure Relief Walkers and the Aircast Pneumatic Walkers. These are effective, but it may present some problems for RA patients because with hand impairments they may be difficult to put on and take off. Where muscle weakness is present in the lower limb they may feel heavy and cumbersome to the patient. This hinders the strategies used so effectively to offload sites of neuropathic ulceration in the diabetic foot (Lavery et al. 1996). Alternatively, lightweight forefoot 'off-loader' boots are available and many of our RA patients use these successfully. Healing is often accelerated in a pain-free or pain-reduced environment.

Debridement, orthoses and off-loader devices may help reduce focal stresses and loading on the ulcer sites, but what role do wound dressings play? It is beyond the scope of this book to consider the many products available. Those that cushion the ulcer, provide an optimal healing environment by absorbing exudates and de-slough are favoured in the Leeds clinic. Bulky dressings, particularly those for interdigital ulcer should be avoided as they may serve to increase local pressures further. Practical issues are just as important for these patients. For example, restricting bathing to keep a wound dry is not necessary as dressings that temporarily seal an ulcer can be used.

Chronic ulceration is a challenge and requires continuous monitoring because the process of healing/deterioration can often be quite subtle. A common sense approach evaluates red flags and assessment of the ulcer volume. Wound-care monitoring systems for the diabetic foot may be employed, but most ulcers associated with RA are mild, so these instruments would lack the sensitivity to detect the subtle changes during the healing process, although none have been formally evaluated for this purpose. Other simple techniques include

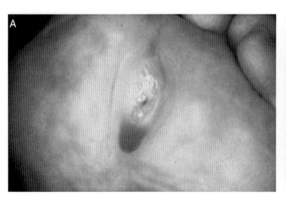
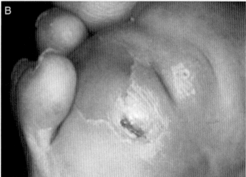

Figure 6.32 An iatrogenic ulcer in rheumatoid arthritis. The callus dilemma. In (A) the callus overlying the 2nd metatarsal head was not debrided and eventually ulcerated underneath the thick plaque of callus. This contrasts with (B), where the callus ulcerated within days of debridement.

having the ulcer photographed and to systematically record features such as amount and colour of any exudate and the state of surrounding tissue. The ulcer volume is often difficult to determine when undermined, and gentle probing is often too painful to undertake. There is a risk of osteomyelitis especially when ulcers extend to bone and radiographs or other imaging modalities are required to detect this. Subtle changes are often difficult to detect when eroded bone sites are involved.

Anecdotal evidence suggests that past and current medication plays a significant role in the development of ulceration and healing. Clinicians managing patients presenting with open wounds should have an understanding of the potential impact of drug treatments on tissue repair and healing. Non-steroidal anti-inflammatory drugs, immunosuppressives and steroids can compromise wound healing and can have a detrimental effect on tissue repair. Patients who are on biologic therapy are at an increased risk of developing infection, which can spread rapidly, as highlighted in Figure 6.33. For this reason, biologic therapy will normally be temporally suspended if a patient develops an ulcer on the foot.

Vasculitis usually involves the foot as part of a generalized vasculitic process (see Chapter 3). Cawley (1987) reported that ulceration on the dorsum of the foot and lower leg are more likely to be vasculitic in origin. However, the clinical review carried out by McRorie et al. (1994) identified studies that estimated that vasculitis (diagnosed primarily on clinical

grounds) has an aetiological role in 18–37% of leg ulcers in RA (Pun et al. 1990, Wilkinson and Kirk 1965). Ulceration in the foot is more likely due to anatomical distortion of the foot where trauma occurs to areas not able to withstand increased repeated pressure (Cawley 1987, McRorie et al. 1994).

Vasculitic ulceration in the leg and foot will normally require a review of the medical management. Frequently, further immunosuppression will be required, including steroids. Anecdotal evidence suggests that intra-venous iloprost may also help healing of vasculitic ulcers.

For management of the high-risk RA foot the above evidence has highlighted the need for good working relationships to be developed between the foot health team and the nursing and medical teams. Regular contact should be maintained between community teams and hospital outpatient departments.

SUMMARY

RA is a complex multisystem disease that requires equally complex multidisciplinary management. The challenges are to co-ordinate this care seamlessly and for everyone concerned, including the patient, to be aware of the others' role. This is particularly important with regard to the foot. This chapter has discussed the important aspects of medical and podiatry management using the available evidence and indicating the optimal points of intervention to minimize disability.

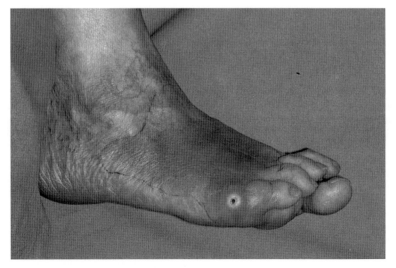

Figure 6.33 Rapid spreading infection in a patient currently on biological therapy. Cellulitis spread to this extent within a 24-h period.

References

American College of Rheumatology Guidelines for the management of rheumatoid arthritis. 2002 update. Arthritis and Rheumatism 2002; 46: 328–346.

Arner A, Lindblom U, Meyerson BA and Molander C Prolonged relief of neuralgia after regional anesthetic blocks. A call for further experimental and systematic clinical studies. Pain 1990; 43: 287–297.

The Big Picture. Arthritis: Research Campaign Arthritis Chesterfield, 2002.

Bansback NJ, Young A and Brennan A The NICE reappraisal of biologics in 2005: what rheumatologists need to know. Rheumatology 2004; 44: 3–4.

Barrett JP Jr Plantar pressure measurements. Rational shoe-wear in patients with rheumatoid arthritis. Journal of the American Medical Association 1976; 235(11): 1138–1139.

Bathon JM, Martin RW, Fleischmann RM et al. A comparison of etanercept and methotrexate in patients with early rheumatoid arthritis. New England Journal of Medicine 2000; 343: 1586–1593.

Bellamy N Clinimetric concepts in outcome assessment: the OMERACT filter. Journal of Rheumatology. 1999; 26(4): 948–950.

Branch VK, Lipsky K, Nieman T and Lipsky PE Positive impact of an intervention by arthritis patient educators on knowledge and satisfaction of patients in a rheumatology practice. Arthritis Care and Research 1999; 12(6): 370–375.

Breedveld FC, Emery P, Keystone E et al. Infliximab in early active rheumatoid arthritis. Annals of Rheumatic Diseases 2004; 63: 149–155.

Brodsky JW, Kourosh S, Stills M and Mooney V Objective evaluation of insert materials for diabetic and athletic footwear. Foot and Ankle International 1998; 9(3): 111–116.

Brown AK, O'Connor PJ, Wakefield RJ, Roberts TE, Karim Z and Emery P Practice, training, and assessment among experts performing musculoskeletal ultrasonography: toward the development of an international consensus of educational standards for ultrasonography for rheumatologists. Arthritis and Rheumatism 2004; 51(6): 1018–1022.

Bukhari MA, Wiles NJ, Lunt M, Harrison BJ, Scott DG, Symmons DP and Silman AJ Influence of disease-modifying therapy on radiographic outcome in inflammatory polyarthritis at five years: results from a large observational inception study. Arthritis and Rheumatism 2003; 48(1): 46–53.

Burns SL, Leese GP and McMurdo MET Older people and ill fitting shoes. Postgraduate Medical Journal 2002; 78: 344–346.

Canoso JJ Aspiration and injection of joints and periarticular tissues. In: Klippel JH, Dieppe PA (eds) Rheumatology, 2nd edn. Mosby, London, 1998; pp. 2.12.1–2.12.12.

Cawley PJ and Morris IM A study to compare the efficacy of two methods of skin preparation prior to joint injection. British Journal of Rheumatology. 1992; 31: 847–848.

Cawley MI Vasculitis and ulceration in rheumatic diseases of the foot. Baillières Clinical Rheumatology 1987; 1(2): 315–333.

Chakravarty K, Pharoah PDP and Scott DGI A randomised controlled study of postinjection rest following intra-articular steroid therapy for knee synovitis. British Journal of Rheumatology 1994; 33: 464–468.

Chalmers AC, Busby C, Goyert J, Porter B and Schulzer M Metatarsalgia and rheumatoid arthritis – a randomized, single blind, sequential trial comparing 2 types of foot orthoses and supportive shoes. Journal of Rheumatology 2000; 27(7): 1643–1647.

Chamberlain MA, Care G. and Harfield B Physiotherapy and osteoarthrosis of the knees: a controlled trial of hospital versus home exercises. International Rehabilitation Medicine 1982; 4: 101–106.

Chandler GN, Jones DR, Wright V and Hartfall SJ Charcot's arthropathy following intra-articular hydrocortisone. British Medical Journal 1959; 2: 952–953.

Chantelau E and Gede A Foot dimensions of elderly people with and without diabetes mellitus – a data basis for shoe design. Gerontology 2002; 48(4): 241–244.

Collis WJMF and Jayson MIV Measurement of pedal pressures. An illustration of a method. Annals of the Rheumatic Diseases 1972; 31: 215–217.

Crawford F, Atkins D, Young P and Edwards J Steroid injection for heel pain: evidence of short-term effectiveness. A randomized controlled trial. Rheumatology 1999; 38(10): 974–977.

Cruz-Esteban C and Wilke WS Non-surgical synovectomy. Bailières Clinical Rheumatology 1995; 9(4): 787–801.

Davys HJ, Turner DE, Helliwell PS, Conaghan PG, Emery P and Woodburn J Debridement of plantar callosities in rheumatoid arthrits: a randomized controlled trial. Rheumatology 2005; 44(2): 207–210.

Day AT, Golding JR, Lee PN and Butterworth AD Penicillamine in rheumatoid disease: a long-term study. British Medical Journal 1974; 1: 180–182.

de Jong Z, Munneke M, Lems WF et al. Slowing of bone loss in patients with rheumatoid arthritis by long-term high-intensity exercise: results of a randomised controlled trial. Arthritis and Rheumatism 2004a; 50: 1066–1076.

de Jong Z, Munneke M, Zwinderman AH et al. Is a long-term high-intensity exercise program effective and safe in patients with rheumatoid arthritis? Results of a randomised controlled trial. Arthritis and Rheumatism 2003; 48: 2415–2424.

de Jong Z, Munneke M, Zwinderman AH et al. Long term high intensity exercise and damage of small joints in rheumatoid arthritis. Annals of the Rheumatic Diseases 2004b; 63: 1399–1405.

Dixon A St.J and Graber J Local injection therapy in rheumatic diseases Eular Publishers, Basle, 1981.

DOH Chronic Disease Management and Self-care. National Sevice Frameworks. A practical aid to implementation in primary care. Department of Health, 2002.

Edwards J, Szczepanski L, Szechinski J et al. Efficacy of B-cell-targeted therapy with Rituximab in patients with rheumatoid arthritis. New England Journal of Medicine 2004; 350: 2572–2581.

Emery P and Seto Y Role of biologics in early arthritis. Clinical and Experimental Rheumatology 2003; 21: 5191–5194.

Falsetti P, Frediani B, Fioravanti A, Acciai C, Baldi F, Filippou G and Marcolongo R Sonographic study of calcaneal entheses in erosive osteoarthritis, nodal osteoarthritis, rheumatoid arthritis and psoriatic arthritis. Scandinavian Journal of Rheumatology 2003; 32(4): 229–234.

Farrow S, Khoshaba B and Scott D Foot involvement, disease activity and disability in rheumatoid arthritis. Rheumatology 2004; 43(Suppl 2): 140.

Faulkner G, Prichard P, Somerville K. and Langman MJ Aspirin and bleeding peptic ulcers in the elderly. British Medical Journal 1988; 297(6659): 1311–1313.

Fitzgerald GA Coxibs and cardiovascular disease. New England Journal of Medicine 2004; 351: 1709–1711.

Foto JG and Birke JA Evaluation of multidensity orthotic materials used in footwear in patients with diabetes. Foot and Ankle International 1998; 19(12): 836–841.

Fransen M and Edmonds J Off-the-shelf orthopedic footwear for people with rheumatoid arthritis. Arthritis Care and Research 1997; 10(4): 250–256.

Genovese MC, Cohen S, Moreland LW, Lium D, Robbins S, Newmark R and Bekker P. Combination therapy with etanercept and anakinra in the treatment of patients with rheumatoid arthritis who have been treated unsuccessfully with methotrexate. Arthritis and Rheumatism 2004; 50: 1412–1419.

Gerber LH Rehabilitation. In: Klippel JH, Dieppe PA (eds) Management of Rheumatic Diseases. Mosby–Year Book, London, 1994; pp. 3.1–3.2.

Gordon P, West J, Jones H and Gibson T A 10 year prospective followup of patients with rheumatoid arthritis 1986–96. Journal of Rheumatology 2001; 28(11): 2409–2415.

Haake M, Buch M, Schoellner C et al. Extracorporeal shock wave therapy for plantar fasciitis: randomised controlled multicentre trial. British Medical Journal 2003; 327: 75–77.

Hakkinen A, Sokka T, Kotaniemi A and Hannonen P A randomized two-year study of the effects of dynamic strength training on muscle strength, disease activity, functional capacity, and bone mineral density in early rheumatoid arthritis. Arthritis and Rheumatism 2001; 44(3): 515–522.

Hammond A The use of self-management strategies by people with rheumatoid arthritis. Clinical Rehabilitation 1998; 12; 81–87.

Hansen TM, Hansen G, Langgaard AM and Rasmussen JO Longterm physical training in rheumatoid arthritis. A randomized trial with different training programs and blinded observers. Scandinavian Journal of Rheumatology 1993; 22(3): 107–112.

Hawkey CJ COX-2 inhibitors. Lancet 1999; 353(9149): 307–314.

Hay SM, Moore DJ, Cooper JR and Getty CJM Diagnostic injections of the hindfoot joints in patients with rheumatoid arthritis prior to surgical fusion. Foot 1999; 9(1): 40–43.

Helliwell PS Use of an objective measure of articular stiffness to record changes in finger joints after intra-articular injection of corticosteroid. Annals of the Rheumatic Diseases 1997; 56(1): 71–73.

Helliwell PS Lessons to be learned: review of a multidisciplinary foot clinic in rheumatology. Rheumatology 2003; 42(11): 1426–1427.

Helliwell PS and Ibrahim G Ethnic differences in the response to disease modifying drugs. Rheumatology 2003; 42: 1197–1201.

Hider SL, Buckley C, Silman AJ, Symmons DPM and Bruce IN Factors influencing response to disease modifying anti-rheumatic drugs in patients with rheumatoid arthritis. Journal of Rheumatology 2005; 32: 11–16.

Hill JA practical guide to patient education and information giving. Baillières Clinical Rheumatology 1997; 11(1): 109–127.

Hochberg MC Role of intra-articular hyaluronic acid preparations in medical management of osteoarthritis of the knee. Seminars in Arthritis and Rheumatism 2000; 30(2 Suppl 1): 2–10.

Hodge MC, Bach TM and Carter GM Novel Award First Prize Paper. Orthotic management of plantar pressure and pain in rheumatoid arthritis. Clinical Biomechanics 1999; 14(8): 567–575.

Hollander JL Arthrocentesis and intra-synovial therapy. In: McCarty DJ (ed.) Arthritis and Allied Conditions, 10th edn. Lea and Febiger, Philadelphia, 1985; 541–553.

Jones A, Regan M, Ledingham J, Pattrick M, Manhire A and Doherty M Importance of placement of intra-articular steroid injections. British Medical Journal 1993; 307: 1329–1330.

Juni P, Nartey L, Reichenbach S, Sterchi R, Dieppe PA and Egger M Risk of cardiovascular events and rofecoxib: cumulative meta-analysis. Lancet 2004; 364: 2021–2029.

Kerry RM, Holt GM and Stockley I The foot in chronic rheumatoid arthritis: A continuing problem. Foot 1994; 4(4): 201–203.

Kirwan JR The effect of glucocorticoids on joint destruction in rheumatoid arthritis. The Arthritis and Rheumatism Council Low-Dose Glucocorticoid Study Group. New England Journal of Medicine 1995; 333(3): 142–146.

Klenerman L The foot and ankle in rheumatoid arthritis. British Journal of Rheumatology 1995; 34(5): 443–448.

Konttinen YT, Santavirta N, Honkanen V, Sandelin S, Schauman L and Gronblad M Systemic lupus erythematosis patient guide: influence on knowledge of the disease. Annals of the Rheumatic Diseases 1991; 50: 900–902.

Krause I, Valesini G, Scrivo R and Schoenfeld Y Autoimmune aspects of cytokine and anti-cytokine therapies. American Journal of Medicine 2003; 115: 390–397.

Kremer J, Genovese M, Cannon GW et al. Combination leflunomide and methotrexate (MTX) therapy for patients with active rheumatoid arthritis failing MTX monotherapy: open-label extension of a randomized, double-blind, placebo controlled trial. Journal of Rheumatology. 2004; 31(8):1521–1531.

Landewe R, Boers M, Verhoeven AC et al. COBRA combination therapy in patients with early rheumatoid arthritis. Arthritis and Rheumatism 2002; 46(2): 347–356.

Lavery LA, Vela SA, Lavery DC and Quebedeaux TL Reducing dynamic foot pressures in high-risk diabetic subjects with foot ulcerations. A comparison of treatments. Diabetes Care 1996; 19(8): 818–821.

Lemmey A, Maddison P, Breslin A et al. Association between insulin-like growth factor status and physical activity levels in rheumatoid arthritis. Journal of Rheumatology. 2001; 28(1): 29–34.

Lorig K Patient education: treatment or nice extra? British Journal of Rheumatology 1995; 34: 703–704.

Madsen OR and Egsmose C Associations of isokinetic knee extensor and flexor strength with steroid use and walking ability in women with rheumatoid arthritis. Clinical Rheumatology 2001; 20(3): 207–212.

Maggs FM, Jubb RW and Kemm JR Single-blind randomised control trial of an educational booklet for patients with chronic arthritis. British Journal of Rheumatology 1996; 35: 775–777.

Masson EA, Stockely I, Veves A et al. Abnormal foot pressures alone may not cause ulceration. Diabetic Medicine 1998; 6: 426–428.

Maxwell SRJ and Webb DJ COX-2 selective inhibitors – important lessons learned. Lancet 2005; 365(9458): 449–451.

McRorie ER, Jobanputra P, Ruckley CV and Nuki G Leg ulceration in rheumatoid arthritis. British Journal of Rheumatology 1994; 33: 1078–1084.

Mengshoel AM, Jokstad K and Bjerkhoel F Associations between walking time, quadriceps muscle strength and cardiovascular disease capacity in patients with rheumatoid arthritis and ankylosing spondylitis. Clinical Rheumatology 2004; 23(4): 299–305.

Mielants H and Veys EM The gut in the spondyloarthropathies. Journal of Rheumatology 1990; 17: 7–10.

Minns RJ and Craxford AD Pressure under the forefoot in rheumatoid arthritis. A comparison of static and dynamic methods of assessment. Clinical Orthopaedics and Related Research 1984; 187: 235–242.

Mitchell MJ, Bielecki D, Bergman AG, Kursunoglu-Brahme S, Sartoris DJ and Resnick D Localization of specific joint causing hindfoot pain: value of injecting local anesthetics into individual joints during arthrography. American Journal of Roentgenology 1995; 164: 1473–1476.

Munneke M, de Jong Z, Zwinderman AH, Ronday HK, van den Ende CHM, Vliet Vlieland TPM and Hazes JM High intensity exercise or conventional exercise for patients with rheumatoid arthritis? Outcome expectations of patients, rheumatologists, and physiotherapists. Annals of the Rheumatic Diseases 2004; 63(7): 804–808.

Murray HJ, Young MJ, Hollis S and Boulton AJM The association between callus formation, high pressures and neuropathy in diabetic foot ulceration. Diabetic Medicine 1996; 13: 979–982.

Neumann VC, Taggart AJ, Le Gallez P, Astbury C, Hill J and Bird HA A study to determine the active moiety of sulphasalazine in rheumatoid arthritis. Journal of Rheumatology 1986; 13: 285–287.

Nordemar R, Ekblom B, Zachrisson L and Lundqvist K Physical training in rheumatoid arthritis: a controlled long-term study. Scandinavian Journal of Rheumatology 1981; 22: 107–112.

O'Dell JR Therapeutic strategies for rheumatoid arthritis. New England Journal of Medicine 2004; 350: 2591–2602.

O'Dell JR, Blakely K, Mallek J et al. Treatment of early seropositive rheumatoid arthritis: a two year double blind comparison of minocycline and hydroxychloroquine. Arthritis and Rheumatism 2001; 44(10): 2235–2241.

O'Dell JR, Leff R, Paulson G et al. Treatment of rheumatoid arthritis with methotrexate and hydroxychloroquine, methotrexate and sulfasalazine, or a combination of the three medications. Arthritis and Rheumatism 2002; 46(5): 1164–1170.

Olsen NJ, Sokka T, Seedhorn CL, Kraft B, Maas K, Moore J and Aune TM A gene expression signature for recent onset rheumatoid arthritis in peripheral blood mononuclear cells. Annals of the Rheumatic Diseases 2004; 63: 1387–1392.

Olsen NJ and Stein M New drugs for rheumatoid arthritis. New England Journal of Medicine 2004; 350: 2567–2579.

Pincus T, O'Dell JR and Kremer JM Combination therapy with multiple disease-modifying antirheumatic drugs in rheumatoid arthritis: a preventive strategy. Annals of Internal Medicine 1999; 131(10): 768–774.

Pratt DJ, Rees PH and Rodgers C Assessment of some shock absorbing insoles. Prosthetics and Orthotics International 1986; 10(1): 43–45.

Pun YLW, Barraclough DRE and Muirden KD Leg ulcers in rheumatoid arthritis. The Medical Journal of Australia 1990; 153: 585–587.

Rall LC, Meydani SN, Kehayias JJ, Dawson-Hughes B and Roubenoff R The effect of progressive resistance training in rheumatoid arthritis. Increased strength without changes in energy balance or body composition. Arthritis and Rheumatism 1996; 39(3): 415–426.

Raynauld J-P, Buckland-Wright C, Ward R et al. Safety and efficacy of long term intra-articular steroid injections in osteoarthritis of the knee. Arthritis and Rheumatism 2003; 48(2): 370–377.

Research Committee of the Empire Rheumatism Council Gold therapy in rheumatoid arthritis. Annals of the Rheumatic Diseases 196120: 315–333.

Riemsma RP, Kirwan JR, Taal E and Rasker JJ Patient education for adults with rheumatoid arthritis. Cochrane Database of Systematic Reviews 2004; 2: 2.

Ronnemaa T, Hamalainen H, Toikka T and Liukkonen I Evaluation of the impact of the podiatrist care in the primary prevention of foot problems in diabetic subjects. Diabetes Care 1997; 20(12): 1833–1837.

Sari-Kouzel H, Hutchinson CE, Middleton A, Webb FMT, Griffin K and Herrick AL Foot problems in patients with systemic sclerosis. Rheumatology 2001; 40: 410–413.

Schwarzer AC, Arnold MH and Brooks PM Combination therapy in rheumatoid arthritis. Baillières Clinical Rheumatology 1990; 4(3): 663–685.

Shrader JA and Siegel KL Nonoperative management of functional hallux limitus in a patient with rheumatoid arthritis. Physical Therapy 2003; 83(9): 831–843.

Smollen JS, Aletaha D and Machold KP Therapeutic strategies in early rheumatoid arthritis. Best Practice and Research Clinical Rheumatology 2005; 19: 163–177.

Spraul M Education – Can it prevent diabetic foot ulcers and amputations. In: Boulton AJM, Conner H and Cavanagh PR (eds) The Foot in Diabetes, 3rd edn. John Wiley and Sons Ltd, 2000; 111–119.

Steiner WA, Ryser L, Huber E, Uebelhart D, Aeschlimann A and Stucki G Use of an ICF model as a clinical problem-solving tool in physical therapy and rehabilitation medicine. Physical Therapy 2002; 82: 1098–1107.

Strenstrom CH, Lindell B, Swanberg P, Harms-Ringdahl K and Nordemar R Intensive dynamic training in water for rheumatoid arthritis functional class II – a long–term study of effects. Scandinavian Journal of Rheumatology 1991; 20(5): 358–365.

Stuart L and Wiles P Patient education and the diabetic foot: a panacea for prevention? The Diabetic Foot 2000; 3: 4.

Stucki G and Ewert T How to assess the impact of arthritis on the individual patient: the WHO ICF. Annals of the Rheumatic Diseases 2005; 64: 664–668.

Symmons DP and Silman AJ Anti-tumor necrosis factor alpha therapy and the risk of lymphoma in rheumatoid arthritis: no clear answer. Arthritis and Rheumatism. 2004; 50(6): 1703–1706.

Thomson F and Masson EA Can elderley diabetic patients co–operate with routine footcare? Age Ageing 1992; 21(5): 333–337.

Tsung BYS, Zhang M, Fan YB and Boone DA Quantitative comparison of plantar foot shapes under different weight-bearing conditions. Journal of Rehabilitation, Research and Development 2003; 40(6): 517–526.

Van der Esch M, Heijmans M and Dekker J Factors contributing to possession and use of walking aids among persons with rheumatoid arthritis and osteoarthritis. Arthritis and Rheumatism 2003; 49(6): 838–842.

Vane JR Inhibition of prostaglandin synthesis as a mechanism of action for the aspirin like drugs. Nature 1971; 231: 232–235.

Verstappen SM, Jacobs JW, Bijlsma JW et al. Five-year follow up of rheumatoid arthritis patients after early treatment with disease-modifying antirheumatic drugs versus treatment according to the pyramid approach in the first year. Arthritis and Rheumatism 2003; 48(7): 1797–1807.

Waxman R, Woodburn H, Powell M, Woodburn J, Blackburn S and Helliwell PS FOOTSTEP: a randomized controlled trial investigating the clinical and cost effectiveness of a patient self-management program for basic foot care in the elderly. Journal of Clinical Epidemiology 2003; 56:1092–1099.

Weinblatt ME, Weissmn BN, Holdsworth DE, Fraser PA, Maier AL, Falchuk KR and Coblyn JS Long-term prospective study of Methotrexate in the treatment of rheumatoid arthritis. Arthritis and Rheumatism 1992; 35: 129–137.

Wilkinson M and Kirk J Leg ulcers complicating rheumatoid arthritis. Scottish Medical Journal 1965; 10: 175–182.

Williams A and Meacher K Shoes in the cupboard: the fate of prescribed footwear? Prosthetics and Orthotics International 2001; 25: 53–59.

Williams A The rheumatoid foot – the essentials. British Journal of Podiatry 2000; November: 123.

Williams JM and Brandt KD Exercise increases osteophyte formation and diminishes fibrillation following chemically induced articular cartilage injury. Journal of Anatomy 1984; 139(4): 599–611.

Wilson A Business organizations' awareness of the communicative properties of footwear: results of a pilot survey on the regulation of footwear with female employee uniforms in a major Polish city. Linguistics Department, Lancaster University, The language of shoes project: Working paper, 2004.

Woodburn J Kinematics at the ankle joint in rheumatoid arthritis, PhD thesis, University of Leeds, 2000.

Woodburn J, Barker S and Helliwell PS A randomized controlled trial of foot orthoses in rheumatoid arthritis. Journal of Rheumatology 2002; 29(7): 1377–1383.

Woodburn J and Helliwell PS Relation between heel position and the distribution of forefoot plantar pressures and skin callosities in rheumatoid arthritis. Annals of the Rheumatic Diseases 1996; 55(11): 806–810.

Woodburn J, Helliwell PS and Barker S Changes in 3D joint kinematics support the continuous use of orthoses in the management of painful rearfoot deformity in rheumatoid arthritis. Journal of Rheumatology 2003; 30(11): 2356–2364.

Woodburn J, Stableford Z and Helliwell PS Preliminary investigation of debridement of plantar callosities in rheumatoid arthritis. Rheumatology 2000; 39(6): 652–654.

Young A, Dixey J, Cox N How does functional disability in early rheumatoid arthritis (RA) affect patients and their lives? Results of 5 years of follow-up in 732 patients from the Early RA Study (ERAS). Rheumatology 2000; 39(6): 603–611.

Young MJ, Cavanagh PR, Thomas G, Johnson MM, Murray HJ and Boulton AJM The effect of callus removal on dynamic plantar foot pressures in diabetic patients. Diabetic Medicine 1992; 9: 55–57.

Chapter **7**

Surgical management of the foot and ankle in rheumatoid arthritis

Mr N J Harris and Mr N Carrington

INTRODUCTION

The foot may be the site of initial presentation in rheumatoid arthritis (RA) and is frequently involved early in the disease process. Over the course of the disease the prevalence of foot pathology is over 85% (Vainio 1956). In fact, it is believed that the feet are involved slightly more often than the hands (Calabro 1962). Disease tends to affect the joints of the forefoot before the midfoot or hindfoot. Ankle involvement is relatively unusual in isolation. Subsequent pain, instability and deformity may necessitate surgical intervention. Manifestations of rheumatoid disease in the soft tissues include tenosynovitis, synovial cysts, and rheumatoid nodules. The surgeon must be able to distinguish these problems from underlying joint disease and operative treatment may be necessary.

GENERAL CONSIDERATIONS

The systemic, polyarticular nature of rheumatoid disease demands a thorough assessment of the whole patient when planning surgical treatment. With few exceptions, medical and non-operative measures should be tried before considering surgical treatment. There may be a role for earlier intervention with synovectomy when disease is severe, to prevent rapid joint destruction. Coughlin (1999) describes a hierarchy of treatment aims based on the stage at which disease presents to the surgeon:

1. Pain relief
2. Prevent deformity
3. Correct deformity
4. Preserve function
5. Restore function.

The main aim is to preserve ambulation and independence. The surgeon should work closely with a multidisciplinary team including rheumatologists, chiropodists, orthotists, physiotherapists and specialist nurses. This ensures all non-operative modalities have been considered, and may aid post-operative rehabilitation.

A good outcome from surgery is more likely if the disease is well controlled pre-operatively. However, the immunosuppressive nature of prednisolone, methotrexate and the TNF and IL-1 antagonists, can all potentially increase the risk of infection and wound dehiscence (Mohan et al. 2003). It is suggested that biologic drugs are temporarily discontinued prior to surgery and attempts should be made to minimize the dose of prednisolone required. However, there is good evidence to suggest continuation of methotrexate is safe (Sany et al. 1993, Grennan et al. 2001). Grennan et al. (2001) showed no increased risk of infection or wound complications if taking methotrexate, but stopping the medication prior to surgery did lead to a flare up in rheumatoid disease in about 5% of patients. The risk of infection can be reduced by the use of antibiotic prophylaxis at the time of surgery, but, despite this, the risk of deep infection is up to five times that of the normal population when arthroplasty is considered. Adrenal insufficiency must also be considered in patients on long-term steroids and additional steroid may be required to cover the stress of more major surgery.

It is vitally important that the surgeon assesses the soft tissues of the foot and ankle carefully. Active vasculitis can increase the risk of infection through poorer wound healing. There may also be elements of vasculopathy or neuropathy, which could threaten successful surgical outcome (see Chapter 3). As a rule, healthy pre-operative soft tissues and careful surgical technique should ensure better outcome.

Finally, it is generally believed that if disease affects the larger proximal joints in the lower limbs, these should be treated prior to the foot, except when there is persistent ulceration in the foot, which might increase the infection risk. Hindfoot surgery for deformity should be performed prior to forefoot surgery, as recurrent forefoot deformity may occur in some cases if this is not adhered to. Bilateral surgery is less well tolerated in rheumatoid arthritis, because of the demand that this places on other joints during mobilization, particularly those of the upper limbs.

FOREFOOT

Metatarsophalangeal joints

The effects of the disease are usually most noticeable in the five metatarso-phalangeal joints (MTPJs). The interphalangeal joints (IPJs) may become diseased, but problems usually arise from contractures and deformity secondary to MTPJ disease. Early symptoms are due to synovitis and effusion, which are present in 65% of patients within the first 3 years (Michelson et al. 1994). In these cases synovectomy of the MTPJs via dorsal incisions is advocated by some surgeons, but with claims that, at best, this is a temporizing measure (Aho 1987). Meticulous technique ensuring excision of all synovium gives short-term satisfactory results in up to 80% of cases (Raunio & Laine 1970).

In about 77% of cases the lesser MTPJs sublux as disease progresses (Vidigal et al. 1975). Loss of capsular and ligamentous integrity due to synovial distension, combined with the dorsiflexion stresses created during ambulation leads to dorsal subluxation of the proximal phalanges with respect to the metatarsal heads. The phalanx can become `locked' on the dorsal surface of the metatarsal and forces from the flexor tendons `push' the metatarsal heads plantarwards. The plantar fat pad, which normally protects the prominent metatarsal heads, is drawn distally as the phalanges sublux. Pressure areas result leading to intractable plantar keratoses or even ulceration. Once joints have subluxed, the surgical solution must be more extensive. There is no role for reduction of these diseased joints and an excision arthroplasty of the lesser MTPJs must be performed (forefoot arthroplasty). This procedure has evolved over a number of years and techniques still differ. However, when performed well it gives reliable relief of symptoms long term. Previous techniques involved excision of the proximal phalangeal bases, sometimes combined with a bevelling of the prominent metatarsal heads (Fowler procedure). However, when done in specialist centres this gave satisfactory results in only 65% of patients (Coughlin 1999). Hoffman's procedure involves excision of the metatarsal heads and this appears to give a more reliable outcome with 89% of results being satisfactory (Mann & Thompson 1984). It is important to recreate the normal metatarsal cascade with gradually shorter stumps from the 2nd to the 5th rays. This reduces the risk of transfer metatarsalgia laterally.

The main complication of this surgery is residual pain or recurrent intractable plantar keratosis (IPK) due to inadequate resection of the metatarsals. These procedures can be performed via plantar or dorsal incisions. The plantar approach allows excision of an ellipse of skin containing ulcers or callosities and can aid reduction of the plantar fat pad. However, there may be difficulties with healing of this wound. Coughlin (1999) recommends two dorsal longitudinal incisions, in the second and fourth web spaces allowing access to all four lesser MTPJs. The risks of a plantar wound are avoided, ambulation may be earlier and evidence suggests that the plantar callosities disappear once the pressure symptoms are relieved (Coughlin 2000). It is important to stress that forefoot arthroplasty is salvage surgery and little active function of these joints is preserved. Silastic replacement of the lesser MTPJs has been attempted, but does not appear to offer any functional benefit over forefoot arthroplasty and carries the additional risks of the implant, and its use is, therefore, not recommended (Coughlin 1999).

There is greater controversy when only one or two lesser MTPJs are affected. It is likely that disease will progress in the remaining joints and Coughlin (1999) recommends excising all four metatarsal heads if two or more are diseased.

Inter–phalangeal joints

In 40–80% of cases the 2nd to 5th toes can develop a hammer deformity, which becomes a claw toe as the MTPJ dorsiflexion contracture worsens (Michelson et al. 1994). This is caused by an imbalance between the intrinsic and extrinsic muscles of the toes. Pressure areas develop over the dorsum of the proximal interphalangeal joints (PIPJs), leading to pain and ulceration. Early hammer-toe deformity can be corrected by manipulation of the joint and insertion of a temporary k-wire across the PIPJ whilst the tissues tighten in extension. However, in most cases a proximal phalangeal condylectomy or PIPJ fusion are required, again using k-wire stabilization. This technique gives consistently good results, but there may be mild recurrence of deformity.

First metatarsophalangeal joint

There is a high incidence of severe hallux valgus deformity in rheumatoid disease. This is due to a combination of disease of the 1st MTPJ and loss of lateral support for the hallux as the lesser toes claw. The deformity destabilizes the 1st ray leading to transfer metatarsalgia laterally. Keller's procedure involves excision of up to 50% of the proximal phalanx at the 1st MTPJ and historically has been performed in large numbers of rheumatoid patients. However, most modern series report dissatisfaction due to a tendency for deformity to recur, as most cases are performed in combination with a forefoot arthroplasty and lateral support for the hallux has been lost.

Silastic 1st MTPJ replacements have also lost popularity due to long-term problems with osteolysis, silicon synovitis, fracture and recurrent deformity. The gold standard treatment is 1st MTPJ arthrodesis. This

provides stability to the first ray in gait and protects the lesser MTPJs from dorsiflexion forces (Mann & Thompson 1984).

Graham has recommended fusion of the valgus joint rather than corrective osteotomy even when only minor joint disease is present (Graham 1994). When performed well fusion rates of 90–100% can be expected with 96% good-to-excellent results (Coughlin 2000). However, meticulous technique is essential for such results. Coughlin (1999) recommends use of conical reamers to provide a convex metatarsal head and concave proximal phalanx, allowing a more precise position for fusion with a larger surface area to encourage healing. The ideal position is 15–20° of valgus, 10–30° of dorsiflexion with reference to the floor and neutral rotation. The upper range for dorsiflexion is more suited to women who wish to wear shoes with higher heels. Fixation must be stable and the use of one or two screws is often supplemented by a dorsal low-profile plate. The main complications arise when a poor fusion position is obtained or non-union occurs. Non-union may be asymptomatic. Union with inadequate valgus causes pressure symptoms over the distal hallux and secondary arthritic changes in the IPJ are common. This joint may then require fusion. Insufficient dorsiflexion leads to plantar pressure at the tip of the hallux, whilst excessive dorsiflexion can cause plantar pressure beneath the metatarsal head (Fig. 7.1).

MIDFOOT

The joints of the midfoot present difficulties for both diagnosis and management. There is a high rate of radiographic involvement, but this does not tally with symptoms (Jaakkola & Mann 2004). Similarly, pain can be difficult to localize in the midfoot and symptomatic joints may go unrecognized. However, there is often structural failure in the midfoot, usually due to rupture of the tibialis posterior tendon and the talonavicular ligament. Collapse of the medial longitudinal arch results in a planus midfoot, usually in combination with a valgus hindfoot deformity.

The rheumatoid disease process in most cases leads to gradual ankylosis of the midfoot, as most of these joints have minimal movement when healthy. This probably explains the low rate of symptoms as ankylosis provides fusion without the need for surgery. The exception to this is the 1st metatarsocuneiform joint, which can develop hypermobility with advanced disease. This may provoke local pain, but can also lead to transfer metatarsalgia as the 1st ray becomes incompetent under load during gait. Other problems arise when severe planus deformity develops creating pressure points. In both these situations, fusion of the

Figure 7.1 Illustrating the typical features of the rheumatoid forefoot with destruction and dislocation of the metatarsophalangeal joints. Surgical treatment has consisted of excision of the lesser metatarsal heads and a realignment and fusion of the great toe.

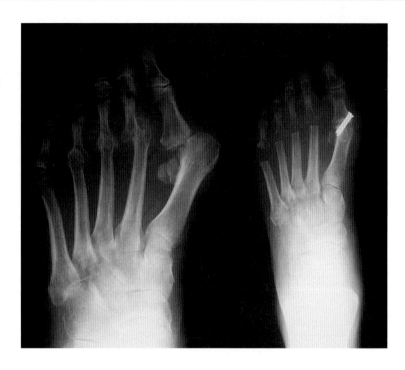

relevant midfoot joints can be attempted, and in the planus foot this may be combined with correction of the deformity. Loss of bone stock may necessitate use of a cortico-cancellous bone graft from the iliac crest to restore the longitudinal arch.

HINDFOOT

Hindfoot involvement is less common than the forefoot, and it usually occurs later in disease progression. The prevalence of disease is 29% for the subtalar joint, 39% for the talo-navicular joint and 25% for the calcaneocuboid joint (Jaakkola & Mann 2004). The problems from hindfoot disease may be due to pain, deformity or both. In most cases, subtalar joint disease combined with interosseous ligament and tibialis posterior tendon rupture lead to a progressive valgus deformity. Varus deformity does occasionally occur, probably in about 5% of cases, usually in sedentary patients due to medially directed forces on the resting foot with the leg externally rotated (Vainio 1956). Varus deformity may also be a consequence of walking strategies used to offload the first ray.

It can be difficult to isolate the precise source of pain since the hindfoot joints are closely related anatomically. Although computerized tomography undoubtedly helps in this respect, there is not always good correspondence between radiological findings and symptoms. Injecting local anaesthetic into selected joints in order to identify the origin of the

pain has been shown to be an effective method of appropriately selecting operative procedures in the hindfoot area in RA (Hay et al. 1999).

Early tenosynovial disease in the tibialis posterior sheath can lead to tendon damage, interstitial tears and elongation. This `functional rupture' leads to dysfunction and planovalgus deformity, despite an apparently intact tendon on ultrasound (U/S) or magnetic resonance imaging (MRI). The tendon may finally rupture fully. Bulky tenosynovitis may lead to tarsal tunnel syndrome with compression of the posterior tibial nerve. Such disease is only encountered rarely in rheumatoid patients, but may be relieved by decompression and debridement of the tendon sheath. With rapid development of a planovalgus mid- and hindfoot deformity, acute rupture of tibialis posterior may be suspected. However, it is not known if reconstruction of the tendon is a good option in this population. In most cases, there will be some associated disease of the hindfoot joints and fusion may be the better option, if non-operative treatment is not tolerated.

The aim when treating hindfoot disease is to restore the normal plantigrade foot position. This may prove challenging owing to contracted lateral soft tissues and loss of bone stock. When disease affects the talonavicular joint in isolation an early fusion of this joint alone can protect the remainder of the hindfoot joints from developing deformity and requiring surgery (Ljung et al. 1992). Most hindfoot movement is eradicated with talonavicular fusion. If there is correctable hindfoot valgus deformity and normal talonavicular and calcaneocuboid joints, then isolated subtalar fusion can be considered. Preservation of two hindfoot joints reduces the risk of secondary ankle degeneration (Jaakkola & Mann 2004). When all three joints are involved, especially when deformity is severe, a triple fusion (talonavicular, calcaneocuboid and subtalar joints) is necessary to achieve correction (Fig. 7.2). This can be challenging surgery, requiring the use of structural bone graft, and extensive internal fixation using screws and plates. However, fusion rates as high as 98% have been achieved with significant pain relief in 94% of cases (Figgie et al. 1993). The caveat to this success is the risk of developing subsequent ankle degeneration requiring fusion, which Figgie et al. noted in 3 of 55 patients at an average of 5 years post triple fusion. It is often necessary to lengthen the Achilles tendon when fusing the hindfoot as a contracture can develop due to the shortened valgus hindfoot deformity.

ANKLE

Ankle involvement is less frequent than disease of the forefoot and hindfoot. Disease is usually in the form of synovitis only with minimal joint destruction or deformity. Adjacent tenosynovitis of the peronei or tibialis posterior may be misinterpreted as ankle joint pathology. As mentioned above, degenerative arthritis in the ankle may occur following hindfoot surgery or secondary to deformity in the hindfoot. Valgus deformity in both the hindfoot and ankle is common. This makes reconstruction complex, with significant lateral shortening of tissues and bone. The surgical options include synovectomy, ankle fusion or ankle replacement. Ankle fusion remains the gold-standard treatment with rates of union up to 93% and good relief of symptoms (Miehlke et al. 1997). The ankle is fused in neutral flexion, with 5° of hindfoot valgus and external rotation to match the contralateral leg. Internal fixation with screws is required and the ankle is usually protected in cast for 3 months until union has occurred. The loss of movement at the ankle can increase stresses in the joints of the hind and midfoot if still present, and degenerative disease may result. When ankle and hindfoot disease coexist three fusion options exist:

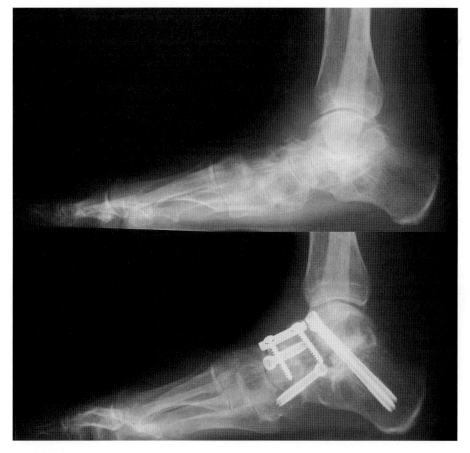

Figure 7.2 Illustrating an X-ray of a patient with a fixed planovalgus deformity. This has been treated with a realignment and triple fusion using a bone graft.

1. Tibio-talo-calcaneal fusion. When the talonavicular and calcaneocuboid joints are free from disease.
2. Tibiocalcaneal fusion. Extensive loss of talus bone stock may necessitate direct fusion of the tibia to the os calcis, often excising the remains of the talus.
3. Pan-talar fusion. When all joints surrounding the talus are diseased.

Poorer functional results are seen for the more complex and extensive fusions.

Ankle arthroplasty has evolved in recent years with modern implants achieving good results beyond 10 years of implantation (Kofoed & Sorenson 1998) (Fig. 7.3). The low demand of the patient with RA makes them good candidates for this surgery.

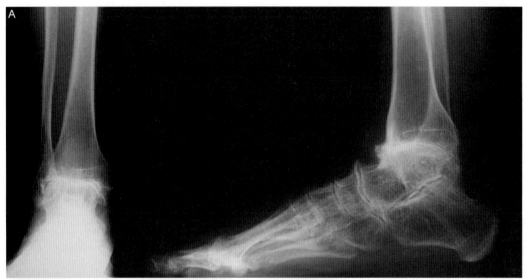

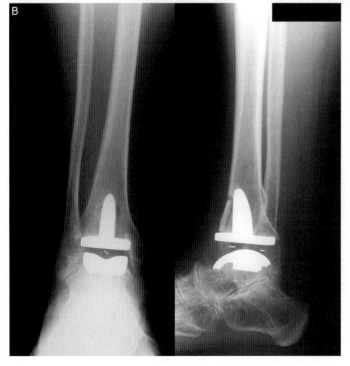

Figure 7.3 Illustrating marked ankle (talo-crural) arthritis (A) and a subsequent ankle arthroplasty (B).

Preservation of joint motion prevents the shift of stresses to adjacent joints encountered with ankle fusion. It also provides an option for better function in pan-talar arthritis, when combined ankle replacement and triple fusion allows preservation of movement. A recent series (Wood & Deakin 2003) showed equivalent survivorship in rheumatoid and degenerative cases at 5 years. The main problems encountered are infection and poor wound healing. Failure of the prosthesis may mean performing a complex fusion or even considering amputation.

SUMMARY

Surgical management of the foot in RA is challenging, but can provide good relief of symptoms in carefully selected cases. Criteria for surgical intervention have yet to be developed and the best way forward at the present time is to organize multidisciplinary foot clinics so that conservative treatment can be optimized and, if this fails, surgical options can be considered. It is important to remember that pain relief, not cosmesis, is the most important aim of surgical intervention.

References

Aho H and Halonen P Synovectomy of MTP joints in rheumatoid arthritis. Acta Orthop Scandinavica Suppl 1991; Suppl 243: 1.

Calabro J 1962 A critical evaluation of the diagnostic features of the feet in rheumatoid arthritis. Arthritis and Rheumatism 5:19–29.

Coughlin M Arthritides. In: Coughlin M, Mann R (eds) Surgery of the Foot and Ankle, 7th edn, Mosby, 1999; pp. 560–645.

Coughlin M Rheumatoid forefoot reconstruction: a long-term follow-up study. Journal of Bone and Joint Surgery 2000; 82A: 322–341.

Figgie MP, O'Malley MJ, Ranawat C et al. Triple arthrodesis in rheumatoid arthritis. Clinical Orthopaedics and Related Research 1993; 292: 250–254.

Graham C Rheumatoid forefoot metatarsal head resection without first metatarsophalangeal arthrodesis. Foot and Ankle International 1994; 15:689–690.

Grennan DM, Gray J, Loudon J et al. Methotrexate and early postoperative complications in patients with rheumatoid arthritis undergoing elective orthopaedic surgery. Annals of the Rheumatic Diseases 2001; 60(3):214–217.

Hay SM, Moore DJ, Cooper JR, Getty CJM Diagnostic injections of the hindfoot joints in patients with rheumatoid arthritis prior to surgical fusion. The Foot 1999; 9: 40–43.

Jaakkola JI, Mann R A review of rheumatoid arthritis affecting the foot and ankle. Foot and Ankle International 2004; 25(12):866–873.

Kofoed H, Sorenson TS Ankle arthroplasty for rheumatoid arthritis and osteoarthritis: prospective long-term study of cemented replacements. Journal of Bone and Joint Surgery 1998; 80B:328–332.

Ljung P, Kaij J, Knutson K et al. Talonavicular arthrodesis in the rheumatoid foot. Foot and Ankle 1992; 13: 313–316.

Mann R, Thompson F Arthrodesis of the first metatarsophalangeal joint for hallux valgus in rheumatoid arthritis. Journal of Bone and Joint Surgery 1984; 66A: 687–691.

Michelson J, Easley J, Wigley F et al. Foot and ankle problems in rheumatoid arthritis. Foot and Ankle International 1994; 15: 608–613.

Miehlke W, Gschwend N, Rippstein P et al. Compression arthrodesis of the rheumatoid ankle and hindfoot. Clinical Orthopaedics and Related Research 1997; 340: 75–86.

Mohan AK, Cote TR, Siegel JN, Braun MM Infectious complications of bidogic treatments of rheumatoid arthritis. Current Opinion in Rheumatology 2003; 15: 179–184.

Raunio P, Laine H Synovectomy of the metatarsophalangeal joints in rheumatoid arthritis. Acta Rheumatologica Scandinavica 1970; 16: 12–17.

Sany J, Anaya J M, Canovas F et al. Influence of methotrexate on the frequency of postoperative infections and complications in patients with rheumatoid arthritis. Journal of Rheumatology 1993; 20: 1129–1132.

Vainio K Rheumatoid foot. Clinical study with pathological and roentgenological comments. Annales Chirurgiae Gynaecologiae 1956; 45(Supplement 1): 1–101

Vidigal E, Jacoby RK, Dixon AS et al. The foot in chronic rheumatoid arthritis. Annals of Rheumatic Diseases 1975; 34: 292–297.

Wood PLR, Deakin S Total ankle replacement. The results in 200 ankles. Journal of Bone and Joint Surgery 2003; 85B(3): 334–341.

Chapter 8

Evaluating care

MEASURES OF DISEASE ACTIVITY, HEALTH STATUS, FUNCTIONAL STATUS AND QUALITY OF LIFE

This section will deal with the various measures that can be applied in clinical practice to quantify the effects of rheumatoid arthritis (RA) in general, in the feet specifically, and their implications for the patient. Outcome measurement is an important facet of modern-day health care. Good measurement enables the practitioner to monitor the natural history of RA in their patients, to inform treatment decisions, and to quantify the effects of the care they provide. It has long been standard practice to undertake a range of assessments at the beginning of an episode of care, but assessing the outcome of treatment requires repeat measures on multiple occasions during the course of the disease, or at least over the episode of care. When outcome measures are used repeatedly, the ongoing record builds over time into an informative database, helpful to individual clinicians in continuing disease management and assessment.

There are a variety of options available to the practitioner wanting to evaluate disease activity, health status, functional status or quality of life, some requiring time-consuming laboratory assessment and considerable expertise, but many requiring no more than photocopied sheets of paper, a pen and some of the patient's time while they sit in the waiting area. The development of these instruments has been particularly thorough in rheumatology and validated tools exist for many applications. We advocate strongly, therefore, that all practitioners involved in the care of the foot in RA should make an effort to record at least a minimum set of such measures for *all* their patients at *every* visit. The availability of the resulting quantitative data is helpful in providing a basis for subsequent audits, as well as contributing to studies of effectiveness and value of services (Higginson & Carr 2001).

This chapter will cover outcome measures ranging from the objective, highly disease-oriented approaches to the more general patient-oriented measures. In the former class, the measures conform closely to the medical model, providing data on specific aspects of the disease process such as disease activity, presence of inflammatory markers, joint destruction and structural change. These measures fit well within the structures/function sections of the ICF classification (see Chapter 1). Objective measures are important and it is right that they form the mainstay of the diagnostic assessment, the clinical review process and tracking chronic disease at the level of the disease process and its immediate effect on impairment.

It is important to recognize, however, that it is a shortcoming of traditional measures such as joint ranges of motion or counts of tender or swollen joints that they can overemphasize the practitioner's model of disease (Dawson & Carr 2001). These medical definitions of disease may not tell the whole story when other patient-specific factors are included and it is also useful to include some insight into the complexity of the patient's own experience of the disease. Within the ICF framework, the domains of activities/participation and the relationship with the environment encompass some of these factors. There is, therefore, a growing acceptance that a combination of objective practitioner-oriented measures and more subjective patient-oriented measures provides a more comprehensive assessment of the broader effects of a chronic disease such as RA (Higginson & Carr 2001). Consequently, it is now recommended that all clinical trials should include some assessment of the patient's perspective of outcome (Garratt et al. 2002) and this is equally the case in good clinical practice.

It is also worth a mention at this point that the measures being discussed in this chapter relate to patient health not to patient satisfaction with services. There is sometimes some confusion over the two concepts, but this chapter will deal only with the measurement of changing health status. There is an entire science built around the specialty of measuring patient satisfaction, and the reader interested in conducting patient satisfaction surveys should consult a more specialized text.

CONCEPTS OF HEALTH STATUS, FUNCTIONAL STATUS AND QUALITY OF LIFE

At the outset it is worth clarifying the terminology involved. This is a field that has evolved rapidly over the past 20 years and, because it crosses disciplinary boundaries, has evolved in the absence of a consistently applied conceptual framework (van Knippenberg & de Haes 1988). As a consequence of this *ad hoc* history there is a tendency for some of the terminology in the field to be used non-specifically or even incorrectly (McKenna & Doward 2004).

In the absence of a uniform standard available for the nomenclature used in this area a series of working definitions are presented here that represent a consensus. This is provided for clarity, although we recognize that some readers will have alternative positions on some these definitions.

It is appropriate to start with a brief discussion about the terms 'health status', 'quality of life' and 'health-related quality of life' as these are terms that are often used interchangeably, and, often erroneously, are even applied to the entire field of subjective or patient-reported heath-status measurement.

Health status/quality of life and its associated group of measures is concerned with the measurement of the experience of illness such as pain, fatigue, disability, and its effects on daily activities and by extension on overall quality of life (Carr 2003). If the concepts of health status, functional status and quality of life are mapped onto the ICF framework (see Table 8.1) then it becomes clear that a measure will be more or less sensitive to the various levels of impairment, activity limitation and participation restriction. Quality of life better represents the centre-right hand side of the schematic, while health status and impairment in body function and structure better reflects the centre-left side. Thus the term quality of life is best used to describe only the broadest effects and impact of disease, where they affect the individual's participation in the activities, roles and relationships required to lead a full and healthy life. By extension, quality of life measures are those measures that quantify the effects of a disease (and other factors) on a broader range of activities, and in the context of the patient's own life (McKenna & Doward 2004).

Measures of the more direct effects of a disease are, more correctly, measures of functioning (e.g. Health Assessment Questionnaire, Foot Function Index), although there may be some overlap depending on the composition of the individual measure.

The term *'health-related quality of life'* is further criticized by some authorities as representing a redundant concept, with proponents of this argument proposing that quality of life is so affected by environmental and social factors that isolating the purely health-related aspects is inappropriate (McKenna & Doward 2004). As health professionals there is a natural desire to

Table 8.1   The component structure of the ICF classification.

	Part 1: Functioning and disability		Part 2: Contextual factors	
Components	Body functions and structures	Activities and participation	Environmental factors	Personal factors
Domains	Body functions Body structures	Life areas (tasks, actions)	External influences on functioning and disability	Internal influences on functioning and disability
Constructs	Change in body functions (physiological) Change in body structures (anatomical)	Capacity executing tasks in a standard environment Performance executing tasks in the current environment	Facilitating or hindering impact of features of the physical, social, and attitudinal world	Impact of attributes of the person
Positive aspect	Functional and structural integrity	Activities participation	Facilitators	not applicable
	Functioning			
Negative aspect	Impairment	Activity limitation Participation restriction	Barriers/hindrances	not applicable
	Disability			

want to focus on the health-related aspects of a disease and so the term has great currency in health care. The authors must agree, however, that there is some logic to the argument that the health-related part is so intertwined as to be inseparable from the whole 'quality of life' concept and so we will use only the terms 'health status', 'functional status' and 'quality of life' in this chapter.

The needs-based model presents quality of life as a highly subjective concept representing the gap between our expectations of our roles and our ability to fulfil them (Carr & Higginson 2001). It follows then that the quantification of quality of life is highly dependent on the perceptions of the individual (i.e. the perception of the gap) and on the ameliorating factors (such as family support) as well as on the actual disease process. Thus, some people with severe disease may report a fairly good quality of life, '. . . at least I am not as bad as my mother was, my husband is great and I still love my work as an artist', while others with less severe disease may report poor quality of life, 'I have become really depressed; I can't play with the kids because of my knees. . . . never mind all the housework'. There is usually, therefore, some relationship between symptoms, disease activity and associated quality of life, but the link is often complex and incomplete (Carr et al. 2001, McKenna & Doward 2004). Quality of life is, therefore, the most highly

individualized concept, with health status and functional status less so. Some recent innovations such as the Personal Impact HAQ (Hewlett et al. 2002) have attempted to bridge this gap by supplementing traditional health-status measures (such as HAQ) with additional factors that attempt to better integrate personal impact into the measure. As a rule of thumb, true quality of life measures are better suited to applications relating to individual clinical decision-making, while measures of disease activity, health or functional status are better suited to analysis by group (Carr & Higginson 2001).

KEY POINTS

- Evaluations of care in research or clinical practice should include a patient oriented measure of the effect of care.
- The terms health status and quality of life are often confused.
- Most of the older patient-completed measures used in evaluating care are functional status or health status measures rather than quality of life measures

MEASURES USED TO EVALUATE DISEASE PROCESS AND THE EFFECTS OF CARE

There are a considerable number of measures used to evaluate progress in RA. Such measures may relate to the systemic effects of the disease, to specific local effects or to broader implications of the disease process. Rheumatologists use a mix of objective and subjective measures, a fact that was incorporated into the American College of Rheumatologists guidelines for the core datasets for both the diagnosis (Felson et al. 1993) and measurement of improvement in RA (Felson et al. 1995).

The American College of Rheumatologists response criteria (20% response – this table can be adapted appropriately to give the ACR50 and ACR70 criteria)

1. ≥ 20% improvement in swollen joint count
2. ≥ 20% improvement in tender joint count
3. ≥ 20% improvement in the least three of the following five measures:
   a. Patient's global assessment of disease activity (100 mm VAS)
   b. Physician's global assessment of disease activity (100 mm VAS)
   c. Patient's assessment of pain (100 mm VAS)
   d. Acute-phase reactant (ESR)
   e. Disability (from HAQ)

For assessment, the accepted ACR criteria include a count of tender and swollen joints (see Chapter 4), a patient-based rating of their own assessment of pain, patient's and physician's global assessments of disease activity, a patient-based assessment of physical function, and laboratory evaluation of at least one acute-phase reactant. This combination of measures has good content validity encompassing the range of features of RA, and all are adequately sensitive to change (responsiveness). Used at baseline, several of these measures have also been shown to predict long-term outcomes in RA, including the severity of physical disability, radiographic damage and mortality rates (Felson et al. 1993).

Measurement of change is also possible when these baseline measures are repeated during the course of the disease. Levels of improvement of 20%, 50% and 70% now form the basis for many treatment pathways and provide meaningful dichotomous outcomes for clinical trials (Felson et al. 1995).

Table 8.2 Core set for longitudinal and observational studies in rheumatology (Molenaar et al. 2000).

Domains	Examples
CORE DOMAINS	
Health status	
'Generic quality of life'	SF-36
Symptoms	Pain scale
Physical function	Health Assessment Questionnaire
Psychosocial function	Social support
Disease process	
Joint tenderness/swelling	Joint counts
Global	Patient assessment of severity
Acute phase reactants	ESR/CRP
Damage	
Radiographic/imaging	Sharp score
Deformity	Radiographic malalignment
Surgery	Total joint replacement
Organ damage	Vasculitis
Toxicity/adverse reactions	
Mortality	
IMPORTANT BUT NOT CORE	
Work disability	Days lost from work
Costs	Direct medical costs

A core set of measures for use in medical rheumatology practice has been suggested by a consensus group at the Outcome Measures in Rheumatoid Arthritis Clinical Trials (OMERACT) conferences and is outlined in Table 8.2. The core set relates only to general rheumatology practice. However, no consensus exists for the foot. In the course of this chapter we will attempt to present some options for the reader intending to assess health outcomes relating to the foot in rheumatology.

To simplify the comparison of like with like, the measures discussed in this chapter will be divided according to whether they are predominantly objective or subjective. Within each of these sections, measures will be further sub-classified so that general measures are dealt with independently of those that relate more specifically to the lower limb.

Objective measures

RA is a systemic disease, so it is appropriate to start this section with some reference to objective and valid measures of systemic disease. Criticism may be levelled at the degree of reliance on these data as they can fail to take into consideration the range of factors contributing to the patient's experience of their arthritis. Notwithstanding such criticism, however, these measures of the rheumatoid disease process remain the mainstay of the medical model and furnish important data for the diagnosis and management of RA. This section will progress from the systemic through the local to the broader effects, covering sequentially laboratory markers of disease activity, imaging measures directed at assessing change in specific joints and tissues, and functional evaluations.

Laboratory markers of disease activity

Acute–phase markers of disease activity The two most commonly used acute phase markers are Erythrocyte Sedimentation Rate (ESR), measured in mm/h, and level of C-reactive protein (CRP), measured in mg/dl (Paulus et al. 1999). CRP assay is more sensitive than ESR to changes in inflammatory levels. Both of these markers are non-specific measures of inflammation and so are not necessarily indicative of disease activity. The two tests are considered complementary, providing a cross check, especially when there is discordance in these non-specific measures and so are used in combination (Wolfe 1997). Plasma viscosity is another useful acute-phase measure, and with some caveats these three reactants can be used interchangeably in the quantification of disease activity (Paulus et al. 1999). As a consequence of their general response to any inflammatory process the acute-phase reactants have a limited role in the *diagnosis* of RA, but will provide a rough indication of current levels of inflammation and are useful for monitoring inflammatory disease (Lane & Gravel 2002, Scott 2000). The ESR (or CRP or PV) (Paulus et al. 1999) can contribute to the gold standard measure of disease activity, the DAS (disease activity score) discussed below (van der Heijde et al. 1990).

Rheumatoid factor Rheumatoid factors are autoantibodies against immunoglobulins, which may have become altered after contact with a sensitizing antigen. The most common rheumatoid factor is an IgM antibody to the immunoglobulin IgG, although other varieties such as IgA are also found. The presence of rheumatoid factor is not in itself diagnostic as low levels can be found in normal people and also in patients with other rheumatic diseases. Conversely, patients negative for rheumatoid factor can present with chronic inflammatory arthritis indistinguishable from RA (Leeb et al. 1998). Nevertheless, the presence of high levels of rheumatoid factor in conjunction with other immunologic assays such as anti-keratin or anti-filaggrin antibodies, is a useful prognostic marker for disease severity and associated features (Scott 2000) (for further details of prognostic factors see Chapter 1).

Imaging joint and tissue change (see also Chapter 5)

The most objective measures of joint and tissue change are those that employ modern imaging techniques to gain the best view of affected tissues. Most imaging techniques that provide clear views will allow for clinician-derived measures of tissue change and these are widespread. The best techniques now also provide quantification of change through measures of tissue volume or lesion size.

Plain X rays (radiographs) remain the first imaging modality to which most people with suspected RA are exposed, although plain radiography is of limited use in early disease because soft-tissue involvement predominates and bony involvement is still minimal. Bony erosions, the main diagnostic feature in RA are typically absent from plain radiographs until 1–2 years, disease duration, although are present in radiographs of feet earlier than in the hands (Devauchelle Pensec et al. 2004). Plain X-ray is more useful, however, in quantifying joint damage in established disease where the degree of damage is better related to functional impairment (Drossaers-Bakker et al. 2000). Radiographs can be quantified using scoring systems such as the Sharp score and Larsen index (Larsen et al. 1977, Sharp et al. 1985). In both of these methods features such erosions and joint space narrowing in a range of joints are quantified using an ordinal scale. The Sharp score includes a broader range of measures and is more time consuming to perform, although it is reported to be marginally more reliable and responsive than the Larsen method (Plant et al. 1994). In the foot, when standardized weight-bearing views are recorded, plain radiography can be of use in quantifying and documenting deformity and mechanical imbalance (Bouysset et al. 2002, Keenan et al. 1991).

Computed tomography (CT) is another imaging modality offering good visualization of bony structures. Modern techniques allow for very high resolution of CT images and 3D reconstructions are also possible in software. CT represents a useful technique for measuring features such as erosions, but its limitations in imaging soft tissues, and requirement for administration of a fairly large dose of radiation, restrict its applicability.

For imaging soft-tissue structures magnetic resonance imaging (MRI) has become the gold standard in recent years (Ostergaard & Szkudlarek 2003). MRI has advantages over CT and plain radiographs in that it differentiates between types of tissue and can be used in conjunction with enhancing agents such as Gadolinium-DPTA to provide excellent contrast between normal and inflamed tissue in structures such as synovial joint linings and tendon sheaths (Bouysset et al. 2003, Weishaupt et al. 1999). It is well suited to early identification of inflammatory arthritis in the clinical setting and MRI of the feet is noted to be particularly sensitive in this regard (Boutry et al. 2003). The latest techniques allow for accurate and objective quantification of features such as synovial volume independent of the clinician, further improving its utility as a research tool (Goldbach-Mansky et al. 2003). The main drawbacks for MRI are the long time required to obtain sequences, the cost and the problems with access to MRI scanners. The physical act of undergoing an MR scan can also be challenging for people with RA, as it is typical for a high-resolution sequence to involve the patient lying motionless in the chamber for more than an hour, often in a physically demanding position. This clearly represents a particular problem for patients with inflammatory joint disease and limits the applications of this modality as a clinical tool. Smaller dedicated 'limb' scanners that are both cheaper and smaller are now emerging, and will probably become the standard MRI tool for musculoskeletal imaging.

As a predominantly 'bedside' clinical tool, high-resolution ultrasound (HRUS) is proving increasingly popular. HRUS offers instant visualization of many of the important features of soft tissue (synovitis, tendonitis) and bony involvement (erosion, joint degeneration) again with no exposure to ionizing radiation, and in a short appointment during which the patient can move, and using equipment that requires little technical support. It is operator-dependent, which introduces a source of error and at present does not offer the same degree of automated quantification of tissue volumes as MRI, rendering HRUS more prone to errors of interpretation (Ostergaard & Wiell 2004). It is, however, more sensitive to detection of bony erosion than plain radiography (Lopez-Ben et al. 2004) and, although more validation studies are required, the undoubted clinical utility of this modality means that in the hands of a skilled operator HRUS offers important insights into the degree of inflammatory involvement and sensitivity to early changes in RA.

Joint counts

Less objective but quick and easy to perform is a simple count of the number of tender and swollen joints (see Fig. 4.4). Ritchie first described this type of approach in 1968, grading joint tenderness in 26 areas on a scale of 0–3, score range 0–78 (Ritchie et al. 1968). Data from some joints were grouped to calculate the total score. Swollen joint counts were added later and

the two approaches are now usually used in tandem, with the original Ritchie index modified considerably. Although subject to some inter-observer variability, this type of test is adequately reliable and has been adopted as part of the core dataset by the ACR (Felson et al. 1993). In general rheumatology practice the count is now usually confined to an assessment of tenderness/swelling in 28 joints, mainly in the upper body. The validity of the joint count assessments has been shown to be only minimally impaired by assessing only 28 joints (Prevoo et al. 1995), and because of the obvious logistical benefits associated with a shortened assessment the shorter version has become widely adopted. Although the truncated joint count provides a quicker, easier assessment important clinical information in the lower limb is neglected. We have experience of a number of patients who have a low swollen and tender joint count, but who can hardly walk because of inflamed joints in the feet and ankles. The Yorkshire Early Arthritis Register, a large multi-centre register of people with RA, requires as part of the assessment protocol for all patients a count of 66 joints for swelling and 68 joints for tenderness.

It may be useful to document affected joints graphically using a manikin, to supplement the simple count described originally by Ritchie (Ritchie et al. 1968). This can be done for the basic 28 joint count or extended to provide better coverage of the lower limb joints. Example manikins are provided in Chapter 4 (see Fig. 4.3).

Functional status

The measurement of functional status is most commonly directed to the measurement of the effects of disease at the level of impairment and activity limitation. Functional status can be measured either objectively or subjectively, with objective measures tending to provide a more specific and abstract quantification of functional capacities, while subjective measures are generally more inclusive and holistic.

The purpose of measuring functional status is to derive quantitative data so that comparisons can be made between the status of different individuals or for a single person over time. As such, measures of functional status should have been subject to a validation process prior to adoption. There are more than 500 instruments available for use in musculoskeletal care, but not all of these will be either suited to every purpose or be of adequate quality to be used with confidence. By the same note it is not appropriate to attempt to devise an instrument *ad hoc*. Without the skills and the capacity to undertake a validation process it is likely that the resulting instrument will contain significant flaws and data arising from its use will not be acceptable to the broader community. The validation processes undertaken for some of the more commonly encountered instruments are discussed later in the chapter, but there are some general principles that can be applied when selecting measures for clinical or research use:

- *Suitability*. The first issue to be addressed is the suitability of a candidate instrument to the purpose for which it is being considered. While this may seem to be a statement of the obvious, researchers have often made the mistake of applying an instrument developed for one clinical population in another, only for the adapted tool to run into significant problems when used out of it is original context. When an instrument is used for the first time in a new population, at least some validation should be undertaken for the new application. There are, however, a number of basic principles that any prospective user should consider when choosing a functional status (or quality of life) instrument (Redmond et al. 2002).

- *Face/content validity*. This is the most basic form of validity and is closely allied to the issue of fitness for purpose as discussed above. Face validity is simply an assessment of whether an instrument will do what one thinks it should do (Katz et al. 2003). It can be difficult to measure face validity formally, although there are techniques such as Delphi and other expert consensus approaches that will allow some evaluation of face validity, and assurance that an instrument does what it is supposed to do.

- *Concurrent validity*. This is an evaluation of how well the instrument performs relative to an existing and well-validated instrument that is considered a gold standard. Assessment of concurrent validity is most commonly undertaken by administering the new instrument at the same time as similar measures that have been previously validated and assessing the degree to which the sets of observations agree (Katz et al. 2003, Redmond et al. 2002).

- *Reliability and responsiveness*. Concepts of reliability and responsiveness are interrelated. Intra-rater reliability is the consistency of repeat measures over time within observers. Inter-rater reliability refers to the consistency of multiple observers when providing ratings of a single subject or group of subjects (Katz et al. 2003, Redmond & Keenan 2002). Responsiveness is the capacity of an instrument to accurately reflect changes over time as they relate to the natural history of the disease or to changes brought about by treatment (Geenen et al. 1995,

Higginson & Carr 2001). Responsiveness is, therefore, significantly affected by test–retest reliability because a less reliable test instrument will be inherently less responsive.

- *Sensitivity and specificity*. These two measures reflect the ability of instruments to differentiate between pathological and normal individuals in the population. To determine the sensitivity and specificity of an instrument the developers will define a cut point reflecting the boundary between normal and abnormal. The sensitivity of an instrument is its ability to identify those who are abnormal (true positives), while its specificity reflects its ability to identify those who are normal (true negatives) (Greenhalgh 1997, Redmond & Keenan 2002).

A brief review of the above features of validity will assist in making appropriate choices for applying functional status measures in the clinical or research settings, although one final note is that instruments are rarely inherently valid or invalid, and their validity must be considered at least in part dependent on the specifics of the situation in which they are being applied. For instance when a clinician must be involved in the ratings, factors such as reliability can be dependent on the individual characteristics of the clinician. Personality, experience, skills, expertise may all influence the reliability, and a conscientious user would make some effort to evaluate the reliability of the instrument in their own clinical setting. Measures of function can also be influenced by interactions with other patient-oriented impairments such as pain, stiffness and fatigue. As a consequence, objective, instantaneous measures may be subject to some short-term variability on the part of the patient. This can further pose problems where these measures are to be used for between-day analyses, such as in therapeutic outcome studies.

Patient-completed measures of functional status draw on the patients' assessment of their own functional capacities. These measures are most often questionnaire based and can include longer-term retrospective elements that serve to dampen down some of the short-term variations. It is of course a disadvantage that these measures are subjective, and coincidental impairments can still influence the data to some degree. Some considerations for choosing a suitable health-status measure are outlined below.

Measurement of functional status is important because these measurements represent useful intermediate outcomes, or milestones quantifying progress towards more final outcomes such as work disability, joint replacement or mortality (Wolfe & Pincus 1999).

Points to consider in assessing a health–status measure for clinical practice (adapted from Higginson & Carr 2001)

1. Are the domains relevant?
2. In what population was it developed and validated?
3. Is the measure valid, reliable, responsive and appropriate – and has this been demonstrated in my proposed field of application?
4. Are there floor and ceiling effects? i.e. is its most relevant range of scores suitable to the degree of impairment/activity limitation in my patient group?
5. Will it measure differences over time and at what power?
6. Who completes the measure? Patients, parents, the health professionals?
7. How difficult is it to complete?
8. How long will it take to complete?
9. Who will need to be trained to use the measure?
10. Who will enter the data and analyse the results?

Functional status is known to be highly variable between groups of patients and so to ensure the valid application of an instrument the clinician must be careful to use a measure suited to the specific patient population. Measures such as the Barthel Index for instance, which is intended for use in a neurological rehabilitation, focuses on significant limitations such as continence, ability to feed oneself, and significant mobility limitations. Such a scale would suit the assessment of functional status in a hospital setting in an area such as stroke rehabilitation, but would clearly suffer from a problematic 'ceiling' effect in a community clinic or rheumatology outpatients setting, where patients would normally be ambulant and functioning at a much higher level.

Other measures of general function or of capacity to perform general activities of daily living (ADL) include the Katz Index, which is measured by a trained clinician observing the performance of ADL tasks.

The Stanford Health Assessment Questionnaire

The Stanford Health Assessment Questionnaire (HAQ) is a measure of general functional status that was designed and validated for use in RA, and has been modified into a number of versions including a UK-specific version (Kirwan & Reeback 1986). It can be self reported by the patient so is easy to administer and has become one of the most widely used functional measures in rheumatology. The HAQ measures difficulties encountered by the patient over the course of the past week, so limiting some of the variation associated with short-term fluctuation in underlying impairments. There are eight categories of function covering 20 activities including dressing and grooming, rising, eating, walking, hygiene, reaching and gripping. The HAQ and subsequent modified versions are well validated and have been shown to provide good reliability and responsiveness, confirming their suitability in therapeutic outcomes studies.

The multidimensional HAQ, first described in 1980, is primarily intended for use in patients with arthritis (Fries et al. 1980). The m-HAQ focuses on five dimensions including physical functioning, discomfort and social factors and also introduces two dimensions (drug/therapeutic toxicity and dollar costs) missing from the measures discussed previously.

The HAQ is generally considered to emphasize the upper limbs over the lower limbs, and only two of the 17 questions relate directly to the lower limb, with a further two of borderline relevance. The HAQ has been validated for self-administration and is widely used in the rheumatology community (Wiles et al. 2001, Wolfe & Cathey 1991), although concerns have been raised regarding its validity in non-RA samples (Tennant et al. 1996). It is considered the gold standard measure of health status in people with RA and is useful at baseline in predicting prognosis as well as measuring change over time (Barrett et al. 2000). The psychometric properties of the HAQ have been evaluated and the scores are deemed to be ordinal rather than interval, rendering it unsuitable for parametric statistical analysis and potentially limiting its use in clinical trials (Tennant et al. 1996). A novel recent modification of the HAQ (the Personal Impact HAQ) has been proposed that converts the HAQ to a true quality of life measure by incorporating patient weightings to the items (Hewlett et al. 2002). This variant, which appears to have good validity and psychometric properties is not yet widely adopted, but offers some benefits over the original.

The HAQ is so widely used in the rheumatology community that it should be considered as part of the core set for any rheumatology foot clinic. It is quick for patients to complete and, despite its limitations in terms of the lower limb, provides a very useful overview of the impact of RA to the practitioner dealing with the foot manifestations.

The MACTAR instrument

Functional status is a highly individual concept and one criticism of generic measures is that they may not reflect the priorities of the patient. The MACTAR patient preference disability questionnaire attempts to address this shortcoming by allowing the RA patient to identify, initially, five functions that they feel are most important and then to report the degree of limitation they experience (Tugwell et al. 1987). The MACTAR questionnaire has been demonstrated to be valid, but the complexity of scoring has limited uptake.

The Steinbrocker scale

Clinician assessed global function in RA was introduced in 1949 by Steinbrocker and the American Rheumatism Association, with a functional classification system that described functional capacity in four classes (Table 8.3).

The Steinbrocker system and the subsequent revision endorsed by the American College of Rheumatologists in 1991 (Hochberg et al. 1992; Table 8.3) have been widely used in the past and are still referred to in the literature. The four class definitions have, however, largely been superseded by more modern instruments capable of providing a more refined picture of functional status.

Table 8.3 The original Steinbrocker classification system.

Class	Definition
I	Ability to carry on full functional activity without handicaps
II	Functional activity adequate to carry out normal activity with discomfort or limited mobility of one or more joints
III	Functional activity adequate to perform little or none of the duties of activity of occupation or self-care
IV	Largely or wholly incapacitated with the patient bed-ridden or wheelchair-bound

The American College of Rheumatologists revised criteria for classification of functional status in rheumatoid arthritis, 1991

Class	Definition
I	Completely able to perform usual activities of daily living (self-care, vocational, and avocational)
II	Able to perform usual self-care and vocational activities, but limited in avocational activities
III	Able to perform usual self-care activities, but limited in vocational and avocational activities
IV	Limited in ability to perform usual self-care, vocational, and avocational activities

Other measures

Functional status can be quantified more objectively through viewing and scoring of specific tasks, or by simple recording of time taken to perform activities. The 'Berg balance test' (Berg et al. 1995) is an example of the former, while the 'Timed get up and go' test or timed 30 m walk are examples of the latter. It is also helpful, especially when considering the impact of RA on the lower limb, to measure some of the basic temporal and spatial parameters of gait, such as gait velocity, cadence, and stride length. This group of observed and measured tests is sometimes referred to as performance tests or rheumatology functional tests (Escalante et al. 2004).

The Berg balance test (Berg et al. 1995) is a broad assessment of functional status that uses performance in a range of 14 tasks to yield an aggregate score. The Berg test emphasizes lower-limb function in standing and standing-related activities, but does not quantify gait directly. It is well validated and may be useful in quantifying function for research purposes, but the lack of evaluation of foot-related function will limit its applicability to readers of this book.

General measures of functional status can be useful in describing the global impact of disease, but the effect of foot pain on global measures can be variable (Chen et al. 2003, Benvenuti et al. 1995). Where care of the lower limb is the primary concern, it is recommended, therefore, that global measures of function are supplemented with lower-limb-specific measures.

Most clinicians involved in foot care will perform gait evaluations routinely and it takes little effort to turn a standard observational gait assessment into useful objective functional data. Such objective measures are useful, as measures such as gait velocity and stride length are closely related to Sickness Impact Profile scores ($r=0.70$ and 0.69 respectively) (Platto et al. 1991) and changes in these objective measures may predate the impact on activities. It is known that patients with RA walk more slowly, have reduced stride length and cadence, and an increased period of double support (Platto et al. 1991). Furthermore, gait velocity has been found to be both particularly useful and one of the more valid of the performance tests (Escalante et al. 2004, Geenen et al. 1995). A more complete analysis of the gait disturbance in RA and how to quantify it can be found in Chapter 2 and Table 8.4.

Most patient-derived measures of functional status or health-related quality of life are self-reporting questionnaires and are largely holistic, and so include factors influenced by the range of the manifestations of RA. Increasingly, however, there is a need to understand the impact of RA on specific body systems or anatomical regions such as the foot, and more specialized measures

Table 8.4 Some of the parameters output from the GaitRite system.

Step time	The time elapsed from first contact of one foot until first contact of the contralateral foot
Cycle time	Time between two successive footfalls of the same foot
Step length	Length of one step (e.g. distance along the line of progression for right heel and subsequent left heel contact points)
Stride length	Length of one complete cycle for one limb (e.g. distance along the line of progression covered by heel contact of successful footfalls of the same limb)
Base of support	Width between the mid point of right and left heels
Single support time	The duration (for each limb) when that limb is weight bearing in isolation
Double support time	The duration (for each limb) when that limb is weight bearing in tandem with the contralateral limb
Swing phase duration	The duration (for each limb) when that limb is non-weight bearing – expressed as a percentage of the gait cycle
Stance phase duration	The duration (for each limb) when that limb is weight bearing – expressed as a percentage of the gait cycle
Step to limb ratio	The ratio of step length to limb length
Toe in/toe out angle	Angle between footfalls and the line of progression
Velocity (raw and normalized)	Distance/time taken. (May be normalized to leg length)
Step count	Number of valid steps
Cadence	Number of steps per minute

have also been developed to address this need. Whether based on whole-body or foot-specific measures, the importance of such instruments is increasingly recognized, with some authors contending that patient-derived data are at least as informative in dictating clinical management as laboratory tests or imaging data (Wolfe & Pincus 1999).

KEY POINTS

- Objective measures are usually scientifically robust but may be removed from the patient's experience of the disease.

- The clinician should be aware of the limitations in a measure, paying attention to the thoroughness with which it has been validated.

- It is usually preferable to use a small battery of measures encompassing a range of objective and subjective measures.

Health–status and quality of life measures

In this rapidly expanding field there are now more than 1200 measures to be found in literature (Garratt et al. 2002). The most commonly used generic measures are the SF-36, the sickness impact profile and the Nottingham health profile (Garratt et al. 2002). The EuroQol EQ-5D (The-Euroqol-Group 1990) is also

popular as it provides a single quotient score that enhances its suitability for clinical trials.

Health-status and quality of life measures are concerned with evaluating the patient's perspective of the disease and its treatment. As we have noted already, they are inherently more subjective than some of the functional status measures outlined in the previous section, but they are an increasingly important adjunct to measures derived from the traditional medical model. Global, generic measures are in the most widespread use because, as well as meeting the basic criteria of established validity discussed earlier, the majority have been designed to provide data that are comparable across diseases and cultural/geographical/ethnic populations. It was the generic measures that first opened this field of evaluation, providing data on the broad implications of disease. There is some advantage in using a global measure still, as data will be available not just for one's own specialty, but for other patient groups as well. As refined versions of the general health status measures have developed in recent years, so too have more specific health-status measures that can be directed towards people with specific diseases or at specific body systems. These address the main shortcoming of the generic measures of health status, namely that they are often less sensitive than would be desirable to the specific effects of a disease process, or to specific regional manifestations.

Measures have been developed that are specific to RA, to disorders of the foot and, recently, to address the requirement for a very precise measure, we have developed and validated the Leeds Foot Impact Scale (Helliwell et al. 2005), a measure specific to the foot in RA.

To ensure that health-status data reflects both the breadth and specifics of a population, it is now considered good practice to supplement the use of a generic measure with one more specific secondary measure (Dawson & Carr 2001, Hawker et al. 1995, Stucki et al. 2003). Some of the more widely used global and specific measures are discussed in the next section.

Generic health status measures

Many generic health-status measures exist, although few are in widespread use. The three most common are the SF-36, the EuroQol EQ-5D and the Sickness Impact Profile. Each has varying strengths and weaknesses, and may be suited to differing purposes.

The Medical Outcomes Survey, Short Form–36 item version, the SF-36 (Ware et al. 1993).   Among the general measures of health status the Medical Outcomes Survey Short Form-36 (SF-36) has gained a high profile through several large studies that have established population norms for a number of countries, and provide comparative data for a range of disorders. This widespread adoption means that the SF-36 allows for comparison of the effects of many disorders with the population norms for unaffected people, and for comparison of the health effects of disorder being studied, with a range of other conditions.

The MOS SF-36 was developed in 1988 by the RAND corporation from a larger survey of the health of the population in the USA.

It is intended to yield a scoring profile rather than a single score, highlighting various aspects of physical and mental status, and quantifying the burden of disease and the effect of treatments (Ware et al. 1993).

The SF-36 consists of 36 individual questions (items) aggregated into eight dimensions:

1. Physical function: the extent to which a person is limited by their health in performing a range of physical activities
2. Impact of physical health on role performance: the extent to physical health affects work or other daily activities
3. Bodily pain: severity of pain experienced and the impact on activities
4. General health: health status combined with perceptions of health relative to others
5. Social functioning: the effect of health or emotional problems on the quality and quantity of social interactions
6. Vitality: perceived levels of energy or fatigue
7. Impact of emotional health on role performance: effects of emotional problems on work or other daily activities
8. General mental health: the extent of feelings of anxiety, depression or happiness

The eight scores are each expressed on a scale of 0–100, where a higher score equates with greater well-being. The eight dimensions can be aggregated into a physical and mental health component summary scores (PCS and MCS).

Three other versions now exist, a revised version of the original SF-36 (SF-36v2), and two shortened versions, the SF-12 and the SF-8.

The validity of the SF-36 has been comprehensively evaluated in a wide range of populations including the USA, UK and Australia (Jenkinson et al. 1994, McCallum 1995), and adapted for use with a variety of languages such as French, German, Dutch, Danish, Italian and others.

The SF-36 is validated for postal surveys and self-completion (McHorney et al. 1994, Shadbolt et al. 1997) and poses few problems for respondents, taking some ten minutes to complete. The scoring of the SF-36 is complex, and Quality Metric, its publishers sell an explanatory manual. Computer-based scoring systems are also available both commercially and in the academic community and are recommended to minimize errors. Licensing is required to use the SF-36 and anyone proposing to use it should be prepared to buy either manual or the appropriate software.

The SF-36 is very widely used worldwide and has been subjected to extensive independent validation studies. Its internal consistency is high, as is the test-retest reliability in all dimensions. It is adequately responsive; although, for disease specific applications, it must be remembered that this is a general health-status measure. The main limitation of the SF-36 relates to its multidimensional nature. It yields data in a maximum of eight dimensions, and in a minimum of two dimensions (as the Mental and Physical Component Scores), which limits its use in outcome studies and health economic analyses.

The EuroQol Group's EQ–5D   The EuroQol group developed a six-point instrument in 1990, modified to the current five-point instrument (EQ-5D) in 1991 (Brooks 1996; The-Euroqol-Group 1990). The EQ-5D is a self-completion instrument yielding a quotient score, with 243 possible health states. The questionnaire employs five descriptive questions addressing health state in five dimensions, answered by trichotomous closed responses.

The five dimensions are: mobility, self-care, usual activities, pain/discomfort and anxiety/depression. A sixth item is a visual analogue scale (presented as a thermometer) through which the respondent reports their perception of their own health (Brooks 1996).

The EQ-5D has been validated in a number of clinical populations (Hurst et al. 1994). It has moderately strong correlation with other measures such as SF-36 and HAQ, although it appears less responsive than the SF-36 and is less responsive than many disease-specific measures used in rheumatology (Carr 2003). Euroqol and SF-36 are comparable in terms of their discriminative ability, although Euroqol is reportedly outperformed on overall performance profile by SF-36 (Brazier et al. 1993, Essink-Bot et al. 1997). Normative data are available for the UK (Kind et al. 1998). The EQ-5D is very quick to complete, and is suitable for self completion or for postal surveys. One deficit of the EQ-5D is the relatively high proportion of missing data noted for the VAS item, with some 6.7% of respondents unable to complete this item (Essink-Bot et al. 1997).

Arguably, the most important factor supporting the use of the EQ-5D is the fact that the descriptive data can be converted into values, and combined to yield a single weighted index score generated from a UK-general population survey. This makes the EQ-5D more suitable than multidimensional measures, such as SF-36, for clinical trials with a single defined outcome, and it is particularly useful for economic studies, as the range of values permits appropriate cost effectiveness analyses.

The Sickness Impact Profile   First described in 1976 (Bergner et al. 1976), and intended for use in population studies, the Sickness Impact Profile (SIP) has been widely used as an outcome of general health status. The 136 items in the SIP are grouped into 12 categories describing different functional behaviours and the instrument measures changes in behaviour and activity due to sickness:

1. Ambulation
2. Body care
3. Mobility
4. Emotional behaviour
5. Social interaction
6. Alertness behaviour
7. Communication
8. Works
9. Sleep and rest
10. Eating
11. Household management
12. Recreational activities.

The SIP has been translated into many languages including French, Dutch and Spanish, and modifications have also been published including a version of the SIP specifically for RA (SIP-RA). The SIP has been comprehensively validated and is suitable for use as a self-completed instrument, or may be administered by an interviewer (Deyo et al. 1982). This is a 136 item survey, however, and, as such, takes in excess of 30 minutes to complete, and 10 minutes to score.

The SIP has been thoroughly validated, the reliability of the SIP is good and test-retest correlations are very high. It has good concurrent validity next to other global status measures, but has been largely superseded by the SF-36, after comparative studies that have recommended the SF-36 over the SIP (Andresen et al. 1998, Beaton et al. 1997). The SIP-RA version has not entered into widespread use in rheumatology as it does not seem to have adequately addressed the limitations of the original, particularly with regard to some lack of responsiveness in musculoskeletal conditions (Carr 2003).

Disease-specific measures of health status and quality of life

The Arthritis Impact Measurement Scale   The Arthritis Measurement and Impact Scale (AIMS) is an arthritis-specific measure first described in 1980 by Meenan et al. that evaluates health status in nine dimensions: mobility, physical activity, dexterity, social role, social activity, activities of daily living, pain, depression and anxiety (Meenan et al. 1980). An expanded version, AIMS2, was described later by the same authors and has been demonstrated to have superior psychometric properties. A shortened version also exists that is less time-consuming to complete, has similar psychometric properties to the original version and is recommended for postal surveys or where time considerations are important. Several other modifications for specific patient groups have been described. While originally developed for use in RA and osteoarthritis, AIMS has also been applied in many other musculoskeletal conditions including psoriatic arthritis, AS and others. It takes the form of self-administered questionnaire requiring between 15 and 30 min to complete, depending on the version (Carr 2003).

The AIMS is widely used and is comprehensive, although there are some problems with some of its wording, in particular over its use of contingent statements. Issues such as these have raised questions over the validity of AIMS, although it has been demonstrated to have moderate good concurrent validity with other functional status measures. AIMS is more responsive than many other measures of generic health or functional status (Carr 2003).

The Rheumatoid Arthritis-specific Quality of Life Instrument   The Rheumatoid Arthritis-specific Quality of Life (RAQoL) instrument represents the latest generation of quality of life/health status measures, which measure quality of life from the patient's perspective, the so-called needs-based approach (McKenna et al. 2004). There are growing numbers of instruments using this approach whereby statements (items) derived from patient interviews are presented in a survey form with dichotomous response options. When correctly constructed, these types of instrument have very strong psychometric properties and allow for comparison between conditions (Doward et al. 2004). The construction process usually involves deriving banks of items from qualitative interviews. These are then carefully mapped so that they provide comprehensive coverage of a range of dimensions of health status.

The RAQoL measure was developed for use in the Netherlands and in the UK, and was initially validated for these populations (de Jong et al. 1997). It is self completed by the patient and takes approximately 5 minutes to complete with little extra time to score as it relies on simple summation of the positive responses. The authors' own initial validation reported good test-retest reliability and moderate concurrent validity, and this has been confirmed independently since (Tijhuis et al. 2001).

One limitation of the RAQoL is that it was developed prior to refinements in some of the statistical techniques used on subsequent measures (Tennant et al. 2004). Since its initial publication it has been noted that the RAQoL, while a significant advance on previous measures, is not unidimensional (Tijhuis et al. 2001), which must be considered a shortcoming.

Region specific measures of health status: the foot
Foot Function Index   Since 1991, the most commonly used measure of foot-specific health status has been the Foot Function Index (FFI). It was originally developed for use with patients with RA undergoing surgery (Budiman-Mak et al. 1991). The FFI has proven so popular that it for some time it has also been used in assessing foot health status in other conditions (Caselli et al. 1997), although the validity of doing this is questionable. The FFI comprises 20 items that aggregate into three subscales: pain, disability and activity limitation. The FFI is validated for self-administration and each item is completed by the respondent indicating their perceived response to a question on a 100 mm visual analogue scale. The scales are anchored at each end with a verbal statement representing the opposite extremes of the dimension being measured. Scores are derived by dividing the scale line into 10 equal segments and assigning a score between 0 and 9 to each

response. The aggregate subscale scores are calculated by dividing the actual score by the maximum possible score on the subscale (Budiman-Mak et al. 1991). Test-retest agreement was reported to be high for the FFI total scores, although it varies for the sub-scales. Concurrent validity is moderate and while the responsiveness was considered appropriate by the original authors, this has been criticized subsequently (Kuyvenhoven et al. 2002).

The FFI is an older measure, and as such was not developed using patient input. As a result it appears to overemphasize disease-related factors at the expense of factors such as footwear, participation restriction psychosocial factors. The use of visual analogue scales has been criticized previously (Essink-Bot et al. 1997), and it is common to find that some patients have difficulty in completing measures based on VAS (Macran et al. 2003). A recent modification of the FFI simplifies the scoring using a five-point scale presented to the patient by interviewer. The simplified version was found to have similar psychometric properties to the original (Kuyvenhoven et al. 2002) and may be better suited to non-RA populations (Kuyvenhoven et al. 2002, Saag et al. 1996).

The Podiatry Health Questionnaire   The Podiatry Health Questionnaire (PHQ) is a fairly new measure that has been designed for use alongside the EQ-5D in evaluating outcomes in podiatry (Macran et al. 2003). It is based on clinician perceptions of disability and limitations, rather than the patient-based approach preferred in the needs model. The PHQ defines six dimensions namely: walking, foot hygiene, nail care, foot pain, worry about feet and impact on quality of life. The PHQ, as does the EQ-5D, uses a visual analogue scale on which the respondent rates their overall foot health status. Content and concurrent validity was assessed in a large sample of more than 2000 patients. For the five trichotomous responses, missing data rates were low at approximately 4%. In common with many other measures employing visual analogue scales, however, completion rates were lower for this item with 10% failing to complete the VAS. The authors report good face validity and good inter-item correlation, but only moderate correlations with EQ-5D and a clinician-assessed health-status score. The PHQ is potentially attractive because of its simplicity and its compatibility with EQ-5D; however, its responsiveness and test-retest reliability has not been established, nor have weightings yet been devised that would allow the development of a quotient score. Further development is required for this measure before we can advocate its use in general clinical practice.

American Orthopedic Foot and Ankle Society foot and ankle rating scales The American Orthopedic Foot and Ankle Society (AOFAS) scales were developed in 1994 to better evaluate the outcome of orthopaedic surgery to the foot and ankle (Kitaoka et al. 1994). There are four scales, one each for the ankle-hindfoot, midfoot, hallux and lesser toes. The scales are completed by clinician interview and one section requires the direct assessment of the clinician. This precludes their use in a self-administered questionnaire, and in intervention studies introduces the possibility for bias.

Of more concern is the fact that the AOFAS have presented no validation of the foot and ankle scales, and one independent report has been highly critical, going so far as to suggest that the scoring of the four scales is susceptible to 'bizarre, skewed behaviour' and recommending that refinements of the scales should be sought (Guyton 2001). The AOFAS scales are widely reported in orthopaedic foot studies so must be acknowledged, although we consider it necessary for this battery of scales to be subjected to far more rigorous validation before we would recommend their use in assessing health status of the foot in rheumatology.

Foot Health Status Questionnaire The Foot Health Status Questionnaire (FHSQ) is a foot-specific measure intended to assess changes in foot-health status associated with surgical and conservative interventions (Bennett et al. 1998). The FHSQ has been subjected to a fairly comprehensive validation process and has already been used in patients with a range of conditions (Bennett et al. 2001). A set of population norms exists for this measure (Bennett et al. 2001).

The FHSQ scores health status in four general health domains derived from the SF-36, and in four foot-specific domains: foot pain, foot function, footwear and general foot health. The FHSQ is similar to the SF-36 outlined previously and, as such, each of the domains yields a score between 0 and 100, with a high score representing good foot health and a low score, poor foot health. It has the same inherent limitations as the SF-36, yielding data in a number of directions and, therefore, being of limited use in clinical trials and health economic analyses. The FHSQ has been directly compared to the FFI in a comparative study and was found to be more sensitive to change (Landorf & Keenan 2002). The FHSQ takes patients approximately 10 minutes to complete, but the scoring can only be undertaken by proprietary software that must be purchased from the author, which may present a barrier to some potential users. It should also be noted that the FHSQ was developed in Australia for an Australian population, and we have encountered some difficulties with comprehension of questionnaire wording in British patients.

The Manchester Foot Pain and Disability Questionnaire This recent addition to the stable of foot-specific, health-status measures shows some promise. It is a measure similar in style to the Euroqol measure comprising 19 short statements with trichotomous responses. It has been subjected to a fairly large-scale validation process (Garrow et al. 2000), including trialling on rheumatology patients and patients in the community setting. It is suitable for self-administration, is quick and easy to score and yields a single index score making it suitable for applications such as clinical trials. There have as yet, been no direct comparisons between the Manchester Foot Pain and Disability Questionnaire (MFPDQ) and any other foot-specific, health-status measures, but the MFPDQ demonstrated good concurrent validity against a more generic measure. At the time of writing there are no normative data on which to make comparisons between normal and pathological patients or between conditions. In a multidisciplinary foot clinic the MFPDQ demonstrated a ceiling effect for patients with RA (Helliwell 2003). At present, we believe that the LFIS, with its needs-based development, supersedes the MFPDQ for patients with RA, but the MFPDQ remains our first choice for evaluating foot health status in our non-rheumatoid patients.

Leeds Foot Impact Scale This measure was the first foot-specific measure to be developed using the needs-based approach (McKenna & Doward 2004) and, as such, is the first patient reported outcome measure for the foot to go beyond basic quantification of foot health status.

The exacting six-stage process involved patients with RA defining the relevant items rather than their practitioners (Helliwell et al. 2005). In stage one 30 patients were selected for qualitative interview and stratified according to age, gender and disease duration. In the needs-based model initial interviews are informal but focused conversations, which are tape-recorded for subsequent transcription. In stage two of the Leeds Foot Impact Scale (LFIS) validation, the transcripts were analysed and content analysis was used to identify eight main themes:

1. Symptoms
2. Mobility
3. Footwear
4. Affects on others/relationships
5. Restrictions (other restrictions not mobility problems)
6. Foot appearance
7. Treatment
8. Emotions.

The research team then selected the potential items based as far as possible on direct quotations from the transcripts. One hundred and thirty-one items were mapped onto the ICF classifications and a fourth foot-specific classification and an initial draft questionnaire was prepared for pilot testing. Stage three involved field-testing for face and content validity and relevance leading to a second 127 item version. The fourth stage consisted of a postal survey involving 288 patients to test the scaling properties of the draft measure, to facilitate item reduction, and to provide preliminary evidence of construct validity and concurrent testing with the Health Assessment Questionnaire (HAQ), the Foot Function Index and Garrow's Manchester Foot Pain and Disability Questionnaire. Responses were subjected to Rasch analysis (Tennant et al. 2004), which provided a basis for reducing a second draft to 63 items. Eighty-five patients then provided test-retest reliability data.

The stages informed the finalization of the LFIS around two subscales, one encompassing the ICF classification of 'Impairments' combined with items relating to footwear or shoes; and one relating to the ICF classifications of activity limitation and participation restriction.

The psychometric properties of the final LFIS are robust. The test-retest reliability is high, yielding an ICC of 0.84. The LFIS also demonstrated good concurrent validity relative to Garrow's MFPDQ. Combined with its verified unidimensionality and needs-based derivation, the LFIS represents the current state-of-the-art in foot specific quality of life measurement for patients with RA.

KEY POINTS

- Health status and quality of life measures can be general or disease specific, and can be whole body or region specific.

- It is usually appropriate to use generic and specific measures in tandem.

- Measures encompassing multiple domains (or dimensions) can be difficult to interept.

- Measures developed for specific populations should not be transferred for use in other populations without re-validation in the new target setting.

Composite measures

As we have noted throughout this chapter, both subjective and objective measures have some limitations. It is not surprising then that the most widely applied meas-

ures in rheumatology practice are composites, comprising both subjective and objective elements. Composite measures quantify disease activity, health status, and response to treatment. Although there are currently no composite measures for the foot in rheumatology, this approach has great benefits for the complex medical manifestations of the systemic effects of RA.

The gold standard for quantifying disease activity in RA has become the Disease Activity Score (DAS), which is a composite measure combining one of the acute phase markers (usually ESR) with a health status measure (100 mm visual analogue scale), the Ritchie index and the number of swollen joints from a 44 joint count (van der Heijde et al. 1990) (see Chapter 4). The original DAS was carefully constructed and so the measure has very good content validity. Twenty potential candidate measures were reduced to four using factor analysis, which are weighted using the formula below to derive a final score:

$$DAS = 0.53938 \times \sqrt{RAI} + 0.06465 \times SW44 + 0.330 \times \ln ESR + 0.00722 \times GH$$

(RAI is the Ritchie articular index, SW44 is the number of swollen joints from a count of 44, lnESR is the log of the ESR using the Westergren method and GH is the General Health score on a 100 mm VAS.)

The original DAS was based on the full Ritchie index and so included a count of 53 joints for assessment of tenderness and 44 joints for assessment of swelling. This original instrument had good validity and high test-retest reliability. A subsequent modification using a reduced joint count was found to be equally valid and less time-consuming to perform, cutting administration time from 10 to 5–6 minutes. The most common application of the DAS is now the 28-joint count version (DAS28) (Prevoo et al. 1995) (Fig. 4.3), which is calculated using the modified formula:

$$DAS28 = 0.56 \times \sqrt{T28} + 0.28 \times SW28 + 0.70 \times \ln ESR + 0.014 \times GH$$

(T28 and SW28 are the number of tender and swollen joints from a count of 28, and lnESR is the log of the ESR using the Westergren method and GH is the General health score on a 100mm VAS as described originally.)

Scores obtained using the original DAS and modified DAS28 methodologies will vary slightly, but can be compared if original DAS scores are converted using the formula:

$$DAS'28' = 1.072 \times DAS + 0.938$$

The DAS score is considered an important and valid enough measure to form the basis of the EULAR response criteria (van Gestel, Haagsma & van Riel 1998).

Change in DAS score from baseline in response to treatment is considered good if the DAS reduces >1.2, a response of between 0.6 and 1.2 is considered moderate and no-response is defined as a change in DAS of <0.2. Threshold values defining low, moderate and high levels of disease activity exist for both the original DAS and DAS28 (see Table 8.5), and thresholds and change scores are currently used to justify eligibility criteria for treatment, and to define treatment outcomes in therapeutic outcomes studies.

Similarly, the American College of Rheumatology response criteria are based on a composite of subjective and objective measures, although the ACR criteria are not weighted in so sophisticated a way as in the DAS28. In the ACR criteria, percentage improvements are itemized for a combination of eight measures as outlined above. Setting a threshold at a given level of change, e.g. 20%, 50% or 70% allows for the definition of dichotomous endpoints for therapeutic outcomes studies that have clinical meaning.

SUMMARY

There can be no doubt that measures for evaluating care are of increasing importance, and that this is an area that should be considered by anyone responsible for providing a foot health service to patients with RA. The variety of options can be bewildering, but as the field matures there is at least a growing acceptance of some basic rules.

The golden rule is undoubtedly that in order to evaluate care meaningfully, it is a minimum requirement that some measurements are taken throughout the case management process. If measures are not made on an ongoing basis, then evaluation of care will continue to be anecdotal and *ad hoc*. The precise choice of which measures to use will be situation specific.

A useful second rule is that measures should be reliable and stable over the short term, as well as having the ability to record clinically meaningful changes.

Preferably the measure should represent the systemic as well as the local aspects of the disease. If the foot health clinic is being provided as part of a general rheumatology clinic, then the practitioner will likely have access to measures that are being collected by the medical team (such as the HAQ or DAS28 scores, joint counts, and radiographic indices). If the foot health rheumatology clinic is separate from the medical clinic, however, it may be necessary for the battery of health-outcome measures to include some systemic measures in addition to those that are foot specific. In this case collating scores such as DAS 28 can be particularly difficult if laboratory results are not available to allow the incorporation of acute phase reactants, and similar problems with access can be found with other medical results, such as those from radiographic reports. In these instances, the foot health practitioner may have to be satisfied with other generic measures such as HAQ scores, which can be derived directly from patients, although this should not preclude some attempt at least to collect some generic measures.

Some attempt should be made to maintain ongoing records and document change in foot posture secondary to RA. Radiographs provide a permanent record, and can be measured to provide some empiric quantification, although, as noted above, access may be problematic depending on circumstances. Digital photographs also provide at least a visual record for comparison over time, although quantification can be unreliable. Goniometric measures are similarly of some limited use and care must be taken not to over-rely on measures that are known to be of suspect reliability. This is particularly important when repeat measures are being used on many occasions over time to document change.

For measures of foot health status/quality of life, the needs-based model has undoubtedly superseded previous practitioner-based models with health-outcome measures that reflect more truly the patient's experience. We would advocate the use of a measure such as LFIS for the RA population, and when similar measures become available for other musculoskeletal foot conditions, we would suggest that they would be preferable to measures derived from the more traditional models. In the meantime, Garrow's MFPDQ serves the purpose well, and with some further validation other measures (such as the PHQ) could also come into contention.

Whichever set of measures are chosen, there are clearly some logistic issues that must be taken into consideration. It is likely that some of the measures will be new to some staff, and so any implementation will require training and role definition, as well as the academic exercise of choosing the set of measures. Some considerations are given below.

Table 8.5 Definition of disease activity using DAS and DAS28.

	Low	Medium	High
DAS	≤ 2.4	>2.4 ≤ 3.7	>3.7
DAS28	≤ 3.2	>3.2 ≤ 5.1	>5.1

Introducing a quality-of-life measure into clinical practice (adapted from Higginson & Carr 2001)

1. Identify a project leader
2. Review measures in use within and outside your organization
3. Involve staff and patients
4. Decide which other outcomes need to be measured
5. Choose a measure
6. Pilot test the measure to assess suitability to your own specific purpose*
7. Prepare and test paperwork
8. Train staff as required
9. Set start date and review points
10. Introduce measure
11. Review
12. Modify administration as required*

*Note: Before any existing measure is adopted, some thought should be given to copyright issues and to the need for re-validation in a specific clinical population. This applies both to the instrument itself and its mode of administration.

This is an area that is still undergoing some development and will likely continue to change rapidly in the near future. It also represents an area where some of the greatest misfit has occurred between mainstream rheumatology and those responsible for the foot health of rheumatology patients. It is in the best interests of our patients to have at least a common currency for communication between the various parties involved, and standardized evaluations represent that currency.

References

Andresen EM, Rothenberg BM, Panzer R, Katz P and McDermott MP Selecting a generic measure of health-related quality of life for use among older adults. A comparison of candidate instruments. Evaluation and the Health Professions 1988; 21(2): 244–264.

Barrett EM, Scott DG, Wiles NJ and Symmons DP The impact of rheumatoid arthritis on employment status in the early years of disease: a UK community-based study. Rheumatology 2000; 39(12): 1403–1409.

Beaton DE, Hogg-Johnson S and Bombardier C Evaluating changes in health status: reliability and responsiveness of five generic health status measures in workers with musculoskeletal disorders. Journal of Clinical Epidemiology 1997; 50(1): 79–93.

Bennett PJ, Patterson C and Dunne MP Health-related quality of life following podiatric surgery. Journal of the American Podiatric Medical Association 1001; 91(4): 164–173.

Bennett PJ, Patterson C, Wearing S and Baglioni T Development and validation of a questionnaire designed to measure foot-health status. Journal of the American Podiatric Medical Association 1998; 88(9): 419–428.

Benvenuti F, Ferrucci L, Guralnik JM, Gangemi S and Baroni A Foot pain and disability in older persons: an epidemiologic survey. Journal of the American Geriatrics Society 1995; 43(5): 479–484.

Berg K, Wood-Dauphinee S and Williams JI The Balance Scale: reliability assessment with elderly residents and patients with an acute stroke. Scandinavian Journal of Rehabilitation Medicine 1995; 27(1): 27–36.

Bergner M, Bobbitt RA, Pollard WE, Martin DP and Gilson BS The Sickness Impact Profile: validation of a health status measure. Medical Care 1976; 19(1): 57–67.

Boutry N, Larde A, Lapegue F, Solau-Gervais E, Flipo RM and Cotten A Magnetic resonance imaging appearance of the hands and feet in patients with early rheumatoid arthritis. Journal of Rheumatology 2003; 30(4): 671–679.

Bouysset M, Tebib J, Tavernier T, Noel E, Nemoz C, Bonnin M, Tillmann K and Jalby J Posterior tibial tendon and subtalar joint complex in rheumatoid arthritis: magnetic resonance imaging study. Journal of Rheumatology 2003; 30(9): 1951–1954.

Bouysset M, Tebib J, Noel E et al. Rheumatoid flat foot and deformity of the first ray. Journal of Rheumatology 2002; 29(5): 903–905.

Brazier J, Jones N and Kind P Testing the validity of the Euroqol and comparing it with the SF-36 health survey questionnaire. Quality of Life Research 1993; 2(3): 169–180.

Brooks R EuroQol: the current state of play. Health Policy 1996; 37: 53–72.

Budiman-Mak E, Conrad KJ and Roach KE The Foot Function Index: a measure of foot pain and disability. Journal of Clinical Epidemiology 1991; 44(6): 561–570.

Carr A Adult measures of quality of life. Arthritis Care and Research 2003; 49(5): 113–133.

Carr AJ and Higginson IJ Are quality of life measures patient centred? British Medical Journal 2001; 322(7298): 1357–1360.

Carr AJ, Gibson B and Robinson PG Measuring quality of life: Is quality of life determined by expectations or experience? British Medical Journal 2001; 322(7296): 1240–1243.

Caselli MA, Levitz SJ, Clark N, Lazarus S, Velez Z and Venegas L Comparison of Viscoped and PORON for painful submetatarsal hyperkeratotic lesions. Journal of the American Podiatric Medical Association 1997; 87(1): 6–10.

Chen J, Devine A, Dick IM, Dhaliwal SS and Prince RL Prevalence of lower extremity pain and its association with functionality and quality of life in elderly women in Australia. Journal of Rheumatology 2003; 30(12): 2689–2693.

Dawson J and Carr A Outcomes evaluation in orthopaedics. Journal of Bone and Joint Surgery – British Volume 2001; 83(3): 313–315.

de Jong Z, van der Heijde D, McKenna SP and Whalley D The reliability and construct validity of the RAQoL: a rheumatoid arthritis-specific quality of life instrument. British Journal of Rheumatology 1997; 36(8): 878–883.

Devauchelle Pensec V, Saraux A, Berthelot JM et al. Ability of foot radiographs to predict rheumatoid arthritis in patients with early arthritis. Journal of Rheumatology 2004; 31(1): 66–70.

Deyo RA, Inui TS, Leininger J and Overman S Physical and psychosocial function in rheumatoid arthritis. Archives of Internal Medicine 1982; 142: 879–882.

Doward LC, Meads DM and Thorsen H Requirements for quality of life instruments in clinical research. Value in Health 2004; 7(Suppl.1): S13–S16.

Drossaers-Bakker KW, Kroon HM, Zwinderman AH, Breedveld FC and Hazes JM Radiographic damage of large joints in long-term rheumatoid arthritis and its relation to function. Rheumatology 2000; 39(9): 998–1003.

Escalante A, Haas R and Del Rincon I Measurement of global functional performance in patients with rheumatoid arthritis using rheumatology function tests. Arthritis Research and Therapy 2004; 6: 315–325.

Essink-Bot ML, Krabbe PF, Bonsel GJ and Aaronson NK An empirical comparison of four generic health status measures. The Nottingham Health Profile, the Medical Outcomes Study 36-item Short-Form Health Survey, the COOP/WONCA charts, and the EuroQol instrument. Medical Care 1997; 35(5): 522–537.

Felson DT, Anderson JJ, Boers M et al. The American College of Rheumatology preliminary core set of disease activity measures for rheumatoid arthritis clinical trials. The Committee on Outcome Measures in Rheumatoid Arthritis Clinical Trials. Arthritis and Rheumatism 1993; 36(6): 729–740.

Felson DT, Anderson JJ, Boers M et al. American College of Rheumatology. Preliminary definition of improvement in rheumatoid arthritis. Arthritis and Rheumatism 1995; 38(6): 727–735.

Fries J, Spitz P, Kraines R, Guy and Holman H Measurement of patient outcome in arthritis. Arthritis and Rheumatism 1980; 23(2): 137–145.

Garratt A, Schmidt L, Mackintosh A and Fitzpatrick R Quality of life measurement: bibliographic study of patient assessed health outcome measures. British Medical Journal 2002; 324(7351): 1417.

Garrow AP, Papageorgiou AC, Silman AJ, Thomas E, Jayson MI and Macfarlane GJ Development and validation of a questionnaire to assess disabling foot pain. Pain 2000; 85(1–2): 107–113.

Geenen R, Jacobs JWG, Godaert G, Kraaimaat FW, Brons MR, Van der Heide A and Bijlsma JWJ Stability of health status measurement in rheumatoid arthritis. British Journal of Rheumatology 1995; 34(12): 1162–1166.

Goldbach-Mansky R, Woodburn J, Yao L and Lipsky PE Magnetic resonance imaging in the evaluation of bone damage in rheumatoid arthritis: a more precise image or just a more expensive one? Arthritis and Rheumatism 2003; 48(3): 585–589.

Greenhalgh T How to read a paper. Papers that report diagnostic or screening tests. British Medical Journal 1997; 315(7107): 540–543.

Guyton GP Theoretical limitations of the AOFAS scoring systems: an analysis using Monte Carlo modeling. Foot and Ankle International 2001; 22(10): 779–787.

Hawker G, Melfi C, Paul J, Green R and Bombardier C Comparison of a generic (SF-36) and a disease specific (WOMAC) (Western Ontario and McMaster Universities Osteoarthritis Index) instrument in the measurement of outcomes after knee replacement surgery. Journal of Rheumatology 1995; 22(6): 1193–1196.

Helliwell P, Allen N, Gilworth G, Redmond A, Slade A and Tennant A Development of a foot impact scale for rheumatoid arthritis. Arthritis Care Research 2005: 53(3): 418–422.

Helliwell PS Lessons to be learned: review of a multidisciplinary foot clinic in rheumatology. Rheumatology 2003; 42(11): 1426–1427.

Hewlett S, Smith AP and Kirwan JR Measuring the meaning of disability in rheumatoid arthritis: The personal impact Health Assessment Questionnaire (PI HAQ). Annals of the Rheumatic Diseases 2002; 61(11): 986–993.

Higginson IJ and Carr AJ Measuring quality of life: Using quality of life measures in the clinical setting. British Medical Journal 2001; 322(7297): 1297–1300.

Hochberg MC, Chang RW, Dwosh I, Lindsey S, Pincus T and Wolfe F The American College of Rheumatology 1991 revised criteria for the classification of global functional status in rheumatoid arthritis. Arthritis and Rheumatism 1992; 35(5): 498–502.

Hurst NP, Jobanputra P, Hunter M, Lambert M, Lochhead A and Brown H Validity of Euroqol – a generic health status instrument – in patients with rheumatoid arthritis. Economic and Health Outcomes Research Group. British Journal of Rheumatology 1994; 33(7): 655–662.

Jenkinson C, Wright L and Coulter A Criterion validity and reliability of the SF-36 in a population sample. Quality of Life Research 1994; 3(1): 7–12.

Katz PP, Pasch LA and Wong B Development of an instrument to measure disability in parenting activity among women with rheumatoid arthritis. Arthritis and Rheumatism 2003; 48(4): 935–943.

Keenan MA, Peabody TD, Gronley JK and Perry J Valgus deformities of the feet and characteristics of gait in patients who have rheumatoid arthritis. Journal of Bone and Joint Surgery 1991; 73(2): 237–247.

Kind P, Dolan P, Gudex C and Williams A Variations in population health status: results from a United Kingdom national questionnaire survey. British Medical Journal 1998; 316(7133): 736–741.

Kirwan JR and Reeback JS Stanford Health Assessment Questionnaire modified to assess disability in British patients with rheumatoid arthritis. British Journal of Rheumatology 1986; 25(2): 206–209.

Kitaoka HB, Alexander IJ, Adelaar RS, Nunley JA, Myerson MS and Sanders M Clinical rating systems for the ankle-hindfoot, midfoot, hallux, and lesser toes. Foot and Ankle International 1994; 15(7): 349–353.

Kuyvenhoven MM, Gorter KJ, Zuithoff P, Budiman-Mak E, Conrad KJ and Post MW The foot function index with verbal rating scales (FFI-5pt): A clinimetric evaluation and comparison with the original FFI. Journal of Rheumatology 2002; 29(5): 1023–1028.

Landorf KB and Keenan AM An evaluation of two foot-specific, health-related quality-of-life measuring instruments. Foot and Ankle International 2002; 23(6): 538–546.

Lane SK and Gravel JW Jr Clinical utility of common serum rheumatologic tests. American Family Physician 2002; 65(6): 1073–1080.

Larsen A, Dale K and Eek M Radiographic evaluation of rheumatoid arthritis and related conditions by standard reference films. Acta Radiologica Diagnosis 1977; 18(4): 481–491.

Leeb BF, Weber K and Smolen JS Rheumatoid arthritis. Diagnosis and screening. Disease Management and Health Outcomes 1998; 4(6): 315–324.

Lopez-Ben R, Bernreuter WK, Moreland LW and Alarcon GS Ultrasound detection of bone erosions in rheumatoid arthritis: A comparison to routine radiographs of the hands and feet. Skeletal Radiology 2004; 33(2): 80–84.

Macran S, Kind P, Collingwood J, Hull R, McDonald I and Parkinson L Evaluating podiatry services: testing a treatment specific measure of health status. Quality of Life Research 2003; 12(2): 177–88.

McCallum J The SF-36 in an Australian sample: validating a new, generic health status measure. Australian Journal of Public Health 1995; 19(2): 160–166.

McHorney CA, Kosinski M and Ware JE Comparisons of the costs and quality of norms for the SF-36 health survey collected by mail versus telephone interview: results from a national survey. Medical Care 1994; 32(6): 551–567.

McKenna SP and Doward LC The needs-based approach to quality of life assessment. Value in Health 2004; 7(Suppl. 1): S1–S3.

McKenna SP, Doward LC, Niero M and Erdman R Development of needs-based quality of life instruments. Value in Health 2004; 7(Suppl. 1): S17–S21.

Meenan R, Gertman PM and Mason JH Measuring health status in arthritis: the arthritis impact measurement scales. Arthritis and Rheumatism 1980; 23(2): 146–152.

Ostergaard M and Szkudlarek M Imaging in rheumatoid arthritis – Why MRI and ultrasonography can no longer be ignored. Scandinavian Journal of Rheumatology 2003; 32(2): 63–73.

Ostergaard M and Wiell C Ultrasonography in rheumatoid arthritis: a very promising method still needing more validation. Current Opinion in Rheumatology 2004; 16(3): 223–230.

Paulus HE, Ramos B, Wong WK, Ahmed A, Bulpitt K, Park G, Sterz M and Clements P Equivalence of the acute phase reactants C-reactive protein, plasma viscosity, and Westergren erythrocyte sedimentation rate when used to calculate American College of Rheumatology 20% improvement criteria or the Disease Activity Score in patients with early rheumatoid arthritis. Western Consortium of Practicing Rheumatologists. Journal of Rheumatology 1999; 26(11): 2324–2331.

Plant MJ, Saklatvala J, Borg AA, Jones PW and Dawes PT Measurement and prediction of radiological progression in early rheumatoid arthritis. Journal of Rheumatology 1994; 21(10): 1808–1813.

Platto MJ, OConnell PG, Hicks JE and Gerber LH. The relationship of pain and deformity of the rheumatoid foot to gait and an index of functional ambulation. Journal of Rheumatology 1991; 18(1): 38–43.

Prevoo ML, van t Hof MA, Kuper HH, van Leeuwen MA, van de Putte LB and van Riel PL Modified disease activity scores that include twenty-eight-joint counts. Development and validation in a prospective longitudinal study of patients with rheumatoid arthritis. Arthritis and Rheumatism 1995; 38(1): 44–48.

Redmond A and Keenan A Understanding statistics: putting p values into perspective. Journal of the American Podiatric Medical Association 2002; 92(5): 115–122.

Redmond A, Keenan AM and Landorf KB Horses for courses: the differences between quantitative and qualitative approaches to research. Journal of the American Podiatric Medical Association 2002; 92(3): 159–169.

Ritchie DM, Boyle JA, McInnes JM, Jasani MK, Dalakos TG, Grieveson P and Buchanan WW Clinical studies with an articular index for the assessment of joint tenderness in patients with rheumatoid arthritis. Quarterly Journal of Medicine 1968; 37(147): 393–406.

Saag KG, Saltzman CL, Brown CK and Budiman-Mak E The foot function index for measuring rheumatoid arthritis pain: Evaluating side-to-side reliability. Foot and Ankle International 1996; 17(8): 506–510.

Scott DL Prognostic factors in early rheumatoid arthritis. Rheumatology 2000; 39(Suppl 1): 24–29.

Shadbolt B, McCallum J and Singh M Health outcomes by self-report: validity of the SF-36 among Australian hospital patients. Quality of Life Research 1997; 6(4): 343–352.

Sharp JT, Young DY, Bluhm GB et al. How many joints in the hands and wrists should be included in a score of radiologic abnormalities used to assess rheumatoid arthritis? Arthritis and Rheumatism 1985; 28(12): 1326–1335.

Stucki G, Ewert T and Cieza A Value and application of the ICF in rehabilitation medicine. Disability and Rehabilitation 2003; 25(11–12): 628–634.

Tennant A, McKenna SP and Hagell P Application of Rasch analysis in the development and application of quality of life instruments. Value in Health 2004; 7(Suppl. 1): S22–S26.

Tennant A, Hillman M, Fear J, Pickering A and Chamberlain MA Are we making the most of the Stanford Health Assessment Questionnaire? British Journal of Rheumatology 1996; 35(6): 574–8.

The Euroqol Group EuroQol: a new facility for the measurement of health related quality of life. Health Policy 1990; 16(3): 199–208.

Tijhuis GJ, de Jong Z, Zwinderman AH, Zuijderduin WM, Jansen LM, Hazes JM and Vliet Vlieland TP The validity of the Rheumatoid Arthritis Quality of Life (RAQoL) questionnaire. Rheumatology 2001; 40(10): 1112–1119.

Tugwell P, Bombardier C, Buchanan WW, Goldsmith CH, Grace E and Hanna B The MACTAR Patient Preference Disability Questionnaire – an individualized functional priority approach for assessing improvement in physical disability in clinical trials in rheumatoid arthritis. Journal of Rheumatology 1987; 14(3): 446–451.

van der Heijde DM, van t Hof MA, van Riel PL et al. Judging disease activity in clinical practice in rheumatoid arthritis: first step in the development of a disease activity score. Annals of the Rheumatic Diseases 1990; 49(11): 916–920.

van Gestel AM, Haagsma CJ and van Riel PL Validation of rheumatoid arthritis improvement criteria that include simplified joint counts. Arthritis and Rheumatism 1998; 41(10): 1845–1850.

van Knippenberg FC and de Haes JC Measuring the quality of life of cancer patients: psychometric properties of instruments. Journal of Clinical Epidemiology 1988; 41(11): 1043–1053.

Ware J, Snow KK, Kosinski M and Gandek B SF-36 Health Survey. Manual and interpretation guide. Boston Health Institute, New England Medical Center, Boston, 1993.

Weishaupt D, Schweitzer ME, Alam F, Karasick D and Wapner K MR imaging of inflammatory joint diseases of the foot and ankle. Skeletal Radiology 1999; 28(12): 663–669.

Wiles NJ, Scott DG, Barrett EM et al. Benchmarking: the five year outcome of rheumatoid arthritis assessed using a pain score, the Health Assessment Questionnaire, and the Short Form-36 (SF-36) in a community and a clinic based sample. Annals of the Rheumatic Diseases 2001; 60(10): 956–961.

Wolfe F Comparative usefulness of C-reactive protein and erythrocyte sedimentation rate in patients with rheumatoid arthritis. Journal of Rheumatology 1997; 24(8): 1477–1485.

Wolfe F and Cathey M. The assessment and prediction of functional disability in rheumatoid arthritis. Journal of Rheumatology 1991; 18(9): 1298–1306.

Wolfe F and Pincus T Listening to the patient: a practical guide to self-report questionnaires in clinical care. Arthritis and Rheumatism 1999; 42(9): 1797–1808.

Chapter **9**

Organizing care

FOOT HEALTH AND MEDICAL SERVICES

There is a large gap between need for foot health services in the UK and their provision (Salvage 1999). Foot pain is highly prevalent and foot-care services have long been underfunded. As a result of the gap between needs and service provision, many people have to make-do; approximately one in ten people with foot pain simply live with it and do nothing, while a further 40% self-manage their painful foot problems independently (Gorter et al. 2001). It is also known that foot problems are substantially under-reported (Gorter et al. 2000, Munro & Steele 1998), and the dearth of accurate and objective figures makes planning and evaluation of foot health services especially difficult.

Only one-quarter of those needing foot health services have adequate access to NHS services (White & Mulley 1989) and while the private sector takes up some of the shortfall in public sector provision, between 30 and 40% of people needing access to foot-care services still lack access to services of any sort (Garrow et al. 2004, Harvey et al. 1997). The discrepancy is greater still in the rheumatology population, with a recent survey of 139 patients attending rheumatology outpatients at a North of England hospital, finding that 89% of this group of patients had foot problems (Williams & Bowden 2004). The inequity in foot health provision to patients with rheumatic disorders has been noted by both rheumatologists and podiatrists (Helliwell 2003, Michelson et al. 1994, Otter 2004).

The foot-health needs for people with rheumatoid arthritis (RA) are highly variable, ranging from no problems or minor demands (such as a need for assistance with foot hygiene or nail care) to a need for expert management of significant structural change or high-risk vasculitic lesions (Helliwell 2003, Korda & Balint 2004).

At the milder end of the spectrum there is considerable scope for patient self-management (Wagner 2000), and many patients can safely rely on self-directed home remedies, over-the-counter medications or alternative therapies. Some will self-manage entirely outside of the umbrella of the formal health-care system, or self-help approaches can be used to supplement patient's mainstream medical care. The potential for self-reliance can lead to a positive situation where, with careful direction and appropriate supervision, the patient can be placed at the centre of the management of the disease process and their foot problems (Waxman et al. 2003) and this shift in emphasis is in line with current health policy (ARMA 2004, Department of Health 2004, 2005). Conversely, care must be taken not to leave patients isolated, or lacking the knowledge required for them to participate in the process safely.

Foot health services in rheumatology can be provided at a range of levels: from 'zero-level' care, where the patient can successfully and safely self-manage; through primary and secondary care; to teaching hospital tertiary care requiring a skilled multidisciplinary team. This philosophy articulates well with latest Chronic Disease Management (CDM) and Long Term Conditions Policy (Department of Health 2004, 2005).

This chapter focuses on services for the majority of patients with RA who will have entered the health-

---

Summary of the Department of Health Long Term Conditions Policy

FULL TITLE
Supporting people with long-term conditions. An NHS and Social Care Model to support local innovation and integration (ref 264799).

STATUS
Policy statement – complements and extends implementation of the National Service Frameworks for Long Term Conditions and Older People.

PURPOSE
- To reduce the reliance on secondary care services, and increase the provision of care in a primary, community or home environment.
- To personalize the care of patients with long-term conditions

KEY ASPECTS OF THE MODEL
- Patients with long-term conditions should be identified

Summary of the Department of Health Long Term Conditions Policy—cont'd

- Patients can be stratified according to need:
  Level 3. Case management for complex needs
  Level 2. Disease specific care
  Level 1. Supported self-care
- Prioritize resources to highly intensive users of services
- Establish community-based multidisciplinary teams
- Develop a local strategy to support self-care.

CONTEXTUAL LINKS
National Service Frameworks for Older People
National Service Frameworks for Long Term Conditions
ARMA Standards of Care
Department of Health Musculoskeletal Services Framework 'A joint responsibility: doing it differently'
National Primary Care Development Team (NPCDT)
National Primary Care Collaborative (NPCC)
National Primary and Care Trust initiative (NATPACT)

KEY ACTIONS FOR IMPLEMENTATION
GENERAL
  Group patients according to need
  Establish available services and needs gaps
  Involve patients and carers
  Establish workforce development programme

LEVEL 3
  Identify patients with complex needs
  Liaise with community matrons/relevant specialists
  Plan integrated service

LEVEL 2
  Develop multi-professional teams
  Identify patients needing disease management
  Create mechanisms for recall/review of patients as appropriate

LEVEL 1
  Develop strategy to support self-care
  Educate people to better manage themselves
  Use local strategic partnerships.

---

care system early in the disease process, at least at the level of primary care. It will not tackle the broader issues of patient access to medical diagnosis or more general public health matters, but will focus on access to adequate foot health services for those who already have a diagnosis. It must be noted, however, that while we will assume, for simplicity's sake, that such patients have had adequate access to *medical* services, the level of foot care input will be highly variable, and many patients may, in the context of their foot health at least, be essentially operating outside the healthcare system, despite receiving direct medical intervention for their rheumatoid disease.

Many patients with rheumatoid arthritis in the UK are monitored on a regular basis in the primary-care setting by their own general practitioner (GP), and those that do not have formal arrangements for shared care will still see their GP on average, some six or seven times a year (Helliwell & O'Hara 1995, Memel & Kirwan 1999). With the advent of GPs with Special Interests (GPwSIs), increasing development of formal shared-care arrangements with hospital specialists, and explicit policy directives such as the Chronic Disease Management/Long Term Conditions Programme, the emphasis has shifted further towards primary care in recent years and continues to be encouraged (ARMA 2004, Department of Health 2004, Hewlett et al. 2000). In the UK NHS model, the GP is regarded as the gatekeeper to other services and so is usually the main entry point to foot health services for the RA patient. The increasing focus on primary care has potential benefits for patients in that this is where most foot health services have been delivered historically, and it should ensure that services are available to the patient within their own community. The GP is also well placed to ensure that foot health services in primary care are articulated with any other disciplines that may be involved in the person's overall health care (Helliwell & O'Hara 1995, Memel & Kirwan 1999). In practice, however, there are some barriers to this ideal. Firstly, it has been suggested that in a medically complex disease such as RA, the training and/or skills of GPs may not prepare them adequately to direct the complex web of services often required by people with RA (Akesson et al. 2003, Badley 1994). This is compounded by an often limited understanding of foot problems (Gorter et al. 2001), and of the scope and capacities of podiatrists and other AHPs in providing foot care for people with RA (Memel & Kirwan 1999). To add a further layer of difficulty there are currently no widely accepted formal assessment and referral pathways for foot problems and their related services in rheumatology patients, and so arrangements that do exist tend to be *ad hoc* and informal in nature (Redmond et al. 2005). As a result, even where excellent foot health services are available, a GP may not have adequate awareness of patient need, practitioner scope or service availability to direct patients toward them (Akesson et al. 2003, Korda & Balint 2004).

The actual provision of foot health/podiatry/chiropody services can be disadvantaged in primary care by legacy systems carried over from decades past. The priority groupings of the 1960s and 70s, where the emphasis was on care for the over 65s, people with diabetes or people taking anticoagulants, should in theory have long been consigned to history (Muir-Gray 1994). In many UK NHS trusts the performance indicators for successful foot health services still emphasize numbers of contacts over quality of service and case-mix, and the old priority groups still exert an influence on the culture if no longer on formal policy (Salvage 1999).

The tension between the breadth of knowledge required for general practice and the specialism required for dedicated rheumatology has already been noted for GPs, but the same issue can also create skill-mix and training issues for departments attempting to serve the foot health needs of patients with RA in primary care. Were comprehensive foot health services to be made available to all patients with RA within the existing NHS climate, there would be a significant shortfall in suitably trained and experienced personnel. As the importance of good foot care in rheumatology becomes an increasingly high profile issue, it is essential that training, specialization and career path shortcomings are addressed. The NHS re-grading exercise offers some opportunities, as does the advent of Extended Scope Practitioner (ESP) roles for AHPs, and the AHP consultant posts (Carr 2001), moves that are being supported to some degree by government-backed initiatives (HEFCE 2001, NATPACT 2003). It is important now that the relevant professions, and especially podiatry, act strategically to ensure that as the demand for disease specific foot care grows the professions are able to meet it (Salvage 1999).

The increasing role of Primary Care Trusts (PCTs) offers considerable potential for purchaser/commissioners to direct services more specifically toward patients in most need, and to ensure that funding flows to support those services that best address the needs of patients. Few PCTs claim to have adequate funds to meet existing obligations, however, and in the absence of strong data for the clinical effectiveness of foot health services in rheumatology, engendering support for new and innovative services is not easy. There is a growing body of evidence for the merits of good foot care in rheumatology (Crawford & Thomson 2003, Woodburn et al. 2002, 2003), and again there is a compelling case that a strategic approach on behalf of the relevant professions to present summaries of available evidence to policy makers, will help substantiate calls for extended services. This requirement is increasingly being included in formal strategy-making (NATPACT 2003).

KEY POINTS

- Most people with RA have extensive foot health needs.
- Rheumatology foot health service provision is patchy in the UK.
- Care of people with long term conditions is increasingly moving into primary care settings.
- Better integration of rheumatology into primary care presents opportunities for better integration of foot health services.

MODELS OF CARE: GETTING THE TIMING OF TREATMENT RIGHT

In providing care for people with foot problems arising from RA it is essential that the full range of medical and patient-related factors, both systemic and local, are considered, and factored into the way that the service is provided. This represents a considerable challenge because a high-quality rheumatology foot health service cannot be a single homogenous entity, but must be a complex, multi-layered service capable of adapting to the changing needs of its patients as they pass through stages of the disease process.

Good service planning recognizes that the needs of the patient will vary over the course of a life-long disease such as RA, and tailors the services required to address those needs as they change during the disease course (ARMA 2004). This adaptive model of service provision is known in rheumatology as the disease staged approach, and fits well with the Department of Health's own Chronic Disease Management and Long Term Conditions models (Department of Health 2004, 2005) (see Fig. 9.1). Using a disease staged approach, the type of treatments provided, skill-mix, case-mix and location of service can be adjusted to best suit the needs of a given stage. Timing of services to disease stages is crucial to the patient, as outcomes can be influenced significantly. Furthermore, getting the timing right fits better with government policy and also allows service planners to maximize their use of resources, prioritizing staff, time and physical assets to those activities most suited to the needs of the patient at a given disease stage.

Some principles suggesting how a responsive disease-staged rheumatology foot-health service can be organized are provided in the rest of this section. We have provided principles rather than a definitive model here because in the absence of a widely accepted or well validated model it would be inappropriate to make firm recommendations. This is espe-

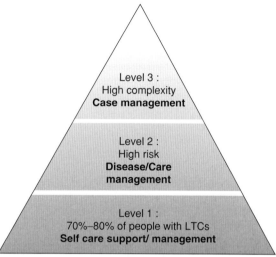

Figure 9.1   The Kaiser Permanente Triangle underpinning the Department of Health, Long Term Conditions model.

cially true when new policy is being launched. We are also mindful that the details of how a rheumatology foot health service can be implemented will be strongly influenced by local factors such as the location of the foot health service in primary, intermediate or secondary care settings; the financial resources and staff available; and parallel services provided locally by other disciplines. The following section is thus intended to provide some governing principles to be adapted to local needs depending on the precise political climate.

Disease staged management: early disease

There are two main priorities for a foot health service providing for patients with early RA: minimizing future joint damage (deformity), and encouraging and enabling patient self-management. This early stage of rheumatoid disease is particularly suited to the first two levels in the Department of Health's Long Term Conditions model: level one, supported self-care, and level two, disease-specific care.

There is a growing body of evidence that these factors may be fairly successfully managed by a combination of medical and local foot health services. The new ARMA standards of care make a recommendation that patients with a new diagnosis of RA are referred for a baseline assessment of foot health needs (ARMA 2004). Early medical intervention and new forms of therapy are proving remarkably successful in managing the systemic effects of early arthritis, with early suppression of inflammatory process leading to reduced rates of joint damage and bony change such as erosions (Breedveld et al. 2004, Emery & Seto 2003). Suppression of inflammation also leads to reduction of impairments and so less limitation of activity or restriction of participation in life roles. The foot particularly, is often involved early in RA (Devauchelle-Pensec et al. 2002) and so good systemic management has a positive effect on the degree of involvement of the foot in the early disease process.

Minimizing the effects in the foot of soft tissue and joint involvement can greatly improve the health status of patients with early RA, maximizing mobility and maintaining many of the physical capacities of people who are often still physically quite able and leading active and demanding lives (Woodburn et al. 2002). The practical application of local therapies will usually be directed towards off loading strategies, particularly in the forefoot (Hodge et al. 1999, Woodburn et al. 2002, 2003).

In the rearfoot, evidence is also accumulating that there are long-term benefits associated with early orthotic therapy in RA (Woodburn et al. 2003). The progressive valgus deformity often seen in later disease seems to respond well to early intervention, with both the associated symptoms and rate of progression positively influenced by orthotic therapy. Work still needs to be done to establish whether there is an economic case for providing orthoses prophylactically for all new cases of RA, and to determine the types of approaches that might be most appropriate, but even based on the current levels of evidence a fairly proactive approach can be justified.

The second priority in early arthritis is to encourage patients to take some responsibility for managing appropriate aspects of their disease. This is proving to be a more contentious area in rheumatology than might initially be expected, however, as the theoretical appeal of health promotion and self-management education appears to translate less well into practical results than would be hoped (Helliwell et al. 1999, Hill 2003, Hill 2001). In a culture where patient empowerment is becoming more important, increasing reliance on health promotion has been advocated by both clinicians and policymakers. The rationale for this is that patients equipped with the necessary information can make informed decisions about their disease, its treatment, and their lifestyles, and so participate more equally with clinical staff in the management of their disease. This approach appears to fail, however, if there is inadequate recognition of complexity of the disease process, the volume of information that patients will need to assimilate, and the emotional burden of coming to terms with a chronic and progressive disease. It is common for patients with newly diagnosed RA to be simply overwhelmed by the amount of information that they are given (Hill 2003), and to receive uncoordinated and sometimes conflicting information from too many sources. The maturation of this field is leading to recognition that, much as the disease needs to be managed according to stage, so does the provision of health promotion information. Again, more work needs to be done to establish optimum timings, but it would seem sensible that foot-health education is undertaken in the period after the patient has had time to reflect on the initial diagnosis, but before the foot problems become irreversible.

Disease staged management: established disease

In this intermediate stage, foot health activities are still directed at minimizing progressive change and palliating symptoms, but the implications of the progression of joint degeneration and structural change become a greater consideration. For service planning, level 1 care is increasingly supplanted by level 2 care aimed at the disease process. The priorities start to shift towards broader outcomes such as maintaining employment or active participation in family roles (Backman et al. 2004, Young et al. 2000). In turn, proactive, preventative treatment approaches will increasingly be supplemented by more reactive, accommodative or palliative interventions. Orthotic interventions will move away from rigid, controlling devices towards hybrid orthoses offering a mix of control and support. Footwear advice may become more relevant as the disease becomes established, when structural change starts to limit the suitability of retail footwear (Williams & Bowden 2004). During this stage the development of secondary features such as areas of raised plantar pressure or the onset of digital deformity may lead to discomfort, or they may lead to the formation of secondary lesions such as corns or callus (Williams & Bowden 2004). Full podiatry services may be required to supplement basic foot care, and insole or padding provision may become more relevant. It is also during this stage that some of the more demanding complications become manifest. A comprehensive rheumatology foot health service will be able to address problems such as vasculitis, ulceration and neuropathy as they arise in more severe disease (Cawley 1987). In the established phase of the disease, management is often anchored in secondary care (in level 2: 'Disease based management' in the Kaiser Permanente Triangle in Fig. 9.1) and the change in this emphasis described in the Long Term Conditions strategy (Department of Health 2005) offers significant opportunity for the development of integrated primary/secondary models for providing foot health services (see later section on Service Provision).

Disease staged management: late stage disease

Regrettably, current experience suggests the effects on the foot will usually become increasingly severe in long-standing RA. The progressive structural changes that occurred initially as part of the inflammatory process enter into a vicious circle where mechanical instability further exacerbates the rate of structural change (Platto et al. 1991, Woodburn et al. 2002). In the late stage foot, subtalar and midtarsal joint subluxation leads to the well-described planovalgus foot posture and marked forefoot deformity. Severely deformed feet may require orthopaedic referral, although many can be managed conservatively (Patsalis 1996). Good links with orthopaedics will smooth referral pathways and ensure the appropriateness of types and timing of referrals. Patients require information about surgical options and careful counselling to ensure that they are able to make informed choices (ARMA 2004). Further data are required on the timing and indication for surgery in both the forefoot and rearfoot; surgical options are discussed in Chapter 7.

Service provision is still rooted in disease-specific management for most patients, but increasing multiple system involvement may require a shift toward a multiservice case-management approach: level 3 in the Long Term Conditions model (Department of Health 2005). Mechanical management of the foot in late stage disease becomes more palliative in approach, and flexible orthoses, often of the 'total contact' type are more widely used in this group than in earlier disease (Hodge et al. 1999). In-shoe orthotics may reduce plantar pain substantially, and advice on, or provision of more specialist footwear becomes more often necessary as disease duration increases (Fransen & Edmonds 1997, Williams & Bowden 2004). Management of the secondary features (corns, callus, nodules, bursae) requires comprehensive podiatry input, with regular treatment the mainstays of footcare. This group of patients may suffer from the diverse secondary features of RA such as the vasculitis, ulceration and soft-tissue lesions noted in Chapter 3, and good footcare will require the input of a clinician with advanced skills and expertise. During the later stages of disease, systemic effects of RA become increasingly important, as cumulative damage to the hands and spine limits the patient's ability to perform basic tasks of foot hygiene and self-care. The diverse nature of the needs of people with late stage RA creates the greatest demand for carefully managed skill mix.

> **KEY POINTS**
>
> - The improvements in the medical management of RA require a review of models of foot health services provision.
> - Foot health services provision needs to be responsive to the varying needs of the patient throughout the course of the disease.
> - There is a role for proactive management in early disease.

SERVICE PROVISION

A growing number of bodies are recommending provision of foot care as a minimum standard for patients with RA (ARMA 2004, Muir-Gray 1994, NWCEG 2002, SIGN 2000).

At present, the majority of foot health service provided to patients with RA is non-specialist and is provided predominantly by allied health professionals (AHPs) and in the primary care environment (Department of Health 2003). Where more specialist rheumatology foot health is provided to people with RA, this usually occurs in the secondary or tertiary sector, even if the services are contracted in from a primary care based trust. Future provision of foot health services in rheumatology will be provided in a changed political climate, reflecting government priorities. An overhaul of the management of long-term conditions is being launched at the time of writing, further embedding chronic disease management in the primary setting (Department of Health 2005). Although the National Service Framework (NSF) for long-term conditions focuses on neurological disease, omitting rheumatology entirely (Department of Health [in press]), the chronic disease management (CDM) and Long Term Conditions initiatives redress this omission to some degree. These two programs provide for the appointment of community-based case coordinators such as community matrons, increasing the emphasis on multidisciplinary care and on integrating specialists and generalists. Integration across professional boundaries is written into the policy, reinforcing the patient-centred approach advocated by the professions themselves in the ARMA standards (ARMA 2004, Department of Health 2004, 2005).

The NHS has been addressing some of these issues as they relate specifically to AHPs through the development of a working group and a self-assessment tool by the National Primary and Care Trust Development Programme (NATPACT). The NATPACT programme

Points to consider: the NATPACT AHP Competency framework, assessing performance in eight areas

- Leadership – service leadership, AHP representation in decision making, developing AHPs.
- Workforce – capacity and capability through recruitment and retention of an appropriate mix of high-quality staff. Skill mix issues, service configuration, and acquisition of advanced skills.
- Corporate governance – aligning services with policy provision of formal criteria for service provision, managerial accountability.
- Clinical governance – provision of evidence-based services, professional and management accountability, active involvement in research and audit, appropriate training and information access.
- Commissioning and service development – involvement of AHPs in the commissioning process, recognition of training needs in Service Level Agreements.
- Performance management – AHPs actively involved in multi-agency and multidisciplinary initiatives, shared understanding of the outcome measures being used.
- Access and choice – AHPs at the heart of challenging traditional ways of working across the NHS, AHP involvement in priority setting, AHP involvement in intermediate care teams, AHP prescribing, single-assessment process, better care pathways, role development, better data collection, evidence for preventative work, proactive collaboration with colleagues.
- Partnership – lead AHPs contribute to planning teams, AHPS are enabled to work across agency and organizational boundaries, AHP participation in delivery of multi-agency, and interdisciplinary education, training and research.

outlines a framework for assessing AHP-based services, for use by PCTs, other commissioners and by the AHP service providers themselves (NATPACT 2003).

NATPACT offers pointers and significant opportunities for more strategic involvement of AHPs and the services they provide in the chronic disease management framework.

A foot health service for rheumatology patients should be able to deal with a spectrum of demand and so should ideally provide services ranging from home assistance with basic foot care, through ongoing foot-care in the primary care setting, to specialist services such as foot orthoses, and management of high-risk foot in the secondary/tertiary setting and as part of a multidisciplinary team. The traditional home of the

relevant disciplines (for example orthotic services in secondary care, podiatry in primary care) can work against cross-boundary working. Some of the Department of Health guidelines for good chronic disease/long-term conditions management are outlined in below.

Features of good chronic disease/long-term conditions management (Department of Health 2004, 2005)

- Stratifying patients by risk
- Involving patients in their care and promoting independence
- Treating patients sooner
- Coordinating care
- Multidisciplinary team working
- Integrating specialists and generalists
- Integrating care across organizational boundaries
- Minimizing unnecessary visits
- Providing care in the least intensive setting and nearer to home

While the basic foot health needs of many patients with RA can be addressed perfectly well by generalists, the complexity of RA and the rapidity of change in its medical management create a requirement for thorough and ongoing post-registration training. It is essential that practitioners involved in the care of the feet are kept up to date with developments in our understanding of the disease process and, more crucially still, with the implications of modern drug management.

In the secondary/tertiary setting it may possible to provide a more specialized foot health service. One important aspect of more specialized foot care in a rheumatology hospital department is the opportunity that is presented for multidisciplinary working. This is important in rheumatology as it becomes possible to address two important limitations that were noted above. On the one side rheumatology patients are often complex medically, and multidisciplinary teams allow the practitioner managing the foot problems to communicate more effectively with, and receive back-up from the patient's rheumatology physician. Conversely, with expertise in dealing with foot problems often limited among rheumatologists, closer contact with foot specialists raises the profile of this neglected aspect of RA patient care in the mind of medical specialists (Korda & Balint 2004).

The relevant foot health services can be readily mapped on to the ICF model. The main requirements are treating impaired body structures and functions, helping overcome existing impairment in body structures and function, limitations in activity and restrictions to participation, and preventing further impairment (Stucki et al. 2003): see Chapter 6.

As such, foot health service provision can fall into five categories:

1. Education and self-management advice, including footwear advice
2. Provision of, or assistance with finding orthoses and footwear
3. General foot care, nail cutting, corn and callus reduction, provision of padding
4. High-risk management of the vasculitic or ulcerative foot
5. Extended scope practice and surgery

These are summarized below but the interested reader is directed to Chapter 6 for a more detailed discussion.

Education and self-management advice

In an era of increased patient empowerment education programmes have become more commonplace. Self-management is known to result in improved health status (Rao & Hootman 2004), but there is conflicting evidence over the merit of formal education programmes for patients with rheumatic disorders. In the inflammatory diseases the measurable benefits are related to short-term effects on drug compliance (Hill et al. 2001) and to psychological factors and impact of disability (Riemsma et al. 2004). Education in RA provides measurable improvement in knowledge, but only small and non-significant changes in objective and health-related quality of life measures (Helliwell et al. 1999, Hill et al. 2001). Nevertheless, education is important in allowing patients to participate in the management process and so provision of information/education is considered a minimum standard in the care of RA (ARMA 2004). Self-care/management is a key pillar of the Long Term Conditions programme and will receive increasing attention as this policy matures. In order for self-care to work, education and information must be supplemented by a practical support system (King's Fund 2004). For general self-care relating to the foot, a comprehensive self management package (the FOOTSTEP programme) has already been described in Chapter 6.

Orthoses and footwear

Foot health departments should provide access to orthotic services for this patient group (Muir-Gray

1994). There is good evidence that foot orthoses are useful in controlling symptoms and in minimizing long-term change (Hodge et al. 1999, Kavlak et al. 2003, Woodburn 2000, Woodburn et al. 2002, 2003). In a Bradford multidisciplinary rheumatology clinic, some 76% of patients required foot orthoses, and 43% replacement footwear (Helliwell 2003), while in a Rochdale audit, the *requirement* (note: *not* the provision) for orthoses and footwear was estimated to be 60% and 51% respectively (Williams & Bowden 2004). Providing rheumatoid patients with off-the-shelf orthopaedic footwear has been demonstrated to improve pain and function (Fransen & Edmonds 1997).

General foot care, nail cutting, corn and callus reduction, provision of padding

Patients with musculoskeletal conditions have long been recognized as having an increased need for a range of basic foot care services (Muir-Gray 1994) with some three-quarters of rheumatology outpatients requiring routine foot care (Williams & Bowden 2004). Arthritis in the hands may make foot care and hygiene tasks difficult (Mann & Horton 1996, Muir-Gray 1994), and hip and knee involvement can make bending to attend to basic foot-care tasks impossible.

Management of the 'high-risk' vasculitic or ulcerative foot

Management of the high risk foot accounts for approximately one-quarter of the Leeds rheumatology foot health clinic's appointments, and in one report of the case profile of multi-system wound care service, rheumatology patients made up 6% of the total caseload (Steed et al. 1993). Prevention and management of lesions in the high-risk foot is an important part of the foot heath service in rheumatology (Korda & Balint 2004) and some provision should be included in service planning.

Extended scope practice and surgery

The advent of the Extended Scope Practitioner (ESP) has created the opportunity for foot health services to be more responsive to patients' needs. The new ESPs are able to access enhanced investigations and can intervene more pro-actively, making amendments to patients' pharmacological management and using injectable steroids (ARMA 2004). There are training issues to be considered that relate to the development of ESPs, but there is great support for extending AHP roles, both from the professions themselves and from within rheumatology (Carr 2001). There is currently no national accredited course so managers do not have a *de facto* standard for ensuring competence, although groups such as the Academic and Clinical Unit of Musculoskeletal Nursing at Leeds run 'M' level modules aimed specifically at allied health professionals working in rheumatology. The Society of Chiropodists and Podiatrists (SCP) has an accredited core syllabus in rheumatology, and the SCP has worked with the Podiatry Rheumatic Care Association to accredit a demanding course, enabling suitably qualified AHPs to undertake injections of joints and soft tissues. Similar arrangements exist with the Chartered Society of Physiotherapists. In 2005, the Arthritis Research Campaign funded the development of an ambitious postgraduate programme, which offers a formal postgraduate qualification in rheumatology care to AHPs, and which should provide an alternative option for accreditation of rheumatology specialist practice. The modular programme, accredited by the University of Brighton, will be relevant to those working in an extended role in rheumatology and will operate primarily on a distance-learning basis, with some attendance at study days, and will be offered across the UK (see http//www.arc.org.uk).

Training issues must be combined with local policy initiatives such as the development of patient group directions (PGDs) for access to a range of prescription only medicines, and access arrangements for diagnostic services. The developing role of ESPs is potentially helpful to patients and exciting for the allied health professions.

The medical complexity of patients with RA, combined with the severity of deformity, require that the surgical care of these patients is usually undertaken in orthopaedic units. Surgical options are discussed in detail in Chapter 7.

WORKING IN A MULTIDISCIPLINARY TEAM

Multidisciplinary care is receiving a great deal of attention at present in both rheumatology and in general health policy (ARMA 2004, Department of Health 2004, 2005). The multidisciplinary model is attractive because it puts patients who have a very complex disease into contact with clinicians with equally specific areas of expertise. Multidisciplinary foot care is well established and of proven benefit in other disciplines such as diabetes (Edmonds et al. 1986), but provision of multidisciplinary foot health services in rheumatology remains patchy.

We have already made the case that most of the foot care provided to rheumatology patients appears to be delivered outside of a multidisciplinary setting. Where foot health services are available, the traditional model is that footcare is provided outside of the rheumatology department, usually by a podiatry, physiotherapy or orthotic department that may or may not even be located within the same trust. Such a situation does not facilitate a 'seamless' service.

A superficial level of multidisciplinary care can be provided by disciplines working independently, as long as they have good lines of communication between them. This model of connected, but not integrated, care probably reflects the most common model for what might be broadly considered multidisciplinary foot health input into rheumatology. This model usually suffices because many rheumatology patients are stable and well-managed medically, and comprehensive local foot health services can be provided largely independently of rheumatology input. For a significant minority of rheumatology patients, however, the complexity and severity of their disease means that better integration between their carers would be of great benefit.

Within a rheumatology multidisciplinary team, rheumatology specialist nurses already play a central role (Redmond et al. 2005), responsible for administering, monitoring and modifying patients' medication, education, and a valuable psychosocial support role. In addition, the multidisciplinary team may include any or all of a physiotherapist, occupational therapist, podiatrist, orthopaedic surgeon, dietician, orthotist, psychologist, pharmacist and social worker.

The therapy professions, specifically physiotherapy, podiatry and occupational therapy (OT) have an important role to play in the overall management of the symptoms and progression of inflammatory arthritis. The main roles for rehabilitation therapies are to help people limit disability through skills training, exercise training, pain management, joint protection programmes, and provision of splints and orthoses (Steultjens et al. 2004). The merit of providing splints as part of a regimen of OT has been demonstrated, and echoes the data for foot orthoses provided as part of podiatric management (Budiman-Mak et al. 1995, Steultjens et al. 2004, Woodburn et al. 2002).

What is the evidence base for multidisciplinary working? Prier et al. (1997) reported that the introduction of a multidisciplinary clinic including nurse, rheumatologist, physical therapist, social worker, dietician, surgeon, psychologist and podiatrist was associated with increased patient satisfaction, improved knowledge and high demand for appointments, but not with measurable gains in quality of life. The experiences of the French are also outlined in two purely descriptive papers in which the desirability of a multidisciplinary service is outlined. No data to support the efficacy of such an approach are provided in either paper, however (Claustre et al. 1979, Simon et al. 1987).

A recent survey of rheumatology secondary/tertiary care departments in the UK found that while 85% of rheumatology departments include rheumatology specialist nurses in the team, and 44% include physiotherapy, only 27.1% include podiatry (Redmond et al. 2005). The provision of foot health services also varies widely with geography, ranging from 65% in Yorkshire and the North East; to 50% in London and the South East; to 25% and 33% in Scotland and Wales. Only half the rheumatology departments in our survey reported having any access to foot heath services for important functions such as nail care and corn/callus reduction. We have criticized the lack of coordination of foot services in rheumatology previously, noting the problems that are created with patient dissatisfaction, and impediment to the development of the service within the medical teams (Helliwell 2003).

A MULTIDISCIPLINARY MODEL OF CARE

The ARMA standards of care for RA call for agreed pathways to be developed between rheumatology and the ancillary services (ARMA 2004) and this is recently echoed in Department of Health Policy (Department of Health 2005).

Five basic principles are outlined in the text box opposite, but in the absence of any proven model we can offer no more than provide some pointers to assist the reader in developing a service appropriate to their local circumstances. Some hints on developing a business plan are given later in the chapter.

The suggested model below is based on the following assumptions:

- Most foot care for rheumatology patients is currently undertaken in primary care, or at least is provided by services based in primary care.
- The spectrum of disease severity is highly variable in RA and so foot health services must cater for patients with a wide range of foot problems.
- The service providing foot health has at least a willingness to train and develop individuals with specialist skills
- Where truly multidisciplinary care is provided for patients with most complex rheumatoid disease, the ideal service setting moves from primary care to the rheumatology hospital department.
- Hospital-based multidisciplinary foot clinics in rheumatology are likely to revolve around the expertise of a few specialized individuals.

Some generic governing principles for organizing a rheumatology foot health service

PRINCIPLE ONE
Patients with complex medical disease such as rheumatoid arthritis (RA) will benefit from a multidisciplinary approach to their foot care.

PRINCIPLE TWO
Rheumatologists often do not understand enough about the foot or about disciplines providing foot care, while foot-care specialists such as podiatrists and orthotists often do not understand enough about the medical aspects of rheumatology. Education is important, and communication of ideas is positive for all professions involved.

PRINCIPLE THREE
A multidisciplinary rheumatology specific foot health service needs to be underpinned by the capacity to provide a comprehensive general foot health service or the demands will outweigh the capacity for provision.

PRINCIPLE FOUR
Providing a multidisciplinary rheumatology foot health service carries skill-mix and training issues. Some formal training and development is needed for specialist clinicians. Clinicians pursuing this type of specialist training provide strong role models for other staff and can be excellent ambassadors for allied health disciplines.

PRINCIPLE FIVE
There is great goodwill between rheumatology and foot health providers, which makes for a positive political climate in which to develop the multidisciplinary services. Commissioning of services is often undertaken by a third party however. Goodwill is not a substitute for a strong business plan.

Multidisciplinary rheumatology foot clinics in primary care

Multidisciplinary care in the form of joint clinics is often impractical and may even be unnecessary, especially given the lower levels of medical demand in rheumatology patients who are being successfully managed in primary care. A more practical solution in this setting is likely to come from initiatives designed to ensure better coordination between disciplines. At the service level, issues to be considered include staff training and education, the development of clear guidelines and pathways for referral, mechanisms to define prioritization of resources, provision of timely and coordinated foot-health services and evaluation of outcomes.

Education and training is crucial in ensuring that staff involved in providing foot health services such as podiatrists, orthotists and physiotherapists understand the medical context of the rheumatic diseases and are familiar with the current standards of care in this rapidly changing field. Similarly, medical staff involved in the care of rheumatology patients will usually benefit from improved education about the foot in health and in the rheumatic diseases. It is our experience that in addition to the obvious educational gains, both sides benefit greatly from the improved professional understanding that goes with cross-discipline education and training.

In the absence of a nationally agreed pathway or guidelines for referral, formal local arrangements are an absolute necessity. As noted above, only 6% of rheumatologists knew of any guidelines for referral to foot health services local to them. In the absence of formal policy, access to foot health services for rheumatology patients will continue to be unnecessarily patchy, and provision of foot health services will be, at best, disjointed and, at worst, nonexistent.

The North West Region's Clinical Effectiveness Group for the Foot and Ankle in the Rheumatic diseases offers some useful pointers for local planning and we have combined their recommendations and our own experiences into the referral/care pathway model seen below.

Suggested referral guidelines
(a) Early disease
- At the time of diagnosis of inflammatory disease, any foot manifestations should be assessed in all patients (by medical/nursing staff or by a podiatrist or other AHP).

- In the absence of foot problems, basic foot-health advice should be given by medical/nursing/AHP staff to provide signposting for future needs, as well as to gently encourage positive foot health and footwear habits in the vulnerable patient. Early foot-health education should be mindful of information overload. Written reinforcement should be provided to ensure that patients have material to refer to if problems arise subsequently.

- There is inadequate evidence at present for the efficacy of any preventative measures, and, in the absence of any foot pathology, no referral into foot health services would be necessary at this stage. If foot problems exist, however, then immediate referral to foot health services is appropriate. In patients with inflammatory arthritis, early inter-

vention improves prognosis and it is appropriate for foot health services to offer a prioritized service to enable timely initiation of foot care for this patient group.

(b) Established disease
- The foot is so often involved in the disease process in rheumatoid arthritis (RA) that it is essential that patients with RA receive regular foot health check ups. It is recommended that foot health is assessed at least annually (by medical/nursing staff or by a podiatrist or other AHP), and that patients are given adequate recourse to services should problems arise. Again, it is appropriate for foot health services to offer a prioritized service to enable timely initiation of foot care should the need arise.

- Structural changes in the foot will usually worsen with increasing disease duration, and the benefit of early mechanical intervention in this patient group is now well documented. Secondary lesions (callus/bursae/nodules) are more common in established disease and indirect problems, such as difficulty with basic foot care or nail cutting, arising from the systemic effects of disease may manifest. While referral to a specialist rheumatology foot health service may be ideal, all of these manifestations can usually be managed satisfactorily by a suitably trained generalist within a primary care clinical setting.

- In a small proportion of patients, however, the severity of the disease process, complexity of secondary features, or the effects of medical therapy may give rise to more sophisticated needs (see 'high risk features in Table 9.1). Where possible, these needs should be addressed by foot health services well integrated with the rheumatology team and provided by practitioners with specialist skills in managing the foot in RA (with acknowledgement to the UK North West Region's Clinical Effectiveness Group).

Table 9.1 outlines how needs in early RA may be mapped onto foot health services that should be provided to these patients.

The definition of formal agreements has obvious benefits in prioritizing resources, and in underpinning the business case for additional resources where appropriate. A wide variation in figures for foot health service provision to rheumatology patients has the potential to provide a useful lever for areas where providing such services has been difficult in the past. Setting out a formal plan can also be helpful in highlighting gaps between need and provision.

Provision of foot care to rheumatology patients in the primary sector will have to reflect the diverse needs of this group of people, ranging from footwear and self-care advice, through basic foot care, management of soft tissue problems, provision of padding and orthoses, and ongoing care of ulceration and other 'high-risk' foot presentations. Most recent policy on managing chronic disease suggests that case-mix profiling to stratify patients according to need or risk is an important first step in implementing effective CDM (Department of Health 2005, King's-Fund 2004). There is considerable scope for a heavily skill-mix-orientated approach here, employing care assistants, registered generalists, and for more complex patient specialists and ESPs/AHP consultants as appropriate. The provision of a multidisciplinary/interdisciplinary service in primary care can be driven by a single service (such as podiatry) and so, to some degree, can be enabled by review of existing working practices.

Multidisciplinary rheumatology foot clinics in secondary/tertiary care

Provision of rheumatology foot health services in secondary care more usually occurs in the context of the rheumatology ward or outpatients department. In this context it is often easier, at least from the logistic perspective, to provide a truly multidisciplinary approach as the centralized hospital location and the likely case profile of rheumatology department patients lends itself better to interdisciplinary working and joint clinics. It must be acknowledged, however, that a joint clinic approach is only targeting the top end of the service pyramid, emphasizing levels two and three. Some mechanism should also exist to enable a hospital-based rheumatology foot clinic to articulate with foot services in primary care so that the wider spectrum of patient needs can be met.

In contrast to the model of adapting an existing primary care service outlined in the previous section, establishing a secondary care rheumatology foot health clinic requires the direct input of both the rheumatology department and the relevant AHP disciplines. It is our experience that there is usually considerable goodwill between all parties, but that a significant limiting factor will be the availability of financial resources. There can be large discrepancies between the desire to provide a service and the capacity to pay for it. Some of the essentials of a good business plan are given in the text box below (adapted from Marshall 2004).

The staff mix of a multidisciplinary foot team in a hospital rheumatology department should include at least a rheumatologist, podiatrist and an orthotist.

It would also be quite appropriate to extend team membership to orthopaedics, physiotherapy and occupational therapy as resources permit. The accommodation requirements for a joint clinic are also significant. A rheumatology foot clinic requires a fairly large room, with at least a 5 m unobstructed area to allow for observation of gait, one or more examination couches, and/or a podiatry/chiropody workstation. Facilities for plaster casting are a minimum and a raised platform is helpful. It is possible for these facilities to be provided on a temporary basis so that the room can also be used by other disciplines, but a dedicated room is preferable.

Once the service is established, some succession planning is imperative, as small teams such as these can be highly dependent on individual personalities

---

Points to consider in developing a business case for a multidisciplinary foot clinic

1. Establish a need for the service:
   a. Use epidemiological data on foot problems related to the local population and different age groups
   b. Use epidemiological data on high-risk groups
   c. Provide existing data on use of services in both primary and secondary care
2. Identify existing resources:
   a. Rheumatology and orthopaedic clinics
   b. Orthotic services
   c. Podiatry services
3. Identify existing costs:
   a. What is the orthotic budget?
   b. What are the podiatry costs for the existing client group
   c. What are indirect costs – if the patient has to make three separate journeys, for example
4. Identify purchasers and providers – you will need to make the case for a combined foot clinic to the major purchaser – the primary care trust
5. Identify benefits:
   No cost implications with improved quality of care
6. Develop business case within this framework
   General points to note:
   - Consider the principles outlined under 'Features of good chronic disease/long-term conditions management' in this chapter.
   - Although the combined multidisciplinary foot clinic will provide a better quality of care arguing this is unlikely to have much impact in a cost limited service. Therefore, the case has to be made by organizing existing services more effectively: this is the basis for the business

Continued on page 202

Table 9.1 Indicators for foot health referral and appropriate associated services in early and established RA.

	Indicators for referral for foot health intervention			
	Localized joints/soft tissue inflammation	Problems affecting the architecture or function of the foot	Secondary lesions (callus/corns/nodules/bursae)	'High-risk' features
Services potentially appropriate to presenting features in early RA.	Foot health advice Footwear advice Local splinting Physical therapies (rest/ice) Padding Functional intervention (functional foot orthoses) Joint or soft tissue injections Periodic review as appropriate	Foot health advice Footwear advice Provision of foot wear Provisions of information re pathological processes occurring Functional foot orthoses Periodic review and monitoring of structural change (at least annually)	Foot health advice Provision of information re pathological processes occurring Cautious reduction of skin lesions if appropriate Self management advice if the patient is able enough Footwear advice Provision of footwear if appropriate Padding/pressure relief Functional intervention (functional foot orthoses) Periodic review (at least annually)	*Not usually applicable in early RA* Baseline can be established if patient attending for other reasons
Services potentially appropriate to presenting features in established RA	as above	as above *plus* Provision of functional foot orthoses (softer materials) Provision of customized footwear Palliation of local lesions secondary to structural change Consideration for surgical intervention	as above *plus* Injection of soft tissue lesions Minimal reduction of callus overlying plantar bursae Monitoring for ulceration	Evaluation of vascular/neurological status – establishment of baselines Integrated care with rheumatology team Capacity to undertake more complex wound care Management self-referral mechanism

> **Points to consider in developing a business case for a multidisciplinary foot clinic**—cont'd
>
> case. An example would be to establish the annual budget for bespoke footwear and use a reduction in that (due to better selection of patients and use of alternative treatments) as one way to fund the improved service. Another would be to introduce a self-management programme for the many elderly people attending for routine podiatry care and to use the savings on the new multidisciplinary clinic.
>
> - Use National targets in your case. Examples are the ARMA standards of care and the NSF for long-term conditions.
> - Use other benefits such as retention of high-quality staff.
> - It may be possible to use waiting times as a lever to introduce this service
> - In the business plan you will need to identify the costs of the project (both capital and running) and match these against the savings identified above.
> - Work together with colleagues. It is possible orthopaedic colleagues would welcome the chance to provide a quality based conservative option
> - Look to other specialties. It is likely that the diabetes service is running such a clinic and it may be possible to graft your new service onto theirs at little extra cost.

for their success. To ensure a level of professional development appropriate to a specialist team it is advisable that arrangements are made for continuing professional development, and for update courses for the foot health specialist to be undertaken jointly with the rest of the rheumatology team (Otter 2004).

A good multidisciplinary rheumatology foot health service is likely to tap into considerable unmet need for foot health services (Prier et al. 1997) and it is our and others' experience that the service will expand rapidly and attract referrals for a range of conditions

(Helliwell 2003, Prier et al. 1997). Robust business planning should pre-empt these potential problems and aid the long-term success of such a venture. As we have noted in the previous chapter, supplementing the initial business plan with careful documentation of patient outcomes will enable the merits of the service to be quantified and the cost-effectiveness evaluated in the long term (Prier et al. 1997).

KEY POINTS

- Multidisciplinary care should be patient facing, i.e. should relate to meeting patient needs rather than reinforcing professional scopes of practice.
- Most services are currently provided in the primary care setting.
- The members of the multidisciplinary team need not be physically present at the same time.
- There is a need for common currency among team members (e.g. assessment protocols, care pathways, standards of care).
- Multidisciplinary and resourcing issues should be considered from the outset.

SUMMARY

There is currently a large gap between need and provision of foot health services to rheumatology patients, generally, and wide geographical variation in what services do exist. The needs of this group of patients are extremely diverse and require services at a variety of levels. Government and professional policy is increasingly supportive of the role of AHPs in providing such care, however, and the combination of diverse needs and developing policy offers exciting opportunities for developing foot health services. There is great scope in the model outlined in this chapter to develop foot health services while building a career structure and developing specialist AHPs. Resource implications should be addressed by a robust business plan at the outset of any new initiatives.

References

Akesson K, Dreinhofer KE and Woolf AD Improved education in musculoskeletal conditions is necessary for all doctors. Bulletin of the World Health Organization 2003; 81(9): 677–683.

ARMA Standards of Care for People with Inflammatory Arthritis. Arthritis and Musculoskeletal Alliance, London, 2004.

Backman CL, Kennedy SM, Chalmers A and Singer J Participation in paid and unpaid work by adults with rheumatoid arthritis. Journal of Rheumatology 2004; 31(1): 47–56.

Badley EM The provision of rheumatologic services. In: Klippel J, Dieppe P (eds) Rheumatology, Mosby, London, 1994.

Breedveld FC, Emery P, Keystone E et al. Infliximab in active early rheumatoid arthritis. Annals of the Rheumatic Diseases 2004; 63(2): 149–155.

Budiman-Mak E, Conrad KJ, Roach KE et al. Can foot orthoses prevent hallux valgus deformity in rheumatoid arthritis? A randomized clinical trial. JCR: Journal of Clinical Rheumatology 1995; 1(6): 313–121.

Carr A Defining the extended clinical role for allied health professionals in rheumatology. Arthritis Research Campaign 2001; proceeedings No 12.

Cawley MI Vasculitis and ulceration in rheumatic diseases of the foot. Baillières Clinical Rheumatology 1987; 1(2): 315–333.

Claustre J, Simon L and Serre H [Rheumatoid foot. Practical podiatric problems]. Revue du Rhumatisme et des Maladies Osteo-Articulaires 1979; 46(12): 673–678.

Crawford F and Thomson C Interventions for treating plantar heel pain. [update of Cochrane Database Syst Rev. 2000;(3): CD000416; PMID: 10908473], Cochrane Database of Systematic Reviews 2003; 3, p. CD000416.

Davys H, Turner D, Helliwel PS,Emery P and Woodburn J A comparison of scalpel debridement versus sham procedure for painful forefoot callosities in rheumatoid arthritis. Rheumatology Diseases 2005; 44: 207–210.

Department-of-Health NHS Chiropody Services Summary Information for 2002–03, England, DH Statistics Division (SD3G), 2003.

Department-of-Health Improving Chronic Disease Management, London, 2004.

Department-of-Health Supporting People with Long Term Conditions, London, 2005.

Department-of-Health National Service Framework for Long Term Conditions, London (in press).

Devauchelle-Pensec V, Saraux A, Alapetite S, Colin D and Le Goff P Diagnostic value of radiographs of the hands and feet in early rheumatoid arthritis. Joint Bone Spine 2002; 69(5): 434–441.

Edmonds ME, Blundell MP, Morris ME, Thomas EM, Cotton LT and Watkins PJ Improved survival of the diabetic foot: the role of a specialized foot clinic. Quarterly Journal of Medicine 1986; 60(232): 763–771.

Emery P and Seto Y Role of biologics in early arthritis. Clinical and Experimental Rheumatology 2003; 21(5 Suppl. 31): S191–S4.

Fransen M and Edmonds J Off-the-shelf orthopedic footwear for people with rheumatoid arthritis. Arthritis Care and Research 1997; 10(4): 250–256.

Garrow AP, Silman AJ and Macfarlane GJ The Cheshire Foot Pain and Disability Survey: a population survey assessing prevalence and associations. Pain 2004; 110(1–2): 378–384.

Gorter K, Kuyvenhoven M and de Melker R Health care utilisation by older people with non-traumatic foot complaints. What makes the difference? Scandinavian Journal of Primary Health Care 2001; 19(3): 191–193.

Gorter K, de Poel S, de Melker R and Kuyvenhoven M Variation in diagnosis and management of common foot problems by GPs. Family Practice 2001; 18(6): 569–573.

GorterKJ, Kuyvenhoven MM and de Melker RA Nontraumatic foot complaints in older people. A population-based survey of risk factors, mobility, and well-being. Journal of the American Podiatric Medical Association 2000; 90(8): 397–402.

Harvey I, Frankel S, Marks R, Shalom D and Morgan M Foot morbidity and exposure to chiropody: population based study. British Medical Journal 1997; 315(7115): 1054–1055.

HEFCE Higher Education Funding Council for England report on research in nursing and allied health professions. Department of Health/HEFCE, London, 2001.

Helliwell PS Lessons to be learned: review of a multidisciplinary foot clinic in rheumatology, Rheumatology 2003; 42(11): 1426–1427.

Helliwell PS and OHara M Shared care between hospital and general practice: an audit of disease-modifying drug monitoring in rheumatoid arthritis. British Journal of Rheumatology 1995; 34(7): 673–676.

Helliwell PS, OHara M, Holdsworth J, Hesselden A, King T and Evans P A 12-month randomized controlled trial of patient education on radiographic changes and quality of life in early rheumatoid arthritis. Rheumatology 1999; 38(4): 303–308.

Hewlett S, Mitchell K, Haynes J, Paine T, Korendowych E and Kirwan JR Patient-initiated hospital follow-up for rheumatoid arthritis. Rheumatology 2000; 39(9): 990–997.

Hill J An overview of education for patients with rheumatic diseases. Nursing Times 2003; 99(19): 26–27.

Hill J, Bird H and Johnson S Effect of patient education on adherence to drug treatment for rheumatoid arthritis: a randomised controlled trial. Annals of the Rheumatic Diseases 2001; 60(9): 869–875.

Hodge MC, Bach TM and Carter GM Novel Award First Prize Paper. Orthotic management of plantar pressure and pain in rheumatoid arthritis. Clinical Biomechanics 1999; 14(8): 567–575.

Kavlak Y, Uygur F, Korkmaz C and Bek N Outcome of orthoses intervention in the rheumatoid foot. Foot and Ankle International 2003; 24(6): 494–499.

Kings-Fund Managing Chronic Disease: what can we learn from the US experience? Kings Fund, London, 2004.

Korda J and Balint GP When to consult the podiatrist. Best Practice and Research in Clinical Rheumatology 2004; 18(4): 587–611.

Mann RA and Horton GA Management of the foot and ankle in rheumatoid arthritis. Rheumatic Diseases Clinics of North America 1996; 22(3): 457–476.

Memel DS and Kirwan JR General practitioners knowledge of functional and social factors in patients with rheumatoid arthritis. Health and Social Care in the Community 1999; 7(6): 387–393.

Michelson J, Easley M, Wigley FM and Hellmann D Foot and ankle problems in rheumatoid arthritis. Foot and Ankle International 1994; 15(11): 608–613.

Muir-Gray J Feet first: Report of the joint department of health and NHS chiropody taskforce, Department of Health, London, 1994.

Munro BJ and Steele JR Foot-care awareness. A survey of persons aged 65 years and older. Journal of the American Podiatric Medical Association 1998; 88(5): 242–248.

NATPACT AHP Significant Issues Group NHS. Modernisation Agency, London, 2003.

NWCEG North West Clinical Effectiveness Group. Guideines for the management of the foot in rheumatic diseases, 2002.

Otter SY, and Cryer J Biologic agents used to treat rheumatoid arthritis and their relevance to podiatrists: a practice update. Musculoskeletal Care 2004; 2(1): 51–59.

Patsalis T, Georgousis H and Gopfert S Long-term results of forefoot arthroplasty in patients with rheumatoid arthritis. Orthopedics 1996; 19(5): 439–447.

Platto MJ, OConnell PG, Hicks JE and Gerber LH The relationship of pain and deformity of the rheumatoid foot to gait and an index of functional ambulation. Journal of Rheumatology. 1991; 18(1): 38–43.

Prier A, Berenbaum F, Karneff A et al. Multidisciplinary day hospital treatment of rheumatoid arthritis patients. Evaluation after two years. Revue du Rhumatisme (English Edition) 1997; 64(7–9): 443–450.

Rao JK and Hootman JM Prevention research and rheumatic disease. Current Opinion in Rheumatology 2004; 16(2): 119–124.

Redmond A, Allen N and Vernon W Effect of scalpel debridement on the pain associated with plantar hyperkeratosis. Journal of the American Podiatric Medical Association 1999; 89(10): 515–519.

Redmond AC, Helliwell PS, Waxman R Provision of foot health servicess in rheumatology in the UK. Rhematology (adance access on-line 2005).

Riemsma RP, Kirwan JR, Taal E and Rasker JJ Patient education for adults with rheumatoid arthritis. Cochrane Database of Systematic Reviews 2004; 2: 2.

Salvage A Feet last? Older people and NHS chiropody services. Podiatry Now 1999; 1: 7–11.

SIGN Scottish Intercollegiate Guidelines Network. Management of Early Rheumatoid Arthritis, 2000.

Simon L, Brun M, Izard MH and Houlez G [Teaching the patients with rheumatoid polyarthritis more about their disease]. Revue du Rhumatisme et des Maladies Osteo-Articulaires 1987; 54(5): 393–395.

Steed DL, Edington H, Moosa HH and Webster MW Organization and development of a university multidisciplinary wound care clinic. Surgery 1993; 114(4): 775–778, discussion 8–9.

Steultjens EMJ, Dekker J, Bouter LM, van Schaardenburg D, van Kuyk MAH and van den Ende CHM Occupational therapy for rheumatoid arthritis. Cochrane Database of Systematic Reviews 2004; 2: 2.

Stucki G, Ewert T and Cieza A Value and application of the ICF in rehabilitation medicine. Disability and Rehabilitation 2003; 25(11–12): 628–634.

Vliet Vlieland TP and Hazes JM Efficacy of multidisciplinary team care programs in rheumatoid arthritis. Seminars in Arthritis and Rheumatism 1997; 27(2): 110–122.

Wagner EH The role of patient care teams in chronic disease management. British Medical Bulletin 2000; 320(7234): 569–572.

Waxman R, Woodburn H, Powell M, Woodburn J, Blackburn S and Helliwell P FOOTSTEP: a randomized controlled trial investigating the clinical and cost effectiveness of a patient self-management program for basic foot care in the elderly. Journal of Clinical Epidemiology 2003; 56(11): 1092–1099.

White EG and Mulley GP Footcare for very elderly people: a community survey. Age and Ageing 1989; 18(4): 276–278.

Williams AE and Bowden AP Meeting the challenge for foot health in rheumatic diseases. Foot 2004; 14(3): 154–158.

Woodburn J, Stableford Z and Helliwell PS Preliminary investigation of debridement of plantar callosities in rheumatoid arthritis. Rheumatology 2000; 39(6): 652–654.

Woodburn J, Barker S and Helliwell PS A randomized controlled trial of foot orthoses in rheumatoid arthritis. Journal of Rheumatology 2002; 29(7): 1377–1383.

Woodburn J, Helliwell PS and Barker S Changes in 3D joint kinematics support the continuous use of orthoses in the management of painful rearfoot deformity in rheumatoid arthritis. Journal of Rheumatology 2003; 30(11): 2356–64.

Woodburn J, Udupa JK, Hirsch BE et al. The geometric architecture of the subtalar and midtarsal joints in rheumatoid arthritis based on magnetic resonance imaging. Arthritis and Rheumatism 2002; 46(12): 3168–3177.

Young A, Dixey J, Cox N How does functional disability in early rheumatoid arthritis (RA) affect patients and their lives? Results of 5 years of follow-up in 732 patients from the Early RA Study (ERAS). Rheumatology 2000; 39(6): 603–611.

Index

Please note that page references to non-textual information such as Figures and Tables are in *italic* print